nding
SUCCESS

rated above and are heartless. So, if the milk of human kindness flows freely in your veins, do a Barnard on yourself and transplant a stone for your heart or at least drain it of the aforementioned m. of. h. k.

Furthermore, your feet should be shod to enable you to ruthlessly trample fellow chasers of Success.

___

ning entry in the
your Chest' Comp.
eceipe for success?".

___

A Lady Macbeth with charm; relatives in high places and money to throw around beside you will be an asset. She will not mind you making Success your mistress because she will enjoy the perks and privileges, reflected glory and envy of others that your dallying will bring more than having a devoted, contented, unambitious husband around the house.

But beware! Mistress Success is a demanding vixen — devouring, destroying and demeaning, while making her ensnared slaves temporarily happy.

Also, once you are with her, you will find yourself isolated on a lonely pinnacle with reaching, scheming hands wanting to dislodge you.

Keep your balance. Stick to the lady and your vantage point with tenacity. Do not bend down to extend a helping hand to another. He may drag you down or climb over your shoulder.

Those whom you've outrun or displaced will curse you, cast aspersions, hurl accusations and discredit you. Grow a thick skin if you already are not kabaragoya-like or go deaf.

Success being flirtatious, hardly dallies long with one man. This is particularly so if you've won her over by foul means or unfair tactics. You have to be prepared to let her go. She needs to, or has got accustomed to changing partners.

With this in mind, exploit your position to the maximum so that when you fall, you can cushion it with a bank account. Alternately, you can break your fall midway by chameleoning yourself.

So here, my friend, is a recipe for success and a bit of advice for achieving it.

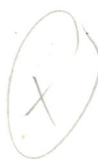

Rescue Emergency Care

This book is dedicated to all those who help others in distress;
and to those who help them in their endeavours

Wherefore by their fruits ye shall know them.
Matthew, *vii*, 20.

Rescue Emergency Care

Edited by
KEN EASTON
OBE, OStJ, MBBS(Lond), DObstRCOG, FRCGP

with a foreword by the late Norman Capener

WILLIAM HEINEMANN MEDICAL BOOKS LTD
23 BEDFORD SQUARE   LONDON   WC1B 3HT

First published 1977

© Ken Easton, 1977

ISBN 0 433 08000 0

Set in Photon Times, printed and bound in
England by R J Acford Ltd, Chichester, Sussex

Contents

Contributors

Hamish Barber MD, FRCGP, DObstRCOG
Norie–Miller Professor of General Practice, University of Glasgow

P J F Baskett BA, MB, BCh, BAO, FFARCS
Consultant Anaesthetist and Chairman of Division of Anaesthesia at Frenchay Hospital, Bristol. Consultant Anaesthetist to the United Bristol Hospitals. Clinical Teacher in Anaesthesia to the University of Bristol

Patrick J Brennan BEM, MIFireE
County Fire Officer, North Yorkshire Fire Brigade

J Peter Bush MBBS(Lond), FRACGP, DMJ
Director of Emergency Services, the Royal Melbourne Hospital, Victoria, Australia. Victorian Police Surgeon. Commissioner, St John Ambulance Brigade, Victoria District

Alfred Dooley BSc Hons(Lond)
was appointed by the Medical Commission on Accident Prevention in 1975 to make a Pilot Study on the evaluation of emergency care, following a varied career in research and development in the chemical industry, wartime inter-service projects, coal utilisation and standardisation, and in agriculture

Kenneth C Easton OBE, OStJ, MBBS(Lond), DObstRCOG, FRCGP
General Practitioner. Chairman, Road Accident After Care Scheme. Member, Medical Commission on Accident Prevention. Divisional Surgeon, St John Ambulance Association

Alison M Elliman BSc, MB, ChB, MRCP
Consultant Paediatrician, West Middlesex Hospital

David O Gibbons MB, MRCP(Lond)
Consultant in General Medicine to the Cornwall Health Area. Late Lecturer and Hon Senior Registrar, Department of Therapeutics, Westminster Hospital and Medical School, London. Medical Registrar, Addenbrooke's Hospital, Cambridge

F John Gillingham MBE, MD(Hon), FRCS, FRCSE, FRCPE, FRSE
Professor of Surgical Neurology, University of Edinburgh. Chairman, Scottish Committee of the Medical Commission on Accident Prevention Consultant Neurosurgeon to the Army in Scotland

P Hatch
Coroner, Western District, North Yorkshire

J F Hindle MBBS, FRCS
Consultant in charge, Emergency Department, Luton and Dunstable Hospital, Luton

E Hoffman MD, FRCS
Consultant Thoracic Surgeon to the Northern Regional Cardiothoracic Surgical Service. Consultant in charge of the Thoracic Surgery Unit at Poole Hospital, Middlesborough. Hunterian Professor, Royal College of Surgeons of England

Ariel F Lant BSc, MB, PhD, FRCP
Professor of Clinical Pharmacology and Therapeutics, Westminster Medical School. Consultant Physician, Westminster Hospital, London

James Lawless MB, ChB
Late Director, Zambian Flying Doctor Service

R F Lea MBE, MIAI, MICAP
Ambulance Training Officer, Yorkshire Regional Health Authority. Member of National Staff Committee (Ambulance)(DHSS)

P S London MBE, FRCS
Surgeon, the Birmingham Accident Hospital. Attending Surgeon, the Robert Jones and Agnes Hunt Orthopaedic Hospital, Oswestry. Hunterian Professor, the Royal College of Surgeons of England

Neil J Macdonald, MB, ChB, DObstRCOG
General Practitioner, Aviemore. Chairman of the Cairngorn Mountain Rescue Association. Advisor to the Cairngorn Sports Development Board Ski Patrol

Henry Matthew MD, FRCP(Edin)
Formerly Consultant Physician, Regional Poisoning Treatment Centre, Royal Infirmary, Edinburgh. Director, Scottish Poisons Information Bureau

S Miles CB, MSc, MD, FRCP, FRCS, MFCM, DTM & H
Surgeon Rear Admiral, Medical Director, Gaelic Healthguard Co Ltd. Chairman, International Trauma Foundation

J R Hanns Pacy MBBS, MD, FRACGP
Hon Director, the Tea Gardens Accident and Emergency Service Foundation. Member of the Emergency Call Committee of the World Organisation of National Colleges, Academies and Scientific Association of General Practice/Family Medicine. Lecturer, Community Medicine, University of New South Wales, Sydney. Member, Research Committee of Preventive Medicine, NSW Faculty, Royal Australian College of General Practitioners. Member of the Road Safety Panel, Australian Medical Association

L W Plewes CBE, MA, MD, FRCSE, FRCS
Consultant (retired) to the Accident and Orthopaedic Service, Luton and Dunstable Hospital

P E A Savage MS, FRCS
Consultant Surgeon, Queen Mary's Hospital, Sidcup, Kent

F W Shakesby
Chief Superintendent, Road Traffic Division, North Yorkshire Police

N A Silverston MB, ChB, MRCGP
General Practitioner. Vice-Chairman, Mid-Anglia General Practitioner Accident Service

Roger Snook MD, MB, ChB
Consultant in Accident and Emergency Medicine, Royal United Hospital, Bath. Accident Medical Officer to the County of Avon Fire Brigade

Alan F Stow MIFireE, AMBIM
Divisional Commander, North Yorkshire Fire Brigade

J C Watts OBE, MC, OStJ, MBBS, FRCS
Consultant Orthopaedic Surgeon, Bedford General Hospital. Formerly

Professor of Military Surgery, Royal College of Surgeons and Royal Army Medical College. Commissioner, Order of St John of Jersusalem

J S M Zorab FFARCS, DA
Consultant Anaesthetist, Frenchay Hospital, Bristol

Foreword

NORMAN CAPENER

The following lines were written by the late Norman Capener, then Chairman of the Medical Commission on Accident Prevention, early in the preparation of this book. They stand here now not only as an introduction but also as a tribute to a major pioneer in the prevention and management of accidental injury.

The Medical Commission on Accident Prevention was set up in 1963 on the initiative of The Royal College of Surgeons of England (Hunt and Marks, 1964). Its purpose is to study the epidemiology of what has become, after heart disease and cancer, the largest cause of mortality and morbidity in the, so-called, advanced civilisations. In children and young adults under 25 years of age, accidents are the principal cause of death. Elsewhere I have outlined this disease as a problem in *ecology* (Capener, 1970), for as the dictionary tells us 'ecology is that branch of biology which deals with the interrelations of organisms and their environment'. Epidemiology is a special aspect of ecology, concerned with the study of the pathological aspects of these interrelations, affecting communities and their individual components. The human disease is trauma, or accidental injury.

In understanding this disease, as with any other, we must study all the factors: its nature, causation, prevention and treatment. The nature of the disease is implicit in the title just given, yet the word accident suggests a chance happening or something that has no obvious cause; in other words those events that are called irreverently 'Acts of God'. These are relatively few in the context of modern civilisation. The causation of accidental injury is dominantly in defects of human behaviour; of architectural and engineering design and maintenance; of

xiii

man's aggressive nature; the faults of his behaviour, whether due to imperfections of training or of vigilance, in response to other human beings and the environment. Accidents, it must be realised, do not always lead to personal injury or material damage. The same accident may cause neither, but equally it may lead to a trivial or serious injury. It may indeed lead to catastrophe or death. Here it is that chance *does* enter; it may determine the severity of the injury, though not the ultimate cause.

Prevention in the modern context requires in childhood, and continuously throughout life, training and vigilance in personal and environmental relationships, good citizenship in the realm of law and order, recognition of risks in personal and environmental associations, and skill in their management with understanding and compassion.

Teamwork of excellence is the practical ideal not only of life, but in prevention and treatment. It is not the purpose here to outline aspects of treatment that belong to the well-established institutions of medical care. There is, however, one aspect of treatment which is of especial importance and which leads rightly to the purpose for which this book is before the reader. It is the whole matter of *community care*; care *for* the community and care *by* the community for its members. This is of extreme importance, not only as a means of rescue for those in calamity, but as a vital part of the educational and so preventive exercise. First, *care* demands knowledge of what to do in emergency; when and how to do it; in other words, it requires training and experience. Second, it demands understanding of causes and effects. Third, care to do the right thing will itself prevent more serious results from the primary injury. Finally, acquaintance with the nature and results of injury will be object lessons in the needs for prevention.

All of this cannot be left to the experts of the statutory or voluntary rescue organisations. All of us, under the conditions of modern mobility on land, sea or in the air, may be far from such rescue services. Then one's life may be in the hands of the nearest passer-by. Lucky we will be if the rescuer has had good training in the principles and practice of first-aid up to modern standards. Such training is one of the big needs in the education of every child and every young adult. This is a matter to which educational authorities should give greater attention.

To conclude: this book has grown from the ideas and work of a group of general medical practitioners who during the past dozen years have developed a scheme of expert immediate care for catastrophies at the roadside and at other accident sites. It has been organised on a voluntary charitable basis and thus is an object lesson to other groups within the community. Not working independently of the statutory organisations, but in collaboration with the police, ambulance and fire services, these doctors act as auxiliaries in the teamwork, supported by a number of hospital specialists. All these doctors cooperate with the lay voluntary first aid organisations, such as the British Red Cross Society and the St John Ambulance Brigade, upon whom the lay population must also depend for their first aid training.

The Medical Commission on Accident Prevention has been privileged to sponsor the earlier years of these medical *Immediate Care Schemes* and recommends this book to the notice of everyone who has concern for the welfare of the injured. Today we all have special responsibility for other peoples' lives.

REFERENCES

Capener, N (1970), The ecology of trauma, *Journal of Clinical Pathology*, **23** (Suppl. Royal College of Pathologists) 4, 1.

Hunt, J and Marks, M (1964), *Accident Prevention and Life Saving*. London: Livingstone.

Introduction

Over the past ten years, the numbers of accident and emergency cases have reached epidemic proportions both in industrialised and in many developing countries. Improved methods of rescue and emergency care have resulted, and these must continue to be perfected and learned—not only by trained personnel but by *all* members of communities at risk. The problems of traffic, industrial and other accidents are international, and intensified by wars and civil disturbance. The response must be equally widespread.

There has been a growing demand for guidance from those increasingly involved in rescue and emergency services: general practitioners, casualty surgeons, regional and area medical officers, senior members of ambulance, police and fire services, and from the armed forces. A great responsibility rests on these groups, whose members must arrange for care at major accidents as well as for the many casualties caused by more everyday hazards. It is encouraging that clinical students have requested such a book as this and the teaching of emergency care as part of their curriculum. And some progress has even been made in educating laymen in the essentials of emergency care, especially in Scandinavia.

The contributors are well known internationally for their work in this field—and to one another through sharing experience—and have already lectured and written extensively on their subjects. The aim of the present book is to bring that experience together as a more permanent record of efforts expended and progress achieved—and, above all as a guide to others. This should provide a firm basis for the further progress needed in the next decade.

While the chapters have been planned to cover a wide field, they do not pretend to be exhaustive. The texts are essentially practical, with references for further reading, instructional aids and useful addresses; there is an appendix showing principal rank badges in the emergency services, and a list of product suppliers. Where the main steps in rescue and resuscitation have been repeated, this is deliberate. They can never be overemphasised. In addition, the authors have sought to answer in advance the oft-repeated questions raised by audiences and correspondents. In these various ways, we hope that readers—nonmedical as well as medical—will be not only informed but also stimulated to play an active part in emergency care.

January 1977   Ken Easton

Don't Quit

When things go wrong, as they sometimes will,
When the road you're trudging seems all uphill,
When the funds are low and the debts are high,
And you want to smile, but you have to sigh,
When care is pressing you down a bit—
Rest if you must, but don't you quit.

Life is queer with its twists and turns,
As every one of us sometimes learns,
And many a fellow turns about
When he might have won had he stuck it out;
Don't give up, though the pace seems slow—
You may succeed with another blow.

Often the goal is nearer than
It seems to a faint and faltering man;
Often the struggler has given up
When he might have captured the victor's cup;
And he learned too late, when night came down,
How close he was to the golden crown.

Success is failure turned inside out—
The silver tint of the clouds of doubt,
And you never can tell how close you are,
It may be near when it seems afar;
So stick to the fight when you're hardest hit—
It's when things seem worst that you mustn't quit.

Author unknown

1

Essentials of Emergency Management

P J F BASKETT and J S M ZORAB

PRIORITIES IN MANAGEMENT

When confronted by a serious emergency, most people react with feelings of anxiety and inadequacy. Only training and practice can overcome this reaction and replace it with the calmness and confidence of knowing what to do and being able to do it.

The first action must always be to assess the condition of the patient and then to render what aid is possible *in the right order of priority*. It may help to bear in mind the following three questions:

(i) *What can I do to preserve this patient's life?*

(ii) *What can I do to reduce the complications arising from this injury or condition?*

(iii) *What can I do to relieve this patient's pain?*

These three questions form the lynch-pins on which all medical aspects of emergency care are founded.

Nevertheless, in the drama and confusion that often surrounds an accident or other emergency, it is only too easy for the inexperienced helper to forget these vital priorities. A calm and confident approach not only brings benefit to the patient but improves the performance and morale of other helpers at the scene.

Let us examine these three questions in more detail.

(i) *What can I do to preserve this patient's life?*

The first priority in emergency management is to assess and, if necessary, treat the respiratory and cardiovascular function of the patient.

This might appear too obvious to require emphasis, but there are numerous instances where this 'obvious' approach has not been fully observed, with disastrous or near-disastrous results. Two examples will serve to reinforce this point.

A patient was admitted to an accident department with a severe compound fracture of the left tibia and fibula. He had no other obvious injuries but did complain of some chest pain. After the initial examination, he was sent for X-ray of his leg and chest. While in the X-ray department he became acutely dyspnoeic and cyanosed. Help was sent for and a tension pneumothorax was diagnosed and relieved just in time. Only then was it realised that a chest injury with two fractured ribs had been sustained.

A pedestrian was involved in a road accident and sustained a head injury together with a fracture and gross laceration of one leg. He was unconscious and bleeding from his laceration. Initial airway care was given and attention then diverted to the leg injury. A few minutes later he was noticed to be blue and pulseless. Examination revealed that he had quietly regurgitated and aspirated stomach contents. Attempts at resuscitation failed. Subsequent autopsy revealed no skull fracture and only a minor brain contusion.

Both these patients had injuries which were not, in themselves, a threat to life. One nearly died and the other did die from complications which were avoidable had the proper priorities in care been maintained.

Questions (ii) and (iii) must always take second place to question (i) but they are, to some extent, interrelated and the relative priorities between them are less clear-cut.

(ii) *What can I do to reduce the complications arising from this injury or condition?*

The answer to this question falls under two headings—general measures and specific measures:

General measures

Good respiratory care will go a long way to reducing subsequent respiratory complications. Avoidance of hypoxia and protection of the lungs from aspiration of blood or stomach contents are the two most important measures. Arrest of active haemorrhage and early intravenous infusion will help to maintain a good circulation.

Specific measures

Careful handling of the injured patient is important so that further damage is not produced. The management of potential fractures of the spine and limbs is dealt with elsewhere and is an important part of the early emergency care.

(iii) *What can I do to relieve this patient's pain?*

Pain relief has been a neglected aspect of accident and emergency work and only recently has it begun to emerge as an important priority in the early stages of management. Pain relief is important, not only for reasons of compassion, but also because pain contributes to the release of catecholamines and, hence, has a deleterious effect on tissue perfusion.

In summary, the first priorities in the management of accidents and emergencies are:

(i) Safeguard life by establishing and maintaining cardio-pulmonary function.
(ii) Prevent complications by general and specific measures.
(iii) Relieve pain.

RESPIRATORY RESUSCITATION

The object of respiratory resuscitation is to improve and maintain the passage of oxygen from the atmosphere to the alveoli. Barriers to effective respiration can be classified as shown in Table I. However, it is probably more useful to consider the subject under the following headings:

(1) Assessment.
(2) Basic airway care.
(3) Suction.
(4) Laryngoscopy and intubation.
(5) Intermittent positive pressure ventilation (IPPV).
(6) Oxygen.

These are purely artificial divisions and are used only for descriptive purposes. The measures actually employed in any particular instance will depend on the condition of the patient and the skill and resources of the operator.

Assessment

Assessment is the first task when faced with a patient in an emergency situation. Only respiratory assessment is discussed here although, in practice, the patient must be assessed as a whole. When making a respiratory assessment the following questions should be considered:

Is the patient in a respirable atmosphere?

Obviously, if he is lying in a gas-filled room or garage, rapid removal to fresh air is essential. In some industrial accidents, this may not be possible and oxygen administration will be necessary at once. This is also true in cases of respiratory distress occurring at high altitude.

Is the patient a normal colour?

The presence of cyanosis should always stimulate the operator to urgent action. But the absence of cyanosis does not mean that all is well. It is now well documented that patients may have markedly reduced arterial oxygen levels without cyanosis being apparent, and many who are injured or have become suddenly ill will be so vaso-constricted that 'paleness' will be the prominent feature of their skin colour. Remember that carbon monoxide poisoning produces the characteristic 'cherry-red' skin colour and that cyanosis is not apparent but these patients are *always* suffering from hypoxia.

Is the patient making respiratory efforts and are those efforts resulting in ventilation of the lungs?

This is the vital question. In many instances respiratory efforts are clearly visible. However, heavy clothing, darkness and difficulty of access can all provide problems. Observation should be supplemented by palpation and by listening.

Where no signs of respiratory efforts can be detected, artificial ventilation should be started at once by whatever method is available.

Where spontaneous efforts are present, it is vital to decide whether they are resulting in effective ventilation of the lungs. *Note that noisy respirations invariably mean partial airway obstruction.* While the operator must do all he can to relieve this obstruction, he can take some comfort from the fact that the obstruction is *partial* and that some air, at least, will be entering the lungs. Silent respiratory efforts *can* mean normal unobstructed respiration but can just as well mean total airway obstruction.

If the patient's clothing and the circumstances permit, check on the movements of the chest and look for 'paradoxical respirations'. In total or severe partial respiratory obstruction, the abdomen will rise as the diaphragm descends but the chest will be drawn in instead of rising at the same time. This 'see-saw' movement of the chest and abdomen is one form of paradoxical respiration and is characteristic of airway obstruction. (It may also be seen where paralysis of the intercostal muscles has occurred, e.g. from a lower cervical or upper thoracic spinal cord lesion.)

Respiratory distress may continue even when a clear airway has been established. Rapid, shallow and jerky respirations should make the operator think of the possibility of interference with the mechanics of ventilation such as pneumothorax or multiple broken ribs—or both. A detailed consideration of the assessment and the management of chest injuries is to be found in Chapter 3 but some repetition seems desirable on this very important topic.

Diagnosis of chest injury can only be made when the chest has been exposed, so removal of some clothes is the first essential. Diminished or absent movement of one side of the chest, accompanied by deviation of the trachea, should lead the operator to suspect a pneumothorax. This can often be confirmed by percussion and auscultation. A unilateral pneumothorax will not usually require immediate treatment and the general condition of the patient must be balanced against the duration of the journey to hospital and the facilities available for resuscitation on the way. Do remember, however, that pneumothorax can be a bilateral condition, and the extreme respiratory distress that results requires immediate treatment.

One of the greatest hazards of chest injuries is the development of a tension pneumothorax. In this condition, air leaks into the pleural cavity through a valve-type lesion with each inspiratory effort. The intrapleural pressure increases, the mediastinum is shifted to the opposite side and collapse of the opposite lung occurs. This potentially lethal complication is a hazard of every chest injury and requires immediate treatment by insertion of an intercostal needle or drain. The institution of IPPV for any chest injury adds to this danger since the air leak will be increased as a result of the positive pressure within the lungs and the progress of the condition will be accelerated.

On examination of the chest, the two sides may move in opposite directions. Alternatively, there may be one segment that is being drawn in when the opposite side expands. This is another form of paradoxical respiration and is due to a breach in the integrity of the chest wall, e.g. from multiple fractured ribs. Minor degrees of paradox that are not accompanied by respiratory distress are acceptable and probably no treatment, other than oxygen administration, is required. Sometimes a degree of fixation of the chest wall may be achieved by apposition of an arm and this may bring some symptomatic relief.

Where marked respiratory distress is apparent, sedation, intubation and IPPV may be required to safeguard the patient's life during transport to hospital. The risks of a developing tension pneumothorax, however, are just as great and the operator must be prepared to insert an intercostal drain if necessary.

From the foregoing paragraphs it can be seen that only the properly trained operator will be in a position to diagnose the cause of respiratory problems of this type and safely institute the appropriate remedies.

Basic airway care

Posture

An unconscious patient is safest in the lateral or semi-prone position (Figs. 1.1 and 2). In this position, airway obstruction from the tongue falling back onto the posterior pharyngeal wall becomes less likely and any stomach contents or blood contaminating the airway will tend to drain from the mouth instead of pooling in the pharynx and, possibly, being aspirated into the lungs. Drainage is improved still further by a combination of the lateral or semi-prone position with a head-down tilt when facilities permit this.

Direct measures

Posture alone will not always be sufficient to overcome airway problems. Where direct measures are required, these are more easily and better performed in the supine position prior to turning the patient.

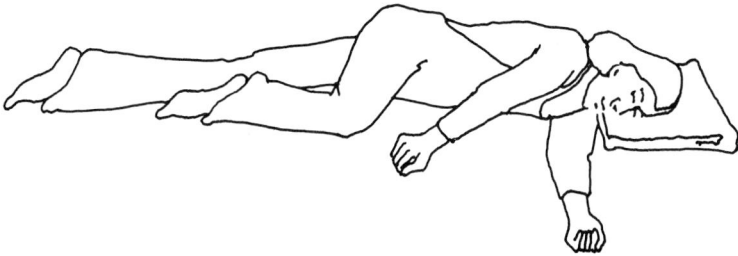

Fig. 1.1.   The Lateral position.

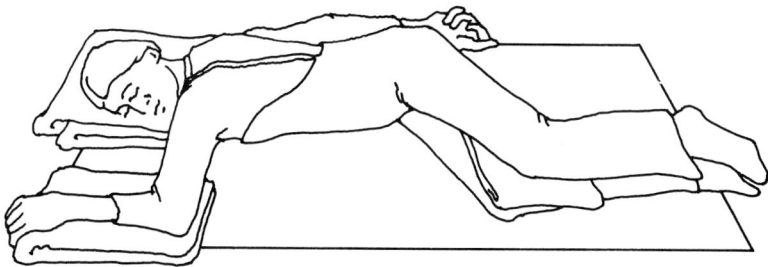

Fig. 1.2.   The semi-prone position.

An examination should be made of the mouth for foreign bodies, particularly dentures and loose teeth. These should be removed together with any solid pieces of stomach contents. Blood and other liquid matter can be cleared to some extent by a finger wrapped in a handkerchief and with the patient's head turned to one side (Fig. 1.3).

In the unconscious patient, the commonest cause of airway obstruction is the tongue. When the head is flexed and the jaw depressed, the tongue comes into contact with the posterior pharyngeal wall and totally closes the air passages (Fig. 1.4). Extension of the head and elevation of the jaw can re-open the airway (Fig. 1.5). **This is probably the most useful and important single manoeuvre in respiratory resuscitation.**

If a simple 'Guedel' oro-pharyngeal airway is available (Fig. 1.6), this will assist in establishing and maintaining unobstructed breathing in the deeply unconscious patient. This airway should be inserted

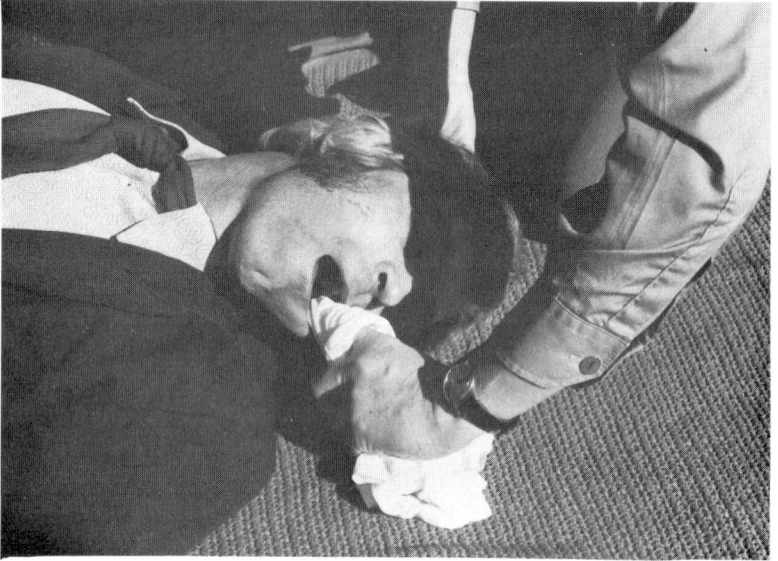

Fig. 1.3.   Clearing the mouth.

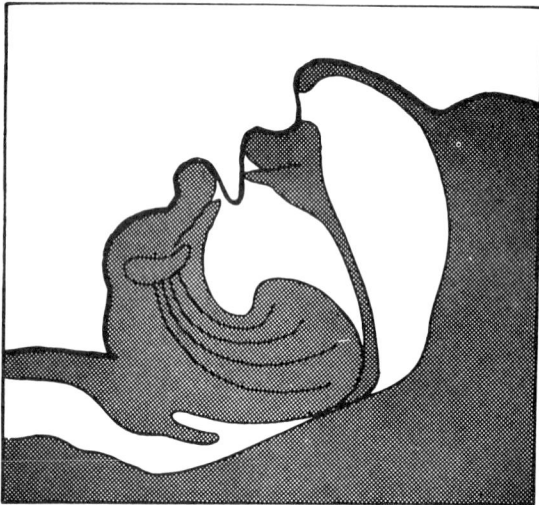

Fig. 1.4.   Obstruction of airway by tongue.

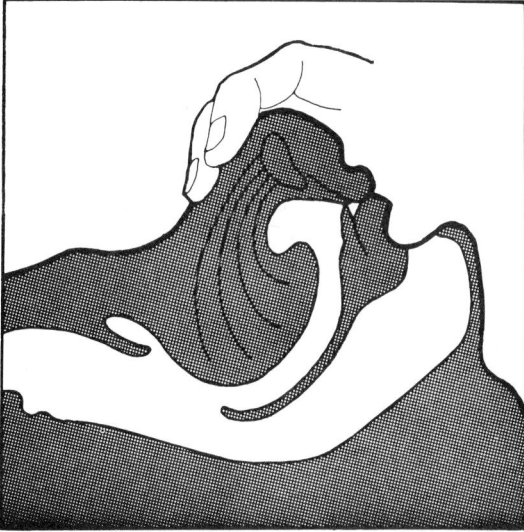

Fig. 1.5. *Reopening of airway by elevation of jaw and extension of head.*

into the mouth in the inverted position and turned as it passes over the back of the tongue into the oro-pharynx (Fig. 1.6). Should the patient resist attempts to insert an oro-pharyngeal airway, it is probably better to try and manage without, as persistence may result in damage to the teeth and is likely to provoke vomiting.

The naso-pharyngeal airway is another simple piece of useful, inexpensive equipment and one that tends to be rather neglected. It is a short piece of curved tubing, designed to pass through the nose into the naso-pharynx, with a flange or other device at the outer end to maintain it in position. A shortened endotracheal tube, with a large safety pin through the outer end, serves very well. A naso-pharyngeal airway has some advantages. Once in position, it will be tolerated at much lighter levels of consciousness than an oral airway; it can be inserted into a patient with a tightly clenched jaw; it provides a ready passage for a suction catheter. Remember, however, that occasionally its passage will produce brisk bleeding into the naso-pharynx which may add to the problems of maintaining the airway! Appropriate sizes, of course, will vary with the patient, but a 7·5 mm or 8·0 mm airway will fit an average adult nose.

If respiratory obstruction persists in spite of this basic airway care, it is probable that the obstruction is at laryngeal level. In these circumstances, further help and equipment are needed with the least possible delay. If total obstruction should supervene, and in the absence of

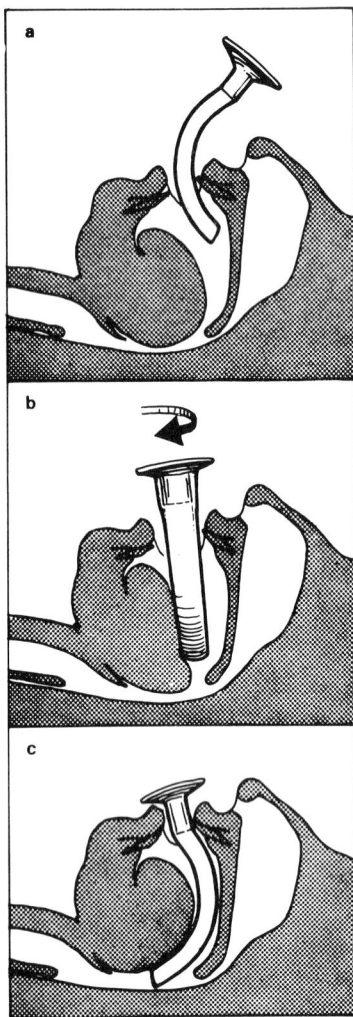

Fig. 1.6.   Insertion of Guedel airway.

a laryngoscope and endotracheal tube, emergency tracheostomy may be life-saving. Certainly there is nothing to lose! Such a situation may arise with a foreign body impacted in the larynx, haemorrhage or oedema occurring in a laryngeal tumour or, occasionally, with laryngo-tracheo-bronchitis or acute epiglottitis in small children.

Suction

Good, portable suction apparatus is very useful in patients whose airways are contaminated by blood, vomit or secretions. Where aspiration has already occurred, intubation and suction down the endotracheal tube may well reduce or prevent pulmonary complications.

The design of portable suction apparatus has improved in recent years. Equipment now available can be divided into four categories according to its power source.

Vacuum operated equipment

For many years it has been possible to modify the inlet manifold of an ambulance engine to make use of the mechanically-induced vacuum. This can be connected to a reservoir bottle and the suction controlled by a tap. The ambulance engine must be running for it to function, and it can only be used for a patient either inside or close to the vehicle.

Compressed gas operated equipment

Venturi devices connected to a source of compressed gas provide another well-tried method of suction. Large gas cylinders reduce the portability of such equipment but recently Laerdal has introduced a very compact venturi sucker based on a disposable cartridge of compressed gas. It is known as the Jet Suction Apparatus (Fig. 1.7) and is used suspended from the operator's neck, leaving the hands free. It is a useful, cheap and effective piece of apparatus.

Manually operated equipment

Foot or hand operated suckers have the advantages of being fully portable and independent of any outside power source. They produce an effective vacuum but can sometimes be difficult to use especially in a moving vehicle. The 'Ambu' foot sucker is probably the best known, being relatively inexpensive and very reliable.

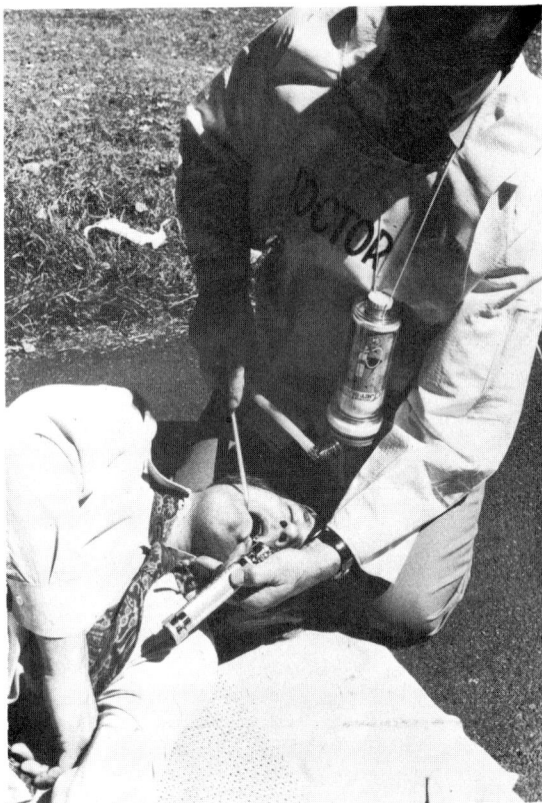

Fig. 1.7.   The Laerdal Jet Suction apparatus (Vickers Ltd).

Electrically operated equipment

The 'Laerdal' battery-operated suction pump is another excellent, though relatively expensive, piece of equipment. It combines portability with compactness and comes complete with re-chargeable battery. It can also be run off any 12 volt supply such as a car or ambulance battery and has an adaptor allowing it to be connected to the mains supply. As with all electrical equipment, regular maintenance is necessary.

Finally, it is worth adding a few words about attachments for the 'business-end' of the sucker. The choice lies between using a flexible catheter or a rigid 'Yankauer' pharyngeal sucker. There is a place for both. Disposable plastic suction catheters can be obtained in various sizes and are essential for sucking down endotracheal tubes. They are also useful for inserting down either oro- or naso-pharyngeal airways or through convenient gaps in the teeth. However, for a good toilet of the mouth and pharynx, the pharyngeal sucker is preferable. The pre-packed plastic version of the 'Yankauer' sucker is the most suitable for emergency work.

Laryngoscopy and intubation (see Guide pp. 16–17.)

The laryngoscope

The laryngoscope is a most useful instrument in its own right and should not just be considered as an aid to intubation. In the unconscious patient, it permits a careful inspection and toilet of the mouth, pharynx and larynx and, if supplemented by a pair of Magill's forceps and a sucker, its proper use will result in an airway known to be free of all foreign materials.

One of the problems of laryngoscopes, especially those infrequently used, is failure of the lighting arrangements at the vital moment. All anaesthetists know how often this can occur, even with instruments maintained by fully-trained staff. Another problem is the substantial cost of the conventional metal folding instrument. These problems have been overcome, to some extent, by the introduction of the fixed blade instrument made in plastic. Fig.1.8 shows a laryngoscope in use. The 'Penlon' laryngoscope has a switch incorporated into the base of the handle and is light, relatively cheap and convenient to use. The Welch Allyn laryngoscope is sold as a discardable plastic shell, with the batteries and light source contained in a special pen-torch that slips into the handle of the shell. The light is transmitted from the torch bulb through a piece of translucent, moulded plastic. The shells come in adult and child sizes and can be washed, though not sterilised. For those who prefer a conventional folding instrument, the 'Laerdal' laryngoscope is of excellent design though more expensive.

Use of the laryngoscope cannot be learned from a textbook. A number of 'models' designed for teaching intubation are now on the market (Fig. 1.8) but they are really no substitute for a real, live patient. Instruction and practice in laryngoscopy (and *practice* is the key word) can usually be arranged on a personal basis by making

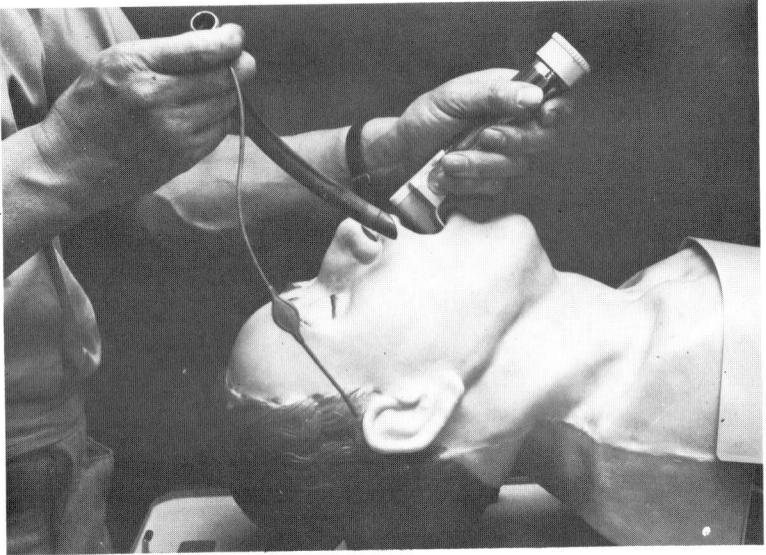

Fig. 1.8.   The Laerdal Adult Intubating model (Vickers Ltd).

contact with a local anaesthetist. This need not be a major, time-consuming undertaking although the distance from home to hospital will be a key factor. Fifteen minutes spent at the beginning of an afternoon operating list is a feasible proposition for many general practitioners and will usually provide the opportunity for using a laryngoscope, if not passing a tube, on a regular basis. Such practice over a period of weeks or months is of far more value than any concentrated tuition. The operator who has mastered the art of laryngoscopy, can easily pass a tube into the trachea when required. The secret of intubation is to become proficient at using a laryngoscope.

Intubation

Many of the problems of providing endotracheal tubes for emergency use have been overcome by recent technical developments. It is now possible to obtain pre-sterilised and pre-packed plastic endotracheal tubes with a long shelf life and containing their own connectors. Cuffed tubes are preferable for emergency use in adults and children over the age of six years and this means a syringe will be needed to inflate the cuff with air. It will also be necessary to occlude the cuff-inflating tube with a clip or a stopper. The plastic, disposable clamp of the Spencer-Wells type can also be used. A selection of tubes will be necessary for the fully equipped kit and four sizes (4·0 mm, 5·5 mm, 7·0 mm and 8·5 mm) will meet most needs.

In the opinion of the authors, disposable items of resuscitation equipment such as tubes, connections, infusion fluids, drip sets and intravenous cannulae should be provided by the local Accident and Emergency Centre. Most of the items mentioned have a long shelf life and are rarely used outside hospital, and this type of cooperation will encourage active participation in emergency care.

Ability to pass an oral endotracheal tube largely rests on the ability to use a laryngoscope. As for laryngoscopy, learning should be on a personal tuition basis. Those who are going to learn the techniques of laryngoscopy and oral intubation, should also try to learn the art of nasal intubation. A nasal endotracheal tube can be passed through either nostril into the naso-pharynx and then guided into the trachea with the help of a laryngoscope. There is, however, an alternative method known as blind nasal intubation, in which no laryngoscope need be used.

In this technique the head is positioned in full extension and rotated slightly to one side. The tube is passed through the nose, aiming the tip at the larynx. By listening to the breath sounds through the tube, one can estimate when the tip lies over the vocal cords and then, by advancing it quickly, it can often be passed into the trachea. This is not an easy technique, and it requires considerable practice, but it may occasionally prove useful where oral intubation is not possible.

For emergency use it is not necessary to have special tubes for nasal intubation, but a word should be said about the length of endo-tracheal tubes. As supplied by the manufacturer, these tubes are invariably too long. If an over-long tube is inserted, there is a strong likelihood of it going into the right main bronchus and leading to left lung collapse. This can be a serious hazard in some patients. Twice the distance from the corner of the mouth to the tragus of the ear is a rough guide for length of an oral endotracheal tube, and a nasal tube will need to be about an inch longer.

What, then, are the advantages of endotracheal intubation?

EQUIPMENT

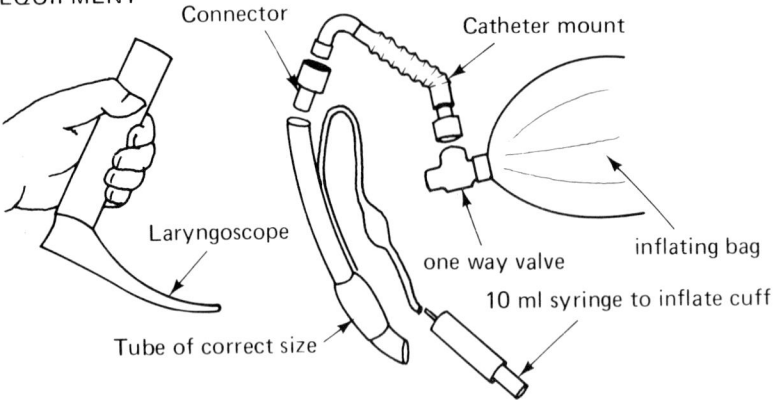

Connector

Catheter mount

Laryngoscope

one way valve

inflating bag

Tube of correct size

10 ml syringe to inflate cuff

Always check
(i) That the equipment fits together
(ii) That the laryngoscope works

Tube sizes
8·0 mm for almost all adults
6·0 mm for 8 - 12 year olds
4·0 mm for 3 - 7 year olds

POSITION IS VITAL

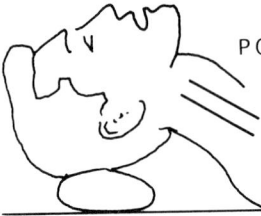
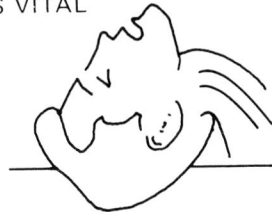

Correct position
Flex neck and extend head on neck;
this straightens the route to the larynx

Incorrect position
Extending the neck
makes things more difficult

LANDMARKS

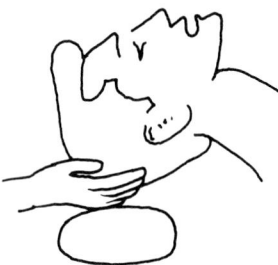
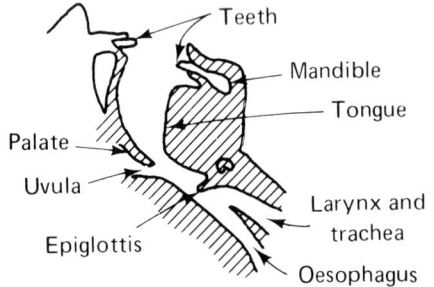

Teeth

Mandible

Tongue

Palate

Uvula

Larynx and
trachea

Epiglottis

Oesophagus

The epiglottis covers the larynx

INTRODUCING THE LARYNGOSCOPE

Hold laryngoscope in <u>left</u> hand

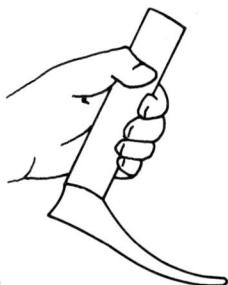

Introduce the laryngoscope to the right
hand side of mouth, deflecting the tongue
to the left and aiming for
the midline at the level of the larynx.

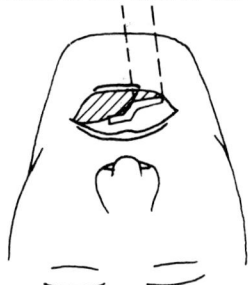

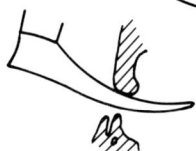

NB Avoid lower lip
by retracting it
out of the way

THE POSITION OF THE LARYNGOSCOPE

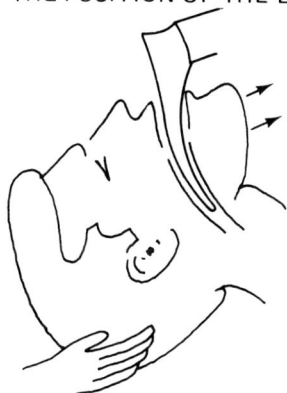

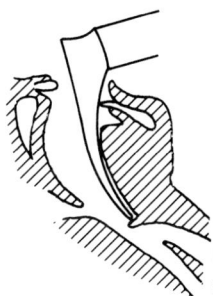

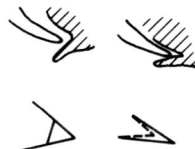

Insert tip of laryngoscope
blade in groove between
epiglottis and tongue to
lift the epiglottis out of
the way and expose the larynx

Draw larynx into line with mouth by
upward and forward lifting of laryngoscope in line with the handle

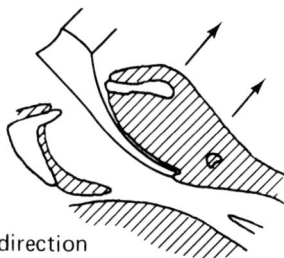

Broken tooth

Lift in this direction

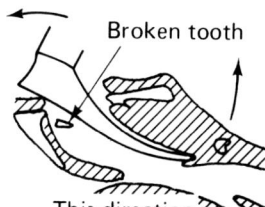

This direction
breaks off the front teeth

(a) It establishes a patent and secure airway.
(b) It protects the patient's lungs from aspiration.
(c) It allows suction of the trachea and main bronchi.
(d) It facilitates IPPV.
(e) It releases a skilled operator from airway management for other duties.

In conscious patients, endotracheal intubation is rarely indicated. Exceptions include patients with severe respiratory paralysis, gross laryngeal obstruction and, occasionally, severe status asthmaticus. But in all these instances, the procedure will be fraught with risks and technical difficulties, and specialist help should be sought if possible. Another exception is the patient with a severe chest injury. This problem is discussed elsewhere.

In the deeply unconscious patient, endotracheal intubation is undoubtedly the method of choice for securing the airway. Indeed, there is little excuse for not doing so if the appropriate skills and equipment are available. The risks and complications of aspiration of vomit alone make this a worthwhile procedure.

This leaves the large and difficult group of patients who are semi-conscious. These are patients who, while unable to safeguard their own airway or to respond to name or command will, nevertheless, offer strenuous resistance to attempts to clear their airway, let alone perform intubation. Such a state usually results from a head injury or from an overdose. Under these circumstances it is wisest to adopt conservative measures for maintaining the airway, while keeping a close watch for any change in conscious level. The patient who is semi-conscious to begin with may rapidly deteriorate. This could indicate active intracranial bleeding so that intubation and IPPV may become necessary in a very short space of time.

Endotracheal intubation, in properly trained hands, is a valuable and, occasionally, life-saving technique. In unskilled hands it can be a menace. Far better to concentrate on good basic airway care than to waste time and inflict trauma by trying to perform a manoeuvre with which one is not familiar. We are a long way behind the United States and many European countries in seeing that our medical students and newly-qualified doctors get adequate *practical* experience in the techniques associated with resuscitation (Editiorial, British Journal of Anaesthesia, 1973).

Intermittent positive pressure ventilation (IPPV)

Expired air ventilation

The efficacy of expired air artificial ventilation has now been established beyond all doubt. One of the major advantages of expired air ventilation is that it requires no apparatus. Many descriptions of the technique have been written but none can compare in value with practical tuition on a training manikin and/or a patient. The principle is simple. Following clearance of the airway, the patient's head is extended and the jaw elevated with one of the operator's hands. The operator then closes the patient's nostrils with the other hand and places his mouth over the patient's mouth (Fig. 1.9). If he now blows into the patient's

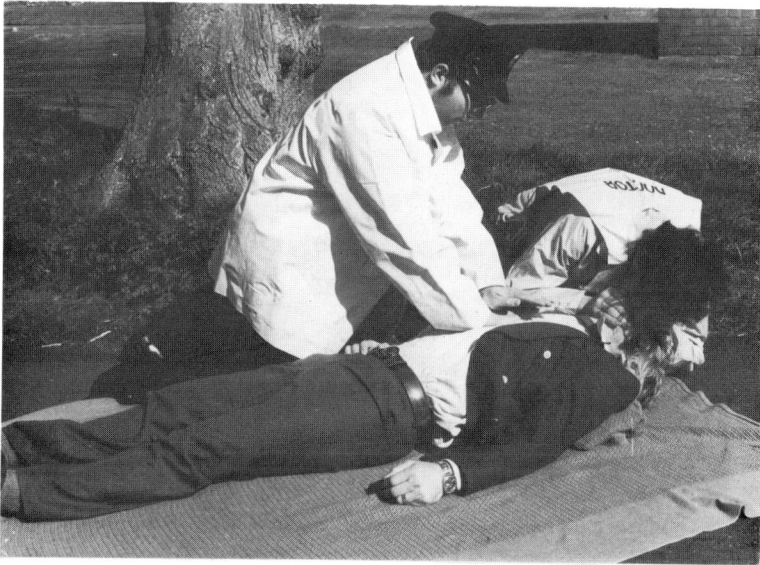

Fig. 1.9.   IPPV coupled with external cardiac massage.

mouth, he should see the chest rise as the patient's lungs are inflated. On removing his mouth, the patient's lungs will deflate and the movement can then be repeated. An alternative method is to hold the patient's mouth closed with the hand elevating the jaw and to blow into the nostrils. When using the technique with small children, it is easier for the operator to use his mouth to cover both the nose and mouth of the child.

Although this technique can be practised without the use of any apparatus, there are a number of simple and cheap devices which may help to increase its efficiency and make it aesthetically more acceptable. A simple pocket mask can be placed over the patient's face and has a small mouthpiece through which the operator can blow. A double airway can be used; with this, one piece is placed in the patient's mouth and the operator blows through the other end. The 'Brook' airway is well known and is used in the same way as the double airway but has a sealing flange to go round the patient's lips and a one-way valve to prevent the patient expiring into the operator's mouth. Expirations are diverted through the side tube Remember, too, that expired air ventilation may also be performed by blowing into the orifice of a properly applied face-mask or into an endotracheal tube.

The normal alveolar oxygen concentration is about 14 per cent. Dead space air has a slightly higher oxygen concentration but expired air ventilation can only supply the patient with sub-atmospheric levels of inspired oxygen (about 16 per cent). There may be occasions when the operator has access to inhaling oxygen but no means of ventilating the patient with it. If the operator inhales oxygen first and then exhales into the patient's lungs, substantially higher oxygen concentrations will be delivered.

The self-inflating bag

In 1957, Ruben and Ruben (1957) described a self-inflating bag for use in resuscitation. Since then a number of similar bags have been manufactured on the same principle. The most useful are the Air Viva Bag (BOC), the Ambu Bag (Ambu) and the Laerdal Resusci Folding Bag (Vickers). The performance of these bags has been reviewed along with a number of others (Redick and colleagues, 1970; Carden and Bernstein, 1970); they have been shown to be effective in use although there is a variation in delivered oxygen concentration when an oxygen supply is connected.

A self-inflating bag can be used either with a face-mask or with an endotracheal tube. It is of the utmost importance to ensure that the apparatus chosen will all connect together. In spite of all efforts at standardisation, a number of different styles and sizes of connector are still being used. The connections of bag, mask, catheter mount and endotracheal tube *must* be compatible. A major advantage of the self-contained kit is that all parts are designed to fit one another. Selection of the face-mask itself is largely a matter of personal preference. Transparent masks which permit close observation of the lips and mouth during use have a lot to commend them.

Using a self-inflating bag with a face-mask for IPPV is not, perhaps, as easy as it might seem. The secret lies in learning how to maintain an airtight fit between the patient's face and the mask at the same time as elevating the jaw and extending the head. This, of course, all has to be done with one hand leaving the other free to squeeze the bag. Fig. 1.10 shows the correct grip to employ but, again, practice

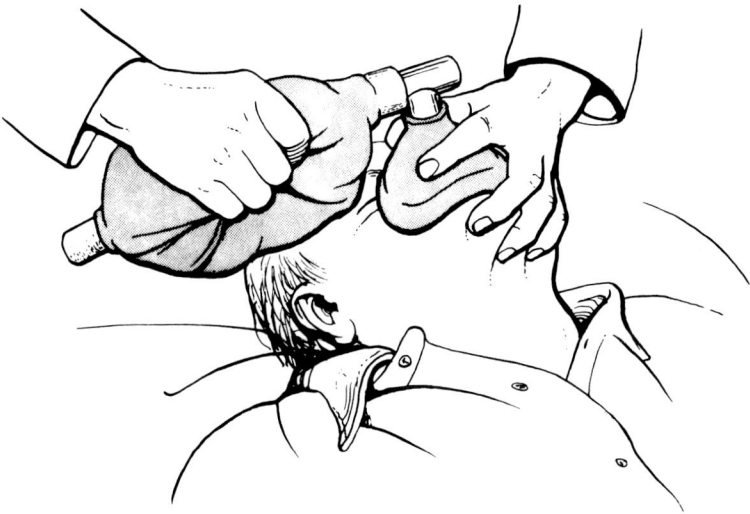

Fig. 1.10.   Use of self-inflating bag and mask.

is necessary. IPPV through an endotracheal tube is simpler (and safer) and, once the tube and bag are connected, the task of ventilation can often be delegated to an unskilled helper.

IPPV on a patient who is making no respiratory efforts of his own presents no problems of timing but when spontaneous respiratory efforts are present, one should try and synchronise squeezing the bag with the patient's own inspiratory effort.

Other methods of IPPV

Where a source of oxygen or compressed air is available, conventional anaesthetic circuits can be used but these are not really suited to emergency work and will not be discussed here. However, several mechanical devices have been designed to provide IPPV in emergencies. One of these, the Stephenson Minuteman, has been standard equipment for a number of ambulance brigades; another similar device, more recently introduced, is the Min-E-Pac . Both of these are designed to inflate the patient's lungs periodically with oxygen. Whilst not wishing to deny the value of these machines in skilled hands, the authors believe that simplicity and flexibility should be the key-note of all resuscitation equipment. For instance, while both the devices are suitable for giving IPPV with oxygen, neither can be used satisfactorily for administering oxygen to the patient with spontaneous breathing.

Expired air ventilation and self-inflating bags are both excellent methods of respiratory resuscitation. **Simple techniques and simple apparatus are the cornerstones on which resuscitation training programmes should be built.**

Indications for IPPV

Teaching methods of IPPV to those involved in resuscitation is one thing; teaching when and where the technique should be used is quite another!

Table I shows a simplified classification of the barriers to effective respiration. Patients in group A would not benefit from IPPV as such—they need a new atmosphere. Patients in group B might benefit from IPPV to some extent for, whereas their own respiratory efforts might be insufficient to overcome their airway obstruction, IPPV might achieve this (IPPV in the management of severe status asthmaticus is an example of this). However, the best treatment for these patients is to relieve their obstruction if possible.

It is the patients in group C who are most likely to need IPPV. Central depression of respiration is most frequently seen as a result of serious head injury, cerebrovascular accident or drug overdose. Respiration may be depressed either in rate or in depth and cyanosis may be apparent. IPPV is always indicated in these patients especially as, although their spontaneous breathing may just be adequate when first examined, they often deteriorate further before reaching hospital.

Acute chest infections in patients with chronic lung disease must also be mentioned here. These patients may be cyanosed, sweating, restless and irritable largely as a result of the underlying hypoxia.

TABLE I

Barriers to effective respiration

A   Unsuitable respirable atmosphere
    (a) Carbon monoxide or other toxic constituents
    (b) Hypoxic environments, e.g. smoke-filled rooms
    (c) High altitude hypoxia
B   Airway obstruction
    (a) Laryngeal and above
    (b) Tracheal and below
C   Failure of bellows
    (a) Central depression
    (b) Interference with mechanics of ventilation

Oxygen administration may produce a transient improvement but, in patients with this condition, who depend on limited hypoxia as a stimulus to respiration, the inspiration of high oxygen concentrations can rapidly lead to respiratory depression. If spontaneous respirations are to be preserved, such a patient needs to be given oxygen concentrations of the order of 24 per cent to 28 per cent. Higher concentrations than these may well produce respiratory depression, in which case IPPV will become necessary.

Interference with the mechanics of ventilation is usually the result of trauma to the chest. The possibility of an upper spinal cord lesion producing partial or total respiratory paralysis has already been mentioned but most problems result from direct chest injuries. The diagnosis and assessment of chest injuries have been mentioned in the section on assessment and are covered in more detail in Chapter 3. The patient whose chest injury is severe enough to cause respiratory insufficiency will undoubtedly need IPPV. It cannot be overstressed, however, that *in the absence of the ability to provide intercostal drainage at a moment's notice* IPPV, in the injured chest, can be a hazardous procedure.

Oxygen

Valuable though it is in all types of respiratory resuscitation, there are problems in having oxygen instantly available. It is, however, carried by almost every ambulance and can be brought to the scene of an emergency very quickly so that, at present, there is little justification for including it as part of an individual's resuscitation kit. This view is strengthened by the increasing adoption of a cylinder of Entonox into resuscitation kits. The prime use of Entonox is, of course, as an analgesic and this is discussed in the section on pain relief. Nevertheless, Entonox does contain 50 per cent oxygen, and that is two and a half times better than atmospheric air!

In many instances where oxygen therapy is required, Entonox will prove to be *more* satisfactory than 100 per cent oxygen because of the pain relief that is simultaneously achieved (Baskett and colleagues, 1973). Examples of this include myocardial infarction and chest injuries. In both instances the relief of pain encourages the patient to make better ventilatory efforts. Even in the unconscious patient, the nitrous oxide element should not deter the operator from using Entonox if the need for oxygen is clear cut. Better to be oxygenated with Entonox than to be hypoxic with air.

Another addition to resuscitation equipment now on the market is a supply of oxygen compressed into a specially made light-weight coil instead of the conventional heavy and expensive cylinder; it comes complete with contents gauge, flowmeter and filling point. The largest coil holds 300 litres of oxygen when factory-filled but can also be filled from a conventional oxygen cylinder when it will hold 200 litres.

The administration of oxygen to the patient needs to be considered in relation to IPPV or spontaneous breathing. With expired air ventilation, it has been suggested that the operator could inhale oxygen first and this would need a mask of some sort. More often a self-inflating bag will be used. Redick and colleagues (1970) and Carden and Bernstein (1970) have studied the percentages of oxygen delivered by bags at different flow rates and with different minute volumes. From their figures it would seem that an oxygen input of 5 – 10 litres per minute will produce inspired oxygen concentrations of from 35 per cent upwards. The longer the expiratory pause, the higher the delivered oxygen concentration will be. The Ambu bag and the Laerdal bag can both easily be modified to take a length of corrugated tubing on the air inlet and this acts as an oxygen reservoir giving even higher delivered oxygen concentrations.

It is worth recording that the Ambu bag and the Laerdal bag can both be used in conjunction with the demand valve system on an Entonox cylinder. If the air inlet of either of these bags is connected to the outlet of the demand valve by a piece of wide-bore corrugated tubing, the self-inflating bag will develop sufficient negative pressure to 'trigger' the demand valve and the bag will fill with Entonox. The indications for ventilating patients with a self-inflating bag and Entonox fall into two groups. One group would be where IPPV with oxygen is indicated and only Entonox is available. Under these circumstances, the value of the 50 per cent oxygen in Entonox must not be overlooked. The other group is where IPPV is indicated in the presence of pain such as a crushed chest injury. Ventilation with Entonox under these circumstances would provide the necessary added oxygen with the benefit of pain relief (Lunn and Kennedy, 1968).

For the spontaneously breathing patient, the self-inflating bag with mask is cumbersome and unnecessary (although it can be used). A cheap disposable mask is preferable and the MC mask (Fig. 1.11) is very suitable. This will deliver about 30 per cent oxygen at 2 litres

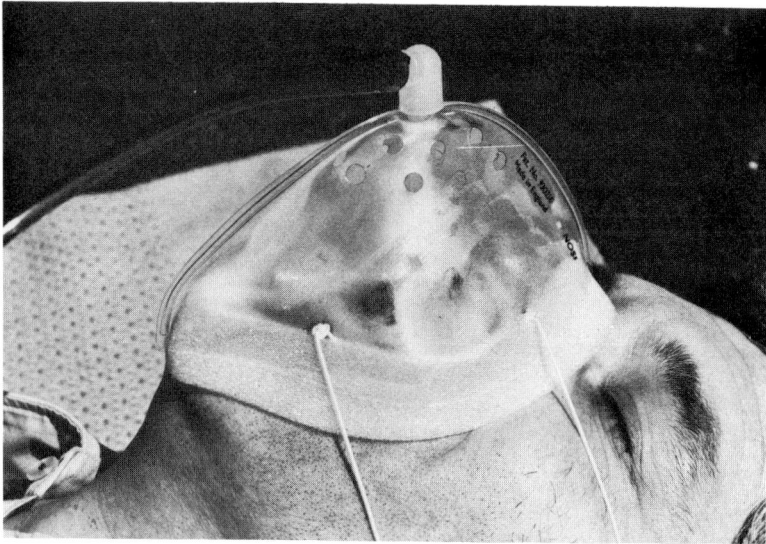

Fig. 1.11.   The MC Oxygen mask.

per minute and about 40 per cent oxygen at 4 litres per minute depending on the patient's tidal volume. Only modest increases are obtained at higher flow rates.

If it is available, oxygen can and should be used in any patient requiring respiratory resuscitation. Almost all of these patients will be hypoxic to a greater or lesser extent and oxygen can only improve their condition. Also oxygen is not only indicated for patients with respiratory problems. Tissue hypoxia will be the result of many cardiovascular emergencies, especially haemorrhage and myocardial infarction. Oxygen (or Entonox) should always be given in these conditions.

Finally, a word of warning regarding fire hazards in the presence of oxygen. Although oxygen is neither inflammable nor explosive, it supports combustion much more readily than air and the same applies to Entonox. So care is needed when using these gases, especially in a confined space. Fire hazards may be caused from sparks, from a cigarette or from electrical equipment. It is not a big risk but one that should be borne in mind.

CARDIOVASCULAR RESUSCITATION

The object of cardiovascular resuscitation is to improve and maintain the circulation of the blood. Almost invariably, in the emergency situation, the basic problem is a reduced cardiac output. As with respiration, however, cardiovascular resuscitation can be considered under some practical headings:

  (i)   Assessment.
  (ii) Basic cardiovascular care.
  (iii) Intravenous infusion.
  (iv) Electrocardiography.
  (v)   Cardiac arrest.

Again, these are purely artificial divisions but are useful for the purposes of description.

Assessment

When assessing a patient from a cardiovascular point of view, attention should be focused on the state of the cardiac output. A simple classification of the causes of a reduction in cardiac output is shown in Table II. While this may be an over-simplification, it provides a useful framework on which to base an emergency cardiovascular assessment.

TABLE II

Causes of reduction in cardiac output

A   Failure of pump
    (a) Congestive cardiac failure
    (b) Myocardial infarction
    (c) Arrhythmias
    (d) Trauma—myocardial injury or haemopericardium
B   Failure of venous return
    (a) Haemorrhage
    (b) Capillary stagnation or pooling

When making such an assessment, think of two questions:

Does the patient have an adequate cardiac output?

The patient who has a good cardiac output will have a good tissue perfusion and this is what really matters. While tissue perfusion cannot be measured directly, the patient who has a peripheral pulse which is regular and of good volume is unlikely to be in any immediate sort of cardiovascular trouble. If, in addition to this, he has reasonably warm and pink extremities, one can rest assured that his tissue perfusion is adequate.

However, do remember that a patient's cardiovascular status can change very rapidly. An early assessment may give no indication for specific therapy but a patient with multiple fractures and a serious abdominal or chest injury can lose blood from the circulation very rapidly. He may have a normal cardiac output when put into the ambulance but this can fall markedly during the journey. He would then arrive at hospital with all the signs and symptoms of acute blood loss. Such a state of affairs can be avoided if the initial assessment takes into full consideration the likely extent and nature of his injury or condition.

In many instances, the patient will be found to display a number of the signs and symptoms of a poor cardiac output. A sweaty, pale and possibly cyanosed skin together with a fast thready pulse is a classical picture. Measurement of the blood pressure is not usually very helpful. It is difficult to take under many emergency conditions and while a low blood pressure may confirm other observations of a reduced cardiac output, a normal blood pressure may simply reflect effective compensatory vaso-constriction. Always be guided by the overall picture, the circumstances of the emergency and the nature and extent of any injuries present.

If the patient does not have an adequate cardiac output, is this due to failure of the pump or failure of the venous return?

Usually the circumstances of an emergency will indicate the underlying cause of any reduction in cardiac output that may be present. Two obvious examples are the road accident victim with evidence of extensive haemorrhage and the patient in his own home who has had a severe myocardial infarction. Both patients will show signs of a reduced cardiac output—the former being due to reduction of venous return as a result of the haemorrhage and the latter due to partial pump failure. Since a rapid intravenous infusion will be beneficial to the former patient but detrimental to the latter, the differentiation is of very considerable importance.

Sometimes this differentiation can be quite difficult. For example, what about the elderly man, involved in a road accident, who is found unconscious and with signs of a reduced cardiac output? Does he have a ruptured liver or spleen with an intra-abdominal bleed or did he have a myocardial infarction and was this the cause of the accident? The differences in the clinical picture may not be very marked but cardiac arrhythmias and congested neck veins are two additional signs in favour of pump failure and against rapid transfusion.

Similar problems of diagnosis may arise with a suspected drug overdose. Signs of a reduced cardiac output may be due to depression of cardiac function from the agent taken or may be due to a failure of the venous return as a result of vasodilatation and capillary pooling. Again, look for arrhythmias and congested neck veins. Early hospitalisation and intensive therapy including measurement of the central venous pressure is needed before specific therapy can be instituted for these sort of problems.

Basic cardiovascular care

Severe reduction of cardiac output leads to a diminished tissue perfusion. The resulting tissue hypoxia causes a metabolic acidosis and the hypoxia and acidosis together may reduce the cardiac output still further. Thus the patient enters into a vicious circle which may lead to his death.

Where pump failure is the cause of the reduction in cardiac output, there is little under the heading of basic cardiovascular care that can improve the situation. However, the administration of oxygen, if available, is always helpful and reduces the ill effects of the poor tissue perfusion. Pain relief is also very important and is dealt with later in this chapter.

Where failure of the venous return—and this usually means haemorrhage—is the main problem, there are some basic measures that may help. Elevation of the legs has stood the test of time and remains a useful manoeuvre. Again, oxygen, if available, should always be used. Active bleeding should be stopped by the application of pressure dressings. This advice applies to limb injuries as well as those elsewhere. *There is no longer any place for the use of the tourniquet in the control of bleeding.* Tourniquets are dangerous and unnecessary relics of a bygone era. Patients can lose a lot of blood from scalp injuries. Pressure dressings are difficult to apply to this area and manual pressure may be necessary to control the bleeding.

Finally, a word must be said about the management of the body temperature. A patient who is allowed to get cold will, unless deeply unconscious, start to shiver. The intense muscle activity of shivering consumes large amounts of oxygen and the patient, who may already be hypoxic, will become still more so. If, on the other hand, over-enthusiastic attempts are made to keep the patient warm, he may become so vasodilated that his compensatory mechanisms will be overcome and a marked fall of blood pressure will result. The sensible course is one of moderation and to keep the patient warm enough to prevent shivering without overdoing it. An inexpensive way of preventing heat loss in an injured patient is by using the so-called 'space blanket' (Fig. 1.12).

Intravenous infusion

What are the indications for putting up a drip under emergency circum-

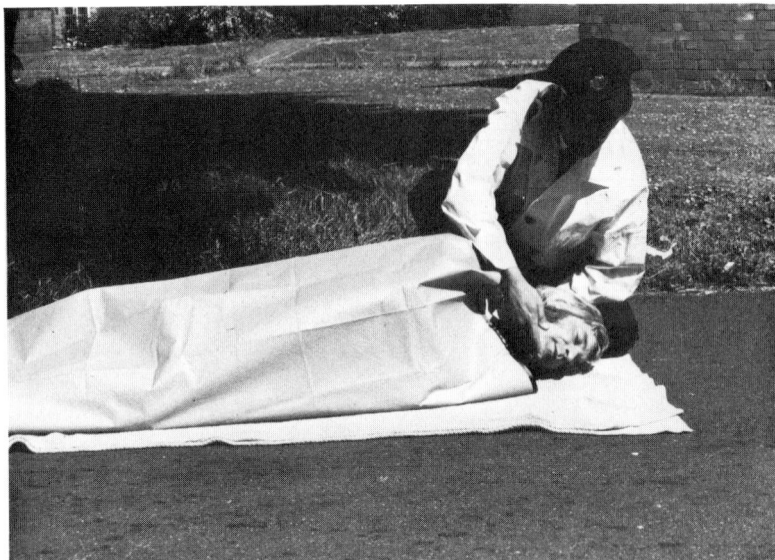

Fig. 1.12.   Space blanket (Sams Bros).

stances before the patient is transferred to hospital? Generally speaking, if a patient needs an intravenous infusion, then the sooner it is started the better. Nevertheless, putting up a drip can take time and there are occasions when delay in transfer will be more detrimental than delay in infusion. The severe head injury with an extradural haemorrhage is a good example. However, most patients who have bled or who are bleeding will need an intravenous infusion. Remember that, apart from visible blood loss, there may be a big occult loss. A fracture of the shaft of the femur usually results in a blood loss of at least 1 litre. If it is compound or comminuted, the loss will be higher. Multiple fractures of the limbs can lead to very substantial losses in blood volume.

Intravenous giving sets should always form part of an emergency kit. Of the versions available the Baxter set incorporates a pumping chamber which is very useful on occasions. Many giving sets are supplied complete with an intravenous needle. These needles, however, are less than ideal for use in emergency conditions. Even in hospital patients, lying in bed with a splinted arm, indwelling intravenous needles have a very short life because the sharp bevel soon cuts through the wall of the vein and the intravenous fluid runs into the tissues. There is now a wide range of needle/cannula sets which allow a plastic cannula to be left in the vein.

The Venflon® comes in several sizes and is sharp enough to be introduced through the skin without difficulty. It is supplied with a bung which allows it to be introduced and 'corked off' until the giving set is ready. This corking off is also useful when a patient is being lifted and moved since the drip set can be disconnected thereby making it less likely that the cannula is pulled out. There is a valvular orifice on the side of the cannula which enables intravenous drugs to be given without having to perforate the latex section of the drip tubing or even have a drip set up at all. Finally, there are two good-sized wings which facilitate fixing the cannula to the skin. Adequate quantities of adhesive strapping are absolutely essential. There are, of course, many other varieties of intravenous cannulae.

The choice of vein for a drip is often dictated by circumstances. If a patient has several veins from which to choose, remember that a forearm or upper arm vein is better than a hand vein or the antecubital fossa. Always avoid using a vein where it crosses a joint if possible and if the limbs are inaccessible, look for the external jugular vein.

The choice of infusion fluid is debatable and of only relative importance. The authors recommend Ringer/Lactate (Hartmann's) solution as being suitable for almost all occasions. It is available in plastic containers which are more manageable than bottles and do not smash when dropped (a not uncommon occurrence in an emergency situation). In addition to Ringer/Lactate solution, a bottle of a plasma expander should be carried such as Macrodex® or Dextraven®. These solutions are, unfortunately, still only available in glass bottles. It is usually more convenient to commence the infusion with the Ringer/Lactate solution and then move on to the plasma expander.

Since many accident patients will subsequently need a blood transfusion, it is important to understand the relationship between the administration of a plasma expander and the cross-matching of blood for transfusion. There is no doubt that the previous administration of a plasma expander does increase the difficulty of cross-matching since the red cells will develop a tendency to rouleaux formation. Nevertheless, *provided the laboratory is aware of the situation*, it is not a big problem. The rule, then, should be—take blood for cross-matching *before* giving a plasma expander. If this is not possible, let the laboratory know that a plasma expander has been given. Do not forget to include blood sample containers in the emergency kit. There should be tubes with an anti-clotting agent for haemoglobin estimations and a plain tube for cross-matching.

Finally, it is essential to emphasise the importance of giving intravenous fluid at an appropriate rate. Most of the patients requiring this treatment will be the victims of accidents. Their blood loss will have occurred very rapidly and, in many instances, will still be occurring. It is largely a waste of time setting up an intravenous infusion if it is then allowed to drip in at the conventional rate of 500 ml over four hours. These patients have lost and are losing their circulating volume very quickly *and it should be replaced quickly.* Therefore insert big cannulae and run the fluid in at a generous rate. The first litre should be through in 20 or 30 minutes at the outside. At times, of course, a faster rate will be indicated.

Electrocardiography

The electrocardiograph (ECG) has a part to play in the initial management of those emergencies that involve acute and potentially dangerous arrhythmias or cardiac arrest. On the other hand, although many general practitioners carry or have access to a portable ECG writer, this instrument will rarely be at the right place at the right time and, because of the limitation imposed by the paper roll, is not suitable for the continuous recording that will usually be required. A more suitable piece of equipment is a portable ECG oscilloscope—commonly known as a cardioscope—but this is not likely to form part of the general practitioner's emergency kit nor should it.

To overcome these problems, a number of areas have now equipped one or more ambulances with both a portable cardioscope and a portable DC defibrillator. These vehicles are variously known as cardiac ambulances, coronary care ambulances and mobile intensive care units. The authors have been associated with one of their own design which is called a Mobile Resuscitation Unit (MRU), the name thus emphasising the two main features, viz. mobility and the general resuscitative nature of the work in which the vehicle is involved. Vehicles of this nature make it possible to provide the advantages of an ECG and a defibrillator, as well as a wide range of other equipment, at the scene of an emergency with very little delay.

While such an arrangement helps to make the equipment available, it makes it necessary to face the problem of who is going to use it.

There are three ways in which this can be tackled and they are not mutually exclusive. One is for the MRU or similar vehicle to be hospital based and to carry a member of the medical or nursing staff who has been trained in resuscitation. Another alternative is to train a number of ambulance men to a standard that will allow them to use the equipment carried. This involves their being able to use and interpret the ECG and to be able to use the defibrillator. The third alternative is for the MRU simply to provide equipment and facilities to a doctor on the spot who has been summoned by a separate arrangement.

At present, there is no right or wrong solution. Much exploratory work remains to be done and the introduction of ECG telemetry whereby the patient's ECG can be transmitted over the ambulance's radio system to the hospital for interpretation is another technique which is being developed and assessed.

Patients who develop acute and potentially dangerous arrhythmias require urgent admission to hospital. With the facilities offered by an MRU the doctor would be in a position to start anti-arrhythmic treatment immediately. Even if this was not required, the early attachment to a cardioscope will enable a close watch to be kept on the heart's rhythm and, should ventricular fibrillation supervene, cardiopulmonary resuscitation can begin at once. Used in this way, a cardioscope, backed by the proper ancillary equipment, helps to safeguard the patient's journey to hospital.

Cardiac arrest

The management of cardiac arrest outside hospital presents many difficulties. Not the least of these is the time scale involved. Unless primary cardiopulmonary resuscitation can be started by someone on the spot, it is unlikely that a resuscitation team that has to be sent for will be able to achieve very much. Nevertheless, cardiac arrest is a *clinical* diagnosis and patients who are said to have arrested may, in fact, have a minimal circulation which is sufficient to extend the time scale. For this reason, efforts at resuscitation should always be made even if the situation — as judged from when the arrest is supposed to have occurred — appears hopeless.

The management of cardiac arrest — whether occurring inside or outside hospital — falls into four phases.

Diagnosis

Cardiac arrest is a clinical diagnosis. The diagnosis rests upon the absence of the carotid (Fig. 1.13) or the femoral pulse. Other signs will be apparent—such as unconsciousness, pallor or cyanosis,

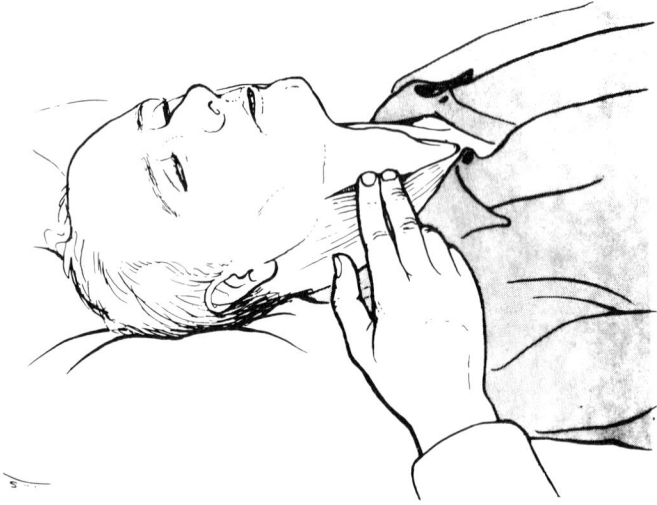

Fig. 1.13.   Palpating the carotid pulse.

stertorous or absent respirations and dilated pupils—but these are consequent upon the arrest and may take some time to appear. The stethoscope plays no part whatever in diagnosing cardiac arrest; it simply wastes valuable time. An ECG, if already connected, may confirm arrest and will be helpful in differentiating between asystole and ventricular fibrillation (see later) but a patient may have an apparently acceptable ECG but an ineffective circulation so that, again, the presence or absence of a pulse is the sign upon which action should be based.

Primary procedures

Once cardiac arrest has been diagnosed, immediate action is necessary. The two vital steps are artificial ventilation, with oxygen if possible, and external cardiac massage.

Artificial ventilation has been dealt with in the previous section but it is worth emphasising that it must be started immediately. Even if all the equipment for intubation is available, initial efforts should be made with expired air ventilation or a bag and mask while the more elaborate equipment is made ready.

External cardiac massage must also begin immediately. The first requirement is for the patient to be lying on a hard surface. Attempts to perform cardiac massage with the patient on a soft mattress are quite useless. Unless a board or tray are readily available to put behind the patient's back, he should be moved onto the ground. External cardiac massage is best done with the operator kneeling beside or astride the patient with his hands placed one over the other and the heel of the bottom hand over the lower one third of the patient's sternum (Fig. 1.9). The action is then one of short, sharp thrusts, keeping the arms straight and allowing the movement to come from the shoulders. Only by doing it in this way can efforts be maintained over any period of time. Practice on some of the manikins now available is helpful in becoming familiar with this technique.

Where the operator is single handed, it will be necessary to alternate between ventilating the lungs and cardiac massage—for every four or five thrusts on the sternum, one inflation of the lungs should take place. The rhythm is depicted in Fig. 1.14. When two operators are

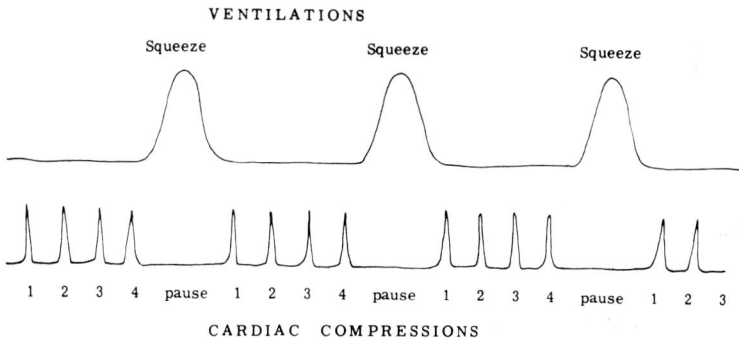

Fig. 1.14.   Rhythm of external cardiac massage and IPPV.

present, the rhythm should be the same with the person performing the massage pausing after every fourth or fifth thrust to allow inflation of the lungs. This coordination is important since, if a thrust on the sternum coincides with an inflation of the lungs, very high intra-pulmonary pressures will be produced. During cardiac massage, brief pauses should be made periodically to check whether a spontaneous cardiac output has returned by feeling for the carotid pulse.

Secondary procedures

A small number of cardiac arrests may revert to a spontaneous rhythm from the primary procedures alone. One particular instance is the basically normal heart that has stopped as a result of acute hypoxia as, for example, in the patient with a total airway obstruction. Relief of the obstruction followed by effective pulmonary ventilation and external cardiac massage will often restore a spontaneous rhythm quite quickly. More usually, however, one has to move on to the secondary procedures to have any chance of success. It may only be possible to do this once the patient has reached hospital but, where an MRU is available, the secondary procedures can be started as soon as the equipment and assistance are available.

The secondary procedures in the management of cardiac arrest are as follows:

(i)   Continue external cardiac massage.
(ii)   Continue and improve artificial ventilation.
(iii) Set up an intravenous drip and start drug therapy.
(iv)   Connect ECG, interpret and defibrillate if necessary.

These procedures and, indeed, the management of cardiac arrest as a whole is covered in detail in a small audio-tape cassette recording and handbook (Zorab, 1972) which, although orientated to hospital management, is eminently applicable to an MRU. These secondary procedures can now be considered in more detail.

External cardiac massage. It is absolutely imperative that this be continued with no more than momentary interruptions throughout the resuscitation period. An occasional pause to check for the return of a spontaneous pulse or to intubate the patient is all that is permissible.

Artificial ventilation. Assuming that artificial ventilation has been started with the expired air method, transfer to a bag and mask should be made as soon as possible and oxygen should be added the moment it is available. If the facilities *and expertise* for endotracheal intubation are present then they should be used but effective ventilation with a bag and mask is far preferable to prolonged, unsuccessful attempts at intubation. Nevertheless, intubation is best when it can be achieved quickly and surely as it ensures a clear airway, makes the addition of oxygen easier, safeguards the lungs from aspiration of stomach contents and enables the operator to transfer the task of IPPV to less skilled hands.

The intravenous infusion and drug therapy. All drugs for restarting the heart must be given directly into the circulation. Attempts to perform intracardiac injections interrupt cardiac massage, require a separate injection for each agent and are not recommended. Intravenous administration combined with good cardiac massage produces excellent results and is the method of choice. Ideally, an intravenous infusion should be started. The infusion fluid is not of great significance and almost any isotonic solution will do. The first drug to be given should be sodium bicarbonate. All patients with cardiac arrest will develop a marked respiratory and metabolic acidosis and the earlier this is treated, the greater the chances of restarting the heart.

Sodium bicarbonate is conveniently used in a strength of 8·4 per cent, as this comes in 100 ml bottles and 1 ml equals 1 mmol. This makes calculation of dosage simple and the authors recommend 50 mmol at once and 30 mmol at intervals of five minutes throughout the peroid of arrest. A disadvantage of 8·4 per cent solution is its short shelf life (3 months), and the 4·2 per cent solution is probably better for keeping in emergency kits. Sodium bicarbonate may be the only drug therapy that is required for, where ventricular fibrillation is diagnosed or suspected, early defibrillation is the treatment of choice. Where defibrillation has failed or where cardiac asystole is present, intravenous adrenaline may be helpful. This is usually supplied in ampoules of 1 : 1000 solution, and 1 ml of this should be diluted with normal saline or water for injection to 10 ml to give 1 : 10 000 solution. One or two ml of this solution will often improve the tone of the heart and increase the chances of a successful defibrillation. The heart in asystole may revert to spontaneous rhythm following intravenous adrenaline or, more usually, it will fibrillate in which case, defibrillation can be used.

Calcium chloride is the only other drug that may be required to restart the heart following cardiac arrest. The heart in asystole can sometimes be very refractory to treatment—even to intravenous adrenaline. Intravenous calcium, by increasing the irritability of the myocardium, is sometimes successful in starting up an asystolic heart or, at least, inducing ventricular fibrillation which, as before, can be treated with defibrillation.

Connecting and interpreting the ECG. The ECG offers both diagnostic assistance and a means of following the effectiveness of treatment. Where cardiac arrest is thought to have resulted from myocardial infarction, many authorities recommend that an initial defibrillation should be attempted without waiting to display an ECG. Subsequent examination of the ECG is, however, helpful in assessing the success or otherwise of treatment and can be useful in deciding on intravenous therapy. Figures 1.15 and 16 show examples of the sort of tracings that might be observed.

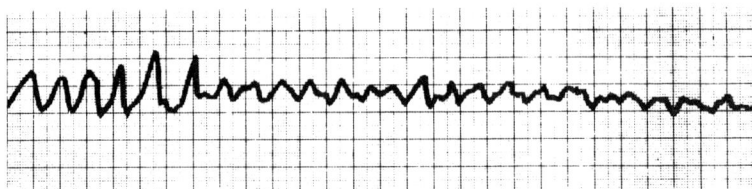

Fig. 1.15.   Ventricular fibrillation.

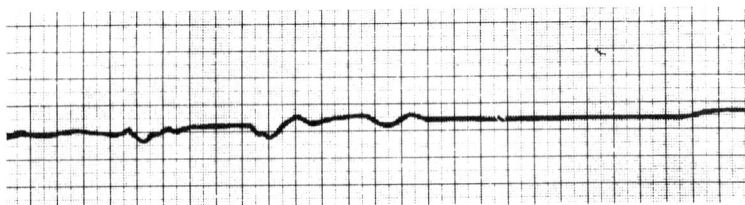

Fig. 1.16.   Cardiac asystole.

Defibrillation has been mentioned a number of times without any details of the technique being given. In ventricular fibrillation, the muscle fibres of the myocardium are contracting in an irregular and uncoordinated manner. By passing an electric shock through the myocardium, a refractory state is produced in all muscle fibres. Once the refractory state is over, a regular rhythm may supervene. It is now customary to use a defibrillator which produces a direct current (DC) shock and this can be delivered through the chest wall. Full instructions are printed on the various instruments available but an outline of the procedure is as follows:

The machine is plugged in and switched on. The external electrodes are connected and the operator is advised to wear a pair of rubber gloves. The charge is set for an initial shock of 200 joules. Electrode jelly is smeared over both electrodes and the machine is switched to 'charge'. One electrode is placed over the lower sternum and the other over the apex beat. Both electrodes must be pressed down hard as they usually incorporate safety switches which only make contact on pressure. The discharge button is pressed and if discharge is effective, the patient will usually give a small jump. *Cardiac massage must then be resumed immediately* and the ECG watched for the return of spontaneous rhythm. If fibrillation persists, further shocks may be given and the charge may be increased up to a maximum of 400 joules.

Failure to defibrillate is always difficult to manage but the following points must be borne in mind:

Has bicarbonate therapy been adequate? Defibrillation is less successful in the presence of acidosis.

Is oxygenation adequate? Myocardial hypoxia militates against successful defibrillation.

Is myocardial tone adequate? Coarse fibrillation (indicating good tone) is easier to reverse than fine fibrillation. More adrenaline may help.

Aftercare

Should the operator have been successful in restarting a patient's heart, it is most important that he should not sit back and think his troubles are over. The heart that has stopped once can easily stop again and this is particularly true in myocardial infarction. Monitoring with a cardioscope is especially useful here but attention must be paid to ventilation and oxygenation. External cardiac massage can break ribs and broken ribs can lead to a pneumothorax. Post-arrest arrhythmias are not uncommon and although the ECG may look reasonable, the cardiac output may be very low. The patient whose heart has been successfully restarted requires maximum vigilance until this task can be taken over by the hospital department.

PAIN RELIEF

The third of the questions posed at the beginning of this chapter was 'What can I do to relieve this patient's pain?' The majority of patients needing emergency care are in genuine pain, often with a very understandable overlay of apprehension and anxiety. The relief of this pain and anxiety is not only a humane act but also carries the extra bonus of improving tissue perfusion in the vasoconstricted victim by reducing the output of catecholamines. Analgesics, however, have their limitations and dangers, and fear of the consequences has often led to the patient being deprived of any pain relief at all.

Pain relief can be considered under the following headings:

(i)   Parenteral analgesics.
(ii) Inhalational analgesics.
(iii) Practical applications.
(iv) General anaesthesia.

Parenteral analgesics

The opiates

Among the opiates and related compounds that are suitable for use in rescue work are morphine, diamorphine, pethidine and pentazocine (Fortral®). All members of the opiate group have basically similar properties. Despite strenuous efforts by the pharmaceutical industry to produce a drug with a better ratio between the therapeutic dose and the dose causing unwanted side effects (therapeutic ratio), the authors believe that morphine remains the most effective member of this group for the combined treatment of pain and anxiety.

The biggest advantage of morphine is that it works. It is a very well proven agent which will almost always produce pain relief and mental sedation provided it is given in a sufficiently large dose. The fit patient in severe pain may need 20–40 mg or even more and these doses are often well tolerated provided the patient is correctly managed. Another advantage of morphine, indeed of all parenteral drugs, is that they are given by injection and do not, therefore, require the cooperation of the patient.

The route of injection, however, is very important. The vasoconstricted patient has poor perfusion of his muscle mass and subcutaneous tissue. Injection into these sites will, therefore, not be absorbed quickly into the circulation and no immediate analgesia will be produced. This lack of effect may lead to further doses being given. When the circulation has improved, the full action of the total doses will become apparent. This has two very undesirable effects. The patient will have been deprived of pain relief when he most needed it and will become maximally and, perhaps, dangerously depressed and insensitive when in the accident department where all the signs and symptoms are needed for diagnosis. For these reasons all parenteral agents should be given by the intravenous route in small incremental doses until the desired effect is achieved. For this purpose, a winged indwelling needle with a short length of flexible tubing and a re-seal injection site is invaluable (Fig. 1.17).

In spite of the effectiveness of the opiates, it is well known that even modest therapeutic doses may depress respiration, the circulation

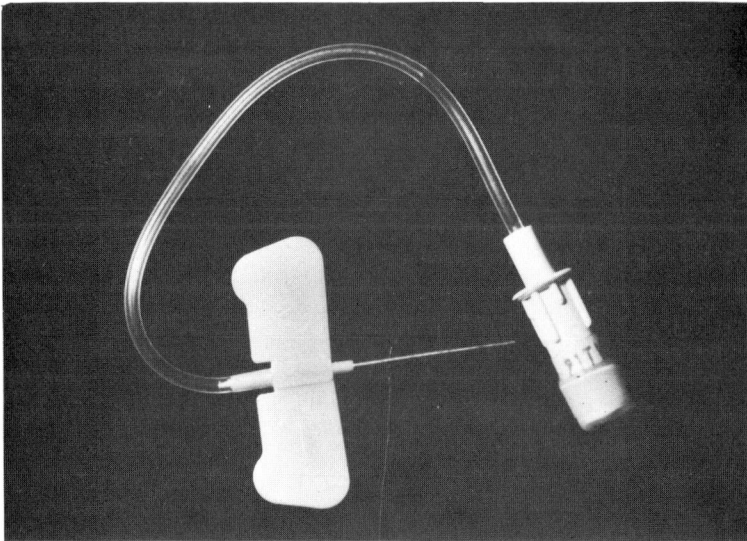

Fig. 1.17.   'Butterfly' indwelling needle (Abbott Laboratories).

and the protective laryngeal reflexes. This depression is accentuated in patients with respiratory embarrassment, e.g. the chest injury, or if there is a reduced cardiac output due to blood loss or pump failure. Although opiates must be used with caution in any seriously ill patient, remember that their depressant actions are usually reduced in the presence of *severe* pain.

Many of the opiates, and morphine in particular, cause constriction of the pupils and sluggishness in their reaction to light. The reaction of the pupils is an important sign in the diagnosis of intracranial compression or damage and masking of these reflexes places the examining doctor at a considerable disadvantage. Indeed, a severe head injury should be regarded as an absolute contraindication to the use of parenteral analgesics.

An injection of morphine or similar drug lasts for a considerable time—up to one or even two hours. This may again embarrass the receiving doctor at hospital by obscuring essential signs and symptoms. Especially vulnerable in this instance is the patient with an abdominal injury who may not complain of pain even though he has sustained a ruptured liver or spleen. Another problem is the emetic property of the opiate group of drugs. The likelihood of nausea and vomiting is increased by a lurching ride in an ambulance. Not only is this distressing for the patient but it is also dangerous in seriously ill cases who may have impaired protective laryngeal reflexes. In the presence of *severe* pain, however, nausea and vomiting are not often seen.

Morphine, diamorphine, pethidine, and most other opiates are, of course, bound by the Misuse of Drugs Regulations, 1973. These specify that they must only be administered under the guidance of a registered medical practitioner, must be kept locked up at all times and be entered in an accurate register maintained for inspection by the authorities. The regulations make it impractical to include these drugs in emergency ambulances or rescue kits. Only pentazocine (Fortral) is exempt from these rules and for this reason it is this drug that is carried by the mobile resuscitation unit (MRU) with which the authors are associated. Even so, it can only be administered by a doctor and cannot be used by paramedical personnel working on their own.

Diazepam

Diazepam (Valium®) is a drug which, although only relatively recently introduced, has already established a place for itself in emergency medicine. It is not a true analgesic in its own right but is a potent, effective tranquilliser and sedative in the apprehensive, restless and uncooperative patient and enhances the action of the specific pain relieving agents. It has a relatively wide therapeutic ratio so that the vital functions of respiration and the circulation are not usually depressed with the therapeutically effective dose which is in the range of 10–20 mg. Obviously, this dose must be reduced in the critically ill patient.

Being a relatively long-acting drug, Diazepam suffers from the same problem as the opiates in that its effect may still be apparent on arrival at hospital and this may present difficulties in diagnosis. Diazepam must, of course, always be given by intravenous injection for the same reasons as other parenteral drugs, and it must be remembered that, given in a sufficiently large dose, it will produce unconsciousness and all the hazards that go with it (see General Anaesthesia).

Inhalational analgesics

Nitrous oxide

Inhalational analgesics have enjoyed widespread popularity in the United Kingdom for the relief of pain in childbirth for many years. Only recently, however, have they been applied in the emergency field. Nitrous oxide is the oldest inhalational analgesic and has stood the test of time. For many years it was used mixed with air but it is now recognized that the inevitable hypoxia that accompanied this technique was unacceptable and consequently nitrous oxide should always be used mixed with oxygen. It was the introduction of nitrous oxide and oxygen premixed in a single cylinder, in a 50 per cent concentration of each gas Fig. 1.18 (Tunstall, 1968), that made this valuable inhalational analgesic so suitable for use in rescue and emergency work (Baskett and Withnell, 1970; Baskett, 1972). The premixed gases are available as Entonox® and are supplied in a cylinder together with a specially designed, portable, demand inhalational unit weighing 6 kg in all.

Nitrous oxide, in a 50 per cent concentration, is a very effective analgesic. Indeed, Parbrook and colleagues (1964) have shown that even 25 per cent nitrous oxide is superior to morphine in a dose equivalent to about 12 mg of morphine in the average adult. Nitrous

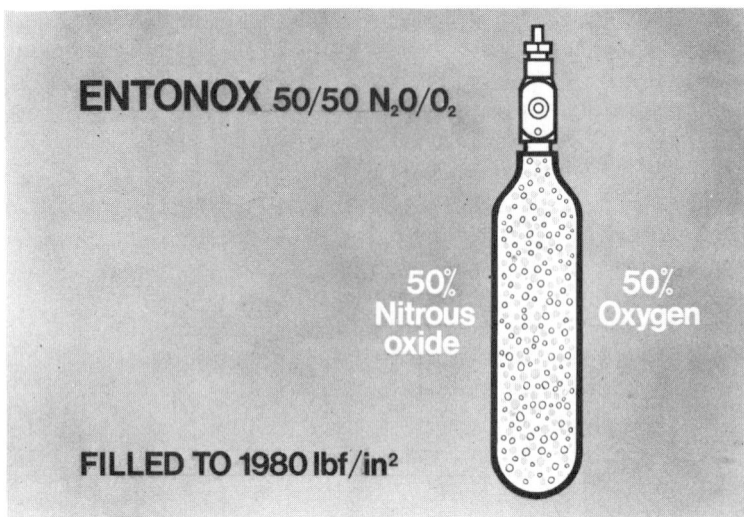

ENTONOX 50/50 N₂O/O₂

50%
Nitrous
oxide

50%
Oxygen

FILLED TO 1980 lbf/in²

Fig. 1.18.   Entonox in cylinder.

oxide is free from depressant and unwanted side effects on the vital functions of respiration and the circulation. Maximal pain relief is achieved about two minutes after beginning inhalation and complete recovery occurs, without any residual analgesia, within the same period of time.

The high oxygen content of Entonox means that it can be used safely and beneficially in patients with vasoconstriction and a low cardiac output. Indeed, if it is used with the demand inhalational unit, a true 50 per cent of oxygen is inhaled. This produces arterial oxygen tensions which compare very favourably with those produced by pure oxygen given under the normal clinical conditions of using a 5 litre flow with a plastic disposable face mask (Baskett and colleagues, 1973).

Entonox can be offered to almost all patients in pain. Exceptions are head injuries with impairment of consciousness and intoxicated patients where there is a primary danger of inhalation of the stomach contents because their protective laryngeal reflexes may be depressed. Maxillo-facial injuries are also usually a contraindication because of the pain inflicted by the initial application of the mask to the face. But, undoubtedly, one of the greatest advantages of Entonox is that,

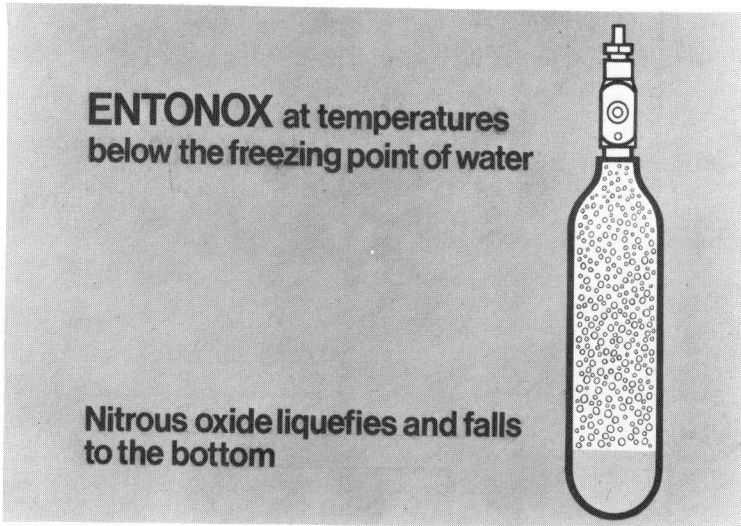

Fig. 1.19.   Entonox. Effect of temperature below freezing point.

provided it is self-administered by the patient, inhalation can be super-vised by trained paramedical personnel without a doctor being present.

With all inhalational analgesics, however, especially if they are administered with a demand apparatus, a certain amount of patient cooperation is required. This is not often a problem but on a few occasions the very apprehensive person may not be able to manage the inhalation correctly. The patient with a chest injury may be reluctant to inhale deeply because of pain and therefore does not get sufficient analgesic mixture to relieve the pain.

While 50 per cent nitrous oxide is an effective analgesic in the majority of patients (Baskett and Withnell, 1970; Baskett, 1972), there are a few instances in which it is not quite potent enough. With Entonox the percentage of nitrous oxide cannot be increased to cope with this extra demand.

Remember that, although Entonox is not an explosive mixture, it does contain 50 per cent oxygen and will, therefore, enhance com-bustion. It must be used with the same precautions as oxygen where cutting equipment is being used to extricate a trapped victim. The gas mixture remains stable and homogenous above a temperature of − 6°C but below this level the nitrous oxide tends to liquefy and falls to the bottom of the cylinder. If the cylinder is now turned on, almost pure oxygen will escape at first, which is safe enough, but as the cylinder empties, the concentration of nitrous oxide will rise at the expense of oxygen until, as the cylinder is just about exhausted, almost pure nitrous oxide is liberated (Fig. 1.19). Entonox, therefore, should only be used in conditions where the temperature is above − 6°C. However, in spite of the well-known British climate, this does not totally invalidate its use!

Methoxyflurane

Methoxyflurane (Penthrane®) is an anaesthetic agent which, like nitrous oxide, when given in subanaesthetic concentration, produces analgesia without unconsciousness. For this purpose the liquid is vaporised in air using a temperature compensated draw-over apparatus such as the Cardiff Inhaler (Major and colleagues, 1967). This device is designed for self administration like Entonox and is even more portable and light in weight. It delivers an inspired concentration of 0·35 per cent V/V which has a similar analgesic potency to 50 per cent nitrous oxide. This fixed concentration does not produce any serious respiratory or cardiovascular depression and the technique of self-administration again means that inhalation can be supervised by trained paramedical personnel without a doctor being present. It can be used in conditions of extreme cold.

However, because the vapour is administered in air, it cannot be used for those patients who need a high inspired concentration of oxygen, e.g. those with chest injuries, respiratory embarrassment, severe blood loss or myocardial failure. Methoxyflurane when used in higher concentrations for anaesthesia has been suspected of causing renal damage in a few instances. The case is by no means proven and problems have not been recorded with the low concentrations used in analgesia. The duration of onset and recovery, while similar to nitrous oxide, is not quite so brisk.

Practical applications

Now that analgesics have been discussed together with their advantages and disadvantages, it is appropriate to consider the following questions:

What should the rescue doctor, operating from his own car, carry with him to provide pain relief at accidents and emergencies?

The authors believe that he should have access to four agents— morphine, pentazocine, diazepam and Entonox. The first three of these he will probably already carry in his own bag but, in the United Kingdom at least, he may choose to rely on the ambulance bringing the Entonox. However, a number of practitioners have found it worthwhile to carry their own Entonox equipment to use before the ambulance arrives, particularly if they practise in a remote area.

What should be carried by the ambulance service?

Every ambulance likely to respond to an emergency call should be equipped with Entonox and the attendants should be fully trained in supervising the use of this apparatus. The fact that in Entonox nitrous oxide is mixed with a high concentration of oxygen makes it, in our opinion, a better choice than methoxyflurane for rescue purposes. In 1972 the Department of Health and Social Security recommended that Entonox be carried in all front-line ambulances. A specially equipped ambulance, like an MRU, which either carries a doctor or provides facilities for local practitioners, should also carry diazepam and penta- zocine. It is not possible for morphine to be included because of difficulties in complying with the regulations of the Misuse of Drugs Regulations.

How should these agents be used in the emergency situations?

As Entonox works effectively in the majority of patients and because it is the safest of all the agents that are available, the authors believe that it should be tried first. The patient should be shown the technique of self-administration (Fig. 1.20) stressing the importance of maintain- ing an airtight fit between the mask and his face, as only if this is achieved will the gas mixture flow from the demand inhalational unit when he inhales. *This technique of self-administration carries with it essential safeguards* because, if the effect of the nitrous oxide is such as to make the patient drowsy, then his grip on the mask will relax, the airtight seal between the mask and his face will be broken and the gas flow will stop. In practice, inhalation tends to

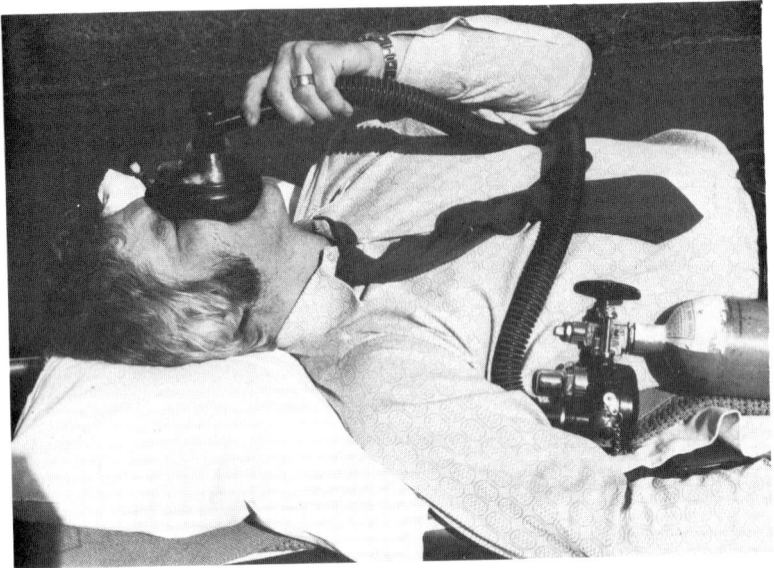

Fig. 1.20.   Self-administration of Entonox.

be intermittent; the patients breathes the gas until his pain is relieved and then has a rest. When the pain returns, he inhales more nitrous oxide.

It is important to remember that, when a painful procedure is planned such as the extrication of a patient from wreckage, Entonox should be inhaled for a full two minutes beforehand to allow it to reach its maximum analgesic effect.

In a few instances, the patient may not be able to cooperate enough to use the apparatus himself. For example, he may have bilateral arm or shoulder injuries or is afraid to inhale deeply because of fractured ribs. Under these circumstances, if a doctor is present, he may help by holding the mask to the patient's face or he can override the demand system by compressing the base of the inhalational unit. Remember, however, that if this is done, the safeguards conferred by self-administration are lost; paramedical personnel should not attempt this manoeuvre.

In a minority of patients, the analgesia provided by 50 per cent nitrous oxide is insufficient or the inhalation is not tolerated. In these patients, incremental doses of 5 mg morphine or 30 mg pentazocine should be given intravenously through an indwelling needle until the desired effects are achieved. If the patient is cooperative, Entonox can be administered simultaneously which reduces the dose of parenteral analgesic required. Should the patient refuse to accept the mask, it is useful to give 5 mg increments of diazepam with the analgesic to allay anxiety and apprehension which often form a large part of the problem.

General anaesthesia

With the modern cutting and rescue equipment now available, it is very rarely necessary for full general anaesthesia to be required at the accident site. The patient can usually be resuscitated and given pain relief, as outlined earlier in this chapter, while specialised rescue equipment is brought to the scene. Indeed, the authors consider that surgical instruments for amputation or other major operative procedures should not be available in the first instance but should have to be sent for from the hospital after the situation has been very carefully assessed. In this way, the unnecessary amputation by the well-meaning enthusiast can be avoided.

Full anaesthesia at the accident site is a hazardous procedure and should only be undertaken by a doctor trained in the specialty and working closely with the rescue teams. Facilities for suction, endotracheal intubation, IPPV and intravenous infusion are all absolutely necessary.

Should general anaesthesia be essential, what agents and techniques are the most suitable?

Ketamine (Ketalar®). Ketamine is a dissociative anaesthetic agent which can be given intravenously in a dose of 2 mg/kg body weight. It is unique amongst anaesthetic agents in that the protective laryngeal reflexes are rarely significantly depressed, so reducing one of the main dangers, viz. inhalation of foreign material.

Diazepam (Valium). Diazepam has already been described. Given in doses of 15–30 mg intravenously, it will induce anaesthesia without undue respiratory or cardiovascular depression. The protective laryngeal reflexes will be impaired.

Alphadione (Althesin®). Alphadione is a steroid anaesthetic which does not depress the respiratory or cardiovascular systems as much as the barbiturate agents. Recovery is rapid and although the drug needs more extensive trials in the accident situation, it promises well in this field. The recommended dose for the average adult patient is between 3·5 and 5·0 ml of the solution.

Nitrous oxide with halothane or trichlorethylene. Davidson and colleagues (1970) have devised a modification of the Entonox apparatus which allows halothane or trichlorethylene to be added to the nitrous oxide mixture and includes provision for artificial ventilation using a self-inflating bag or bellows.

In the authors' opinion, ketamine is the agent of choice where it is impossible to gain access to the head and airway. If access is possible, then ketamine, diazepam or alphadione can be used as an induction agent and anaesthesia can be maintained using the David-son apparatus. For a very brief general anaesthetic, alphadione may be recommended as the sole agent.

TRAINING IN EMERGENCY MANAGEMENT

The first approach to teaching and training in any subject is to define the target audience and then to set out the objectives that are to be achieved.

When this approach is applied to training in emergency management, the target audience can be subdivided into three major groups:

(i)   The doctor.
(ii) The ambulance man (and other paramedical workers).
(iii) The general public.

Having defined the target audiences, what are the learning objectives? These will, of course, vary with each of the audience groups but the variation will mainly be one of degree. A training course being planned for any one of the audience groups could be based on the learning objectives listed below with the course content being varied to suit the particular audience:

(a) Ability to provide emergency medical treatment including cardiopulmonary resuscitation, pain relief and specific therapy related to the patient's injury or condition.

(b) Knowledge of the supporting ambulance services, their vehicles and equipment, and the facilities of the local Accident and Emergency centre.

(c) Familiarity with police procedures at accident sites.

(d) Knowledge of the type and capabilities of the cutting and jacking apparatus carried by the local fire brigade.

(e) Ability to use a two-way radio and knowledge of the communication resources of the police and ambulance services.

(f) The pre-arranged plans of action to be followed in the event of a major public disaster in the area.

The training methods required in order to achieve these learning objectives for the three different audience groups can now be considered.

The doctor

Rescue work cuts across the usual divisions between the classical specialties of medicine and demands of the operator not only special knowledge and skills, but also the ability to apply these in difficult and unfamiliar outside surroundings. How, then, is the enthusiastic doctor —for enthusiast he must be—to find the teaching and training that will allow him to fulfil the learning objectives that have been listed?

Teaching can be broadly divided into three categories:

(i)   Large group teaching such as courses, seminars and symposia.

(ii) Small group or personal tuition.

(iii) Individual study.

Large group teaching

The postgraduate department or postgraduate centre of the District General Hospital should form the focus of the majority of courses and symposia in Emergency Management. These centres are usually the responsibility of the clinical tutors who are the people to contact and urge towards providing courses in accident and emergency work. It is vital that such courses are not too much biased towards hospital treatment by hospital specialists. A mass of X-rays or a detailed account of a surgical procedure, however interesting, is not the relevant information that the audience requires.

Anaesthetists should play a leading part in initiating and teaching on such courses. The management of emergencies is based, in the first instance, on the provision of resuscitation and pain relief and this, of course, is primarily the province of the anaesthetist.

The authors have run such a course annually since 1967. While the major part of the course is devoted to the medical management of a wide variety of emergency conditions, the following additions to the programme have been made as a result of feedback questionnaires issued to successive audiences:

(a) Radio and other forms of communication.
(b) The integrated activities of the emergency services including a demonstration of the management of a mock accident.
(c) An exhibition of rescue and resuscitation equipment.
(d) Talks and discussion led by general practitioners actively engaged in rescue work themselves.

In order to produce a course on these lines, it has been necessary to seek help from several quarters. Apart from talks by doctors actively engaged in the field of immediate care the majority of medical teaching has come from consultants and senior registrars in various specialties including anaesthesia, orthopaedics, neuro-, general and thoracic surgery and ophthalmology. In addition the cardiologists and general physicians have contributed. In all cases the practical aspects of emergency care in the home, the factory or on the road have been emphasised.

In addition to teaching contributed from medical sources, the emergency services have been extremely helpful in providing training and information to doctors interested in emergency work and, indeed, have often been instrumental in starting a medical emergency and rescue service by making the initial contact with the local practitioner or hospital. All three of the emergency services have contributed in this way.

In the event of a major incident the police stress the importance of their regulations and procedures in preventing further accidents. If the doctor arrives unidentified, dressed in a dark suit, parks his car in the way of oncoming traffic and behaves as if he is the only important person on the scene, then he is more likely to be a hindrance than a help and may well be a positive danger. He will soon find that cooperation is not all it might be and that his popularity is at a low ebb with everyone.

If, on the other hand, he attends the incident in a car identified by an appropriate flashing light, parks well into the side some distance ahead of the accident site and carries his equipment to the scene wearing a reflective jacket labelled DOCTOR (Fig. 1.7) then he will find everyone anxious to help.

Instruction and advice of this nature can easily be incorporated into a course either as an illustrated talk or by practical demonstrations.

The fire brigade are masters of technique when it comes to extricating trapped victims from a variety of situations. Like the police, they are very willing to take part in organised courses and in demonstrations. On some occasions, the authors have arranged for mock accidents to simulate a trapped driver and this allowed the fire brigade to demonstrate their cutting and other equipment and led to useful discussions on such topics as fire hazards in the presence of oxygen and Entonox.

It is, however, the ambulance service with which the doctor will have the closest contact and anyone intending to take up this work must make himself known to the ambulance officers and acquaint himself with their base station, vehicles and equipment, call-out procedures and radio arrangements. Members of the ambulance service have a substantial contribution to make to training courses, especially in the field of communications. Many services now have talk-through facilities from the ambulance to the nearest hospital accident department or intensive therapy unit. It may even prove possible for the doctor to link a two-way radio in his own car into the ambulance network. The subject of communications is dealt with in more detail in Chapter 15.

Small group or personal tuition

The *fundamental, practical aspects of emergency management can only be properly taught by small group or personal tuition* and this most important part of training cannot be replaced by any number of theoretical courses. The District General Hospital offers an unparalleled source of clinical material for practical training. Members of the anaesthetic and accident and emergency departments can provide individual tuition in basic airway care, laryngoscopy, endotracheal intubation, artifical ventilation and intravenous cannulation with a wide variety of patients. Here the trainee can actually use the resuscitation equipment available and decide which is best suited to his own particular use.

In order to see and practise the management of cardio-pulmonary resuscitation, a few days attachment with the resuscitation registrar (Marshall, 1966; Eltringham and Baskett, 1973) responsible for cardiac arrest calls will offer very useful experience. The value of this first hand training cannot be overemphasised and it is to be hoped that every anaesthetic and accident and emergency department will try to offer this tuition on request to doctors engaged in immediate care work in the area.

Individual study

In addition to organised courses and personal tuition, a number of doctors will wish to do some individual study. The range of study materials is not as great, perhaps, as one would wish. One of the authors (JSMZ) has prepared a small tape recording and booklet (Zorab, 1972) on the management of cardiac arrest and although this is aimed primarily at hospital medical officers, much of it may prove useful to the doctor engaged in emergency work outside hospital. Jointly the authors have also produced another tape recording with slides on the use of Entonox in the Ambulance Service (Zorab and Baskett, 1970), and the Medical Recording Service of the Royal College of General Practitioners has a number of similar audiovisual aids that cover the emergency management of a wide range of conditions.

The ambulance man

The ambulance men remain the backbone of the medical side of the emergency services. In recent years, a number of them have emerged from the category of professional first-aiders and have become highly skilled exponents of resuscitation. Recommendations by the Department of Health and Social Services for a period of in-hospital training have done much to upgrade the general standard in the service. Certain centres have gone far beyond these recommendations and have demonstrated clearly that selected men can absorb a detailed knowledge of resuscitation and can competently perform such technical skills as endotracheal intubation, intravenous cannulation and infusion, and electrical defibrillation of the heart (Gearty and colleagues, 1971).

At Frenchay Hospital, Bristol, a training scheme has been instituted for selected men who have been seconded fulltime in two categories, one month training or six months training. Both groups receive theoretical and practical instruction in the accident centre; anaesthetic, operation and recovery rooms; intensive therapy and coronary care units; general wards; post-mortem room; and with the cardiac arrest service.

One month training

Those training for one month concentrate their practical work on:
Basic airway care.
Oxygen and Entonox therapy.
Hand ventilation with a bag and mask.
Assistance with intravenous infusions.
Connecting a patient to a cardioscope.
Preparing an electrical defibrillator for use.
Emergency care of soft tissue injuries and fractures.
The preparation of drugs.

Six months training

The men training for six months, in addition to the above, receive a full training in:
Endotracheal intubation.
Intravenous cannulation.
Electrical defibrillation.

They naturally have a greater depth of both theoretical and practical instruction in all varieties of accidents and medical emergencies.

Whilst on the course, the trainees staff the Frenchay Mobile Resuscitation Unit which attends selected emergency calls where their special skills and equipment are thought to be needed. In this vehicle a 'one-month man' is always teamed with a 'six-months man', and frequently an anaesthetist and/or a nurse from the intensive therapy unit travel as well to amplify the team and to give 'on-site' tuition.

After satisfactory completion of the course, including an examination, the men are awarded a certificate and those who have trained for six months are given, for their personal use on duty, a resuscitation bag containing equipment for intravenous infusion, a laryngoscope and endotracheal tube and a manual inflating bag. They are given permission to use the infusion and endotracheal equipment for a period of six months after 'graduating' and approval is only renewed after satisfactory completion of a refresher course and further examination.

Gradually it is hoped to upgrade the general standard of ambulance men's skills and build up a nucleus of very competent men to lead the resuscitation teams in a first class service throughout the area.

In some areas, hospital nurses accompany the emergency ambulance on its calls and have proved highly successful in working with ambulance men. At St Jans Hospital in Bruges, Belgium, selected male nurses, who have been specially trained, now work with doctors in providing an excellent resuscitation service for accidents and medical emergencies (Tytgat, 1972). At Frenchay Hospital, Bristol, nurses from the intensive care unit often travel with the MRU and nave proved very valuable. Their training should be orientated towards resuscitation techniques and familiarity with the accident scene, broadly along the same lines as those for the doctor. Many nurses find this new aspect of their work interesting and the project has helped us towards realising the underlying concept of bringing intensive care outside the hospital to the accident or emergency and providing that care throughout the period of transit (Binning, 1970).

The general public

No single advance in emergency care could bring as much benefit as the ability of each member of the general public to provide basic resuscitation and first aid. The simple act of placing all unconscious patients in the lateral or semi-prone position and clearing their airway would probably save more lives than any dramatic advance in medicine. Is this an impossible ideal? Can such an enormous task be taken on and, if so, how and by whom?

The Scandinavian countries and parts of Northern Europe have already made great strides towards achieving such an ideal. Classes in resuscitation and first aid are a compulsory part of the educational programme. A wide and increasingly sophisticated range of training aids are used and the school classes are reinforced with programmes on radio and television. In Denmark, special mobile teams tour the countryside giving demonstrations of simple resuscitation techniques. Gradually a state of awareness of their responsibilities is being created in the populations so that they feel it their duty to their fellow countrymen to learn the simple skills of emergency medical care.

One section of the population which is more accessible for tuition than the rest is the motoring public. In some countries it is now necessary to acquire a certificate of competence in first aid and resuscitation to qualify for a driving licence. In any road accident the first person on the scene is most likely to be another driver and there is, therefore, a great deal of sense in singling out this section of the population for 'compulsory' first aid training.

Health education of this nature and on this scale would, undoubtedly, be a major undertaking. Teaching loads of all medical workers would need to be increased and new teachers would have to be trained. But this challenge should be accepted. Together with modern methods of educational technology, a great deal could be accomplished.

RESCUE AND EMERGENCY CARE SCHEMES

Some emergency services have confined themselves to a particular specialist field such as road traffic accidents or patients with myocardial infarction. The reason for this is usually that the enthusiasm and drive that resulted in the service being started has stemmed from either an accident surgeon or a cardiologist. It has now become clear that the primary skills required by any emergency service are those of cardiopulmonary resuscitation and pain relief. Additional skills will, of course, be required to handle, for example, chest injuries, poisonings, fractures and cardiac arrhythmias, but these can be built upon the primary skills.

For these reasons, the authors believe that emergency services should be organised to cater for the resuscitation of *all* emergency patients, regardless of their illness or injury and that anaesthetists have an important part to play in the organising and training, as well as the staffing, of these services in conjunction with other participating disciplines.

There is, however, another aspect to be considered in the overall organisation of rescue and emergency care schemes. In rural areas, hospitals are often so far away from the scene of the emergency as to make primary attendance by a hospital based service completely impractical. It is in these rural areas that the general practitioner, operating from his own car and working in a roster with his colleagues, has frequently demonstrated that he can form the basis of the rescue and emergency service. The number of these general practitioner schemes is increasing rapidly in the United Kingdom and these doctors should be able to count on their local District General Hospital for the relevant part of their training. They should also be able to obtain a supply of disposable items of equipment such as endotracheal tubes and intravenous cannulae from the hospital and replace these as they are used. Through personal tuition sessions the general practitioner can build up a close relationship with his hospital colleagues which contributes to providing a high standard of care for the patient throughout his treatment.

In urban areas, however, the problem is different. The sheer difficulties of getting about through the traffic in our towns and cities in an ordinary car makes it virtually impossible for the general practitioner to provide a reliable service in this environment. District General Hospitals are usually situated in the urban precincts and the ambulance service can usually be at the scene in a matter of a few minutes. A scheme with which the authors are associated seems to work well for urban and semi-urban calls. A special ambulance—the Frenchay Mobile Resuscitation Unit or MRU—is based at the hospital and the ambulance men spend their time at the hospital engaged on their training programme as outlined in the previous section. The MRU is fully equipped to enable the operators to carry out all forms of cardiopulmonary resuscitation. The ambulance base calls out the MRU to those cases where it is felt that resuscitation and other skills may be needed. The MRU is despatched together with an anaesthetist and, sometimes, a nurse (Baskett, in preparation). This plan is similar to those pioneered by Poulsen and Lysgaard (1968) in Denmark, Ahnefeld and Kilian (1972) in West Germany, Lust (1972) in Belgium, Lund (1972) in Norway and others.

COORDINATION IN RESCUE AND EMERGENCY CARE WORK

Organised rescue and emergency services are really still in their infancy although they are developing rapidly. A coordinating mechanism is needed to receive, sift and disseminate information on new methods, techniques, apparatus and training schemes and, at the same time, authoritatively represent those involved in this work.

In the United Kingdom, The Medical Commission for the Accident Prevention (see the Introduction of this book) has formed an Immediate Care Committee to take on this role. This committee has representatives from each region of the country who can act as a two-way link between the grass roots and the centre. In Denmark, an organisation called Interescue (Rormark, 1972) performs a similar function.

On an international scale, the International Institute for Emergency First Aid has been set up in Bruges with the object of providing a forum for the exchange of information and ideas between nations, setting standards of competence for the emergency services and initiating pilot trials of new schemes, techniques and equipment involved in emergency work. It is hoped to establish research fellowships in the subject to investigate special problems. Symposia are held each year to include such topics as training methods, methods of service organisation, techniques of resuscitation and the design and function of the hospital accident and emergency centre.

REFERENCES

1. Ahnefeld, F. W. and Kilian (1972), Organisation of the treatment of emergency patients inside and outside hospital, *Folia St Jan*, p. 23, published by St Jans Hospitaal, Brugge, Belgium.
2. Baskett, P. J. F., and Withnell, A. (1970), The use of Entonox in the Ambulance Service, *Brit. Med. J.*, **2**, 41.
3. Baskett, P. J. F. (1972), The use of Entonox in the Ambulance Service, *Proc. Roy. Soc. Med.*, **65**, 7, 1.
4. Baskett, P. J. F., Eltringham, R. J. and Bennett, J. A. (1973), Pain relief and oxygen therapy, *Anaesthesia*, **28**, 4, 449.
5. Baskett, P. J. F., Diamond, A. W., Johnston, R. and McKenna, T. (1976), (in preparation).
6. Binning, R. (1970), Ambulance for intensive care, *Proc. 3rd Asian and Australasian Congress of Anaesthesiology*. Butterworth and Co. (Australia).
7. Carden, E. and Bernstein, M. (1970), Investigation of the nine most commonly used resuscitator bags, *J.A.M.A.*, **212**, 589–592.

8. Davidson, J., Beddard, J. B., Bennett, J. A. and Whitford, J. H. W. (1970), A new technique for Flying Squad Anaesthesia, *Brit. J. Anaes.*, **42**, 465.

9. Editorial (1973), *Brit. J. Anaesth.*, **45**, 5.

10. Eltringham, R. J. and Baskett, P. J. F. (1973), Experiences with a hospital resuscitation service, *Resuscitation*, **2**, 57–68.

11. Gearty, G. F., Hickey, N., Bourke, G. J. and Mulcalny, R. (1971), Prehospital Coronary Care Service, *Brit. Med. J.*, **3**, 33–5.

12. Lund, I. (1972), Experiences with a doctor–manned ambulance service in Oslo, *Folia St Jan*, p. 9, published by St Jans Hospitaal, Brugge, Belgium.

13. Lunn, J. N., Kennedy, B. R. (1968), Pain relief for crushed chests, *Brit. Med. J.*, **2**, 828.

14. Lust, P. (1972), Discourse on the 900 system, *Folia St Jan*, p. 108, published by St Jans Hospitaal, Brugge, Belgium.

15. Major, V., Rosen, M. and Mushin, W. W. (1967), Concentration of methoxyflurane for obstetric analgesia by self-administration inhalation, *Brit. Med. J.*, **2**, 1554.

16. Marshall, R. D. 1966, A year of resuscitation, *Anaesthesia*, **21**, 86.

17. Parbrook, G. D., Rees, G. A. D. and Robertson, G. S. (1964), Relief of post-operative pain—comparison of 25 per cent nitrous oxide and oxygen.mixtures with morphine, *Brit. Med. J.*, **2**, 480.

18. Poulsen, H. and Lysgaard, A. (1968), Aspects of Resuscitation— Emergency Aid Organisation, *Acta Anaesth. Scandinav.*, Suppl. **XXIX**.

19. Redick, L. F., Dunbar, R. W., MacDougall, D. C., and Merket, T. E. (1970), An evaluation of hand-operated self-inflating resuscitation equipment, *Anaes. and Anal.: Curr. Res.*, **1**, 28–32.

20. Rørmark, A. (1972), On rescue—technical investigation and training, *Folia St Jan*, p. 69, published by St Jans Hospitaal, Brugge, Belgium.

21. Ruben, H. and Ruben, A. (1957), Apparatus for resuscitation and suction, *Lancet*, **ii**, 373–4.

22. Tunstall, M. E. (1968), Implications of pre-mixed gases and apparatus for their administration, *Brit. J. Anaesth.*, **40**, 675.

23. Tytgat, R. (1972), Organisation of the accident system in Belgium, *Folia St Jan*, p. 85, published by St Jans Hospitaal, Brugge, Belgium.

24. Zorab, J. S. M. and Baskett, P. J. F. (1970), Entonox in the Ambulance Service, British Oxygen Company. (Audio-tape and slides.)

25. Zorab, J. (1972), The management of cardiac arrest, London: Churchill Livingstone. (Audio-tape and handbook.)

Guide to intubation (pp. 16–17) is adapted from the Royal Free Intubation Trainer booklet; acknowledgement is made to Dr J. E. Boys, Dr M. Emery and Dr T Hilary Howells.

2

Head and Spinal Injuries—Care at the Site of the Accident

F JOHN GILLINGHAM

Over the past twenty years the pattern of injuries to the central nervous system has changed radically in the Western Hemisphere, largely due to the rapid increase of vehicle population on the roads. In the Head and Spinal Injuries Research Unit at the Royal Infirmary of Edinburgh over 19 000 patients have been admitted during the past fifteen years. In 1963, 664 were treated and this had risen to 1543 in 1969, without increasing our catchment area at all.

In 1967, anxious about this rapid escalation, we set up a prospective computer study to analyse 800 facts on each patient, not only to determine how better to prevent accidents but also to look at other problems which were causing concern. It was evident that there were reasons for disquiet in respect of patient care at the site of accident, during transportation, on arrival in hospital, in the hospital itself and during convalescence and rehabilitation. At the road-side or other accident site, the prevention of a second 'accident', almost as important as the prevention of the first, seemed to demand urgent consideration, e.g. the care of the airway, control of bleeding and blood replacement, splinting of suspected spinal dislocation or fracture and thoughtful, speedy transportation. Much of the information which came out of the computer study confirmed these anxieties and pointed to their solution. As was to be expected, a change in our organisation and improvements in continuing education appeared urgent.

Tables I–III show the steady annual increase in admissions but also the important fact that most accidents tend to occur, in Edinburgh at any rate, at periods when medical, nursing and ancillary staff are least available, e.g. the summer months, at weekends and after five in the evening when a half or even two thirds are off duty. A complete reappraisal of duty rosters including secretarial and records departments was, therefore, necessary.

TABLE I

Monthly admissions to Ward 20,
Royal Infirmary of Edinburgh,
1963 – 1968.

	1963	1964	1965	1966	1967	1968
January	58	64	70	84	96	102
February	39	55	62	77	77	132
March	44	69	79	100	102	154
April	59	71	89	121	111	154
May	65	82	93	128	110	162
June	53	63	101	126	127	178
July	71	66	78	104	108	159
August	44	87	98	102	106	189
September	35	106	81	111	104	129
October	64	103	92	91	116	158
November	65	69	88	104	94	121
December	64	87	80	108	138	126
Totals	661	922	1011	1256	1289	1770

TABLE II

Day	Total admissions per day	Average admissions per day	
Sunday	157	2·9	
Monday	159	3·0	
Tuesday	144	2·7 ⎱	least number of
Wednesday	144	2·7 ⎰	admissions per day
Thursday	152	2·8	
Friday	174	3·3	
Saturday	234	4·5	largest number of admissions per day

TABLE III
Daily times of admission to Ward 20,
Royal Infirmary, 1967.

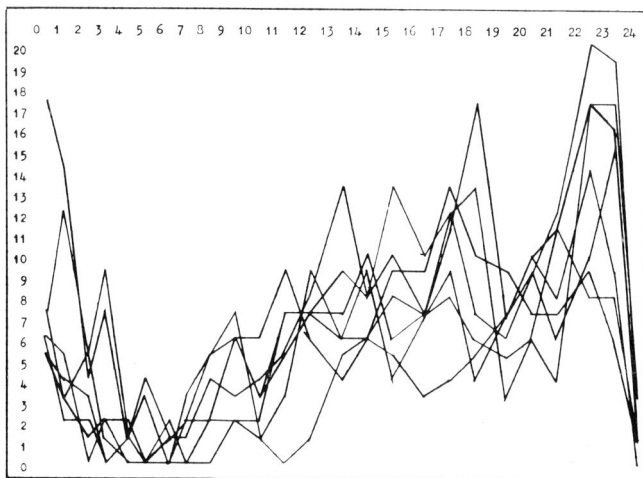

MODE OF INJURY

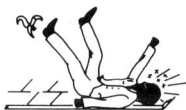

FALL ON SAME LEVEL   = 215 ← MINOR = 185 / MOD. = 26 / SEVERE = 4

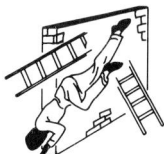

FALL FROM A HEIGHT   = 210 ← MINOR = 159 / MOD. = 30 / SEVERE = 21

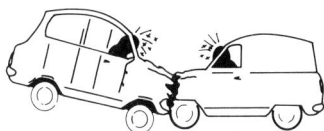

TRAFFIC ACCIDENTS   = 440 ← MINOR = 321 / MOD. = 75 / SEVERE = 44

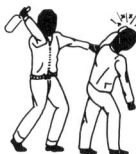

ASSAULT   = 123 ← MINOR = 111 / MOD. = 12 / SEVERE = 0

Fig. 2.1.

MODE OF INJURY

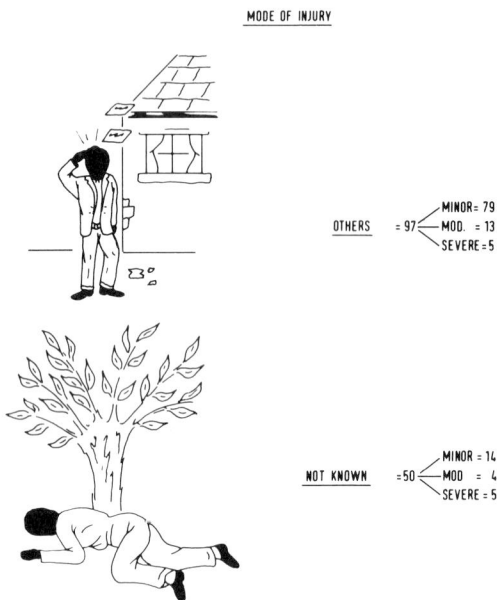

OTHERS = 97 — MINOR= 79 / MOD. = 13 / SEVERE = 5

NOT KNOWN = 50 — MINOR = 14 / MOD = 4 / SEVERE = 5

Fig. 2.2.

Figures 2.1 to 2.3 show the main causes of brain injury and its severity. Minor injury is measured by the loss of consciousness for less than five minutes, moderate injury by unconsciousness for less than 24 hours and severe injury by periods of unconsciousness for over 24 hours.

TYPES OF INJURY

If immediate and continuing care of the brain-injured is to be effective, it is essential to understand the dynamic pathology of head injury and the events which immediately follow.

There are two types of head injury: crush injury in which loss of consciousness is unusual, and the more common and important acceleration or deceleration injury which is usually associated with concussion. Crush injuries are relatively infrequent and they will not be considered further here.

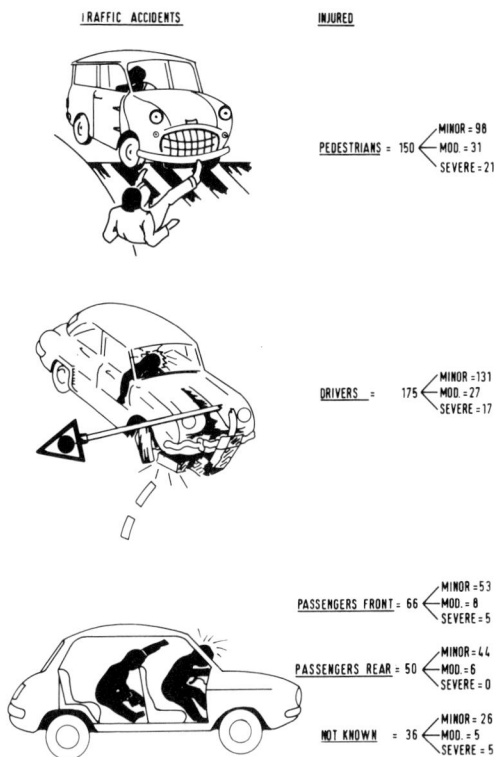

Fig. 2.3.

Acceleration and deceleration injuries are essentially similar in their effect upon the head. In the case of direct injuries, compression distortion of the skull is maximal at the site of the blow, and immediately on the opposite side there is a tensile type of deformation. If fracture occurs, it may be immediately subjacent to the site of the injury, or, because of distortion, some distance from it. It is this type of skull distortion, with or without skull fracture, which is responsible for tearing of the middle meningeal vessels, the usual cause of extradural haematoma.

The extent of underlying injuries of the cerebral cortex and its blood vessels is dependent on the severity of these deformations, probably from local negative pressure effects, and coup and contre-coup injuries are partly accounted for in this way. They may be minimal, so that the patient completely recovers in a few days or, at the other extreme, they may be very severe with instantaneous death, or coma for many years. There are, of course, all grades of severity between. The brain substance as a whole is relatively incompressible and therefore subjected to transmitted distortion stresses, which in the more serious injuries are responsible for the scattered haemorrhages in the white matter that are occasionally seen at autopsy.

However, the common source of brain injury is from rotational and linear acceleration forces which occur when the head is suddenly accelerated or decelerated in space. As we shall see later, these forces determine direct injury to the brain and its superficial blood vessels, the cortical veins and arteries. Of greater significance is indirect injury to the important basal brain structures, from distortion of their fibre connections, and stretching of the perforating branches of the circle of Willis (their blood supply) which occurs as a result of the sudden cerebral displacements of rotational and linear acceleration forces.

The commonest sites of laceration and contusion in acceleration and deceleration injuries are the inferior surfaces of the frontal lobes, and the anterior aspect of the temporal lobes in the region of the lesser wing of the sphenoid, the result of positive pressure in forward rotation and negative pressure injury in backward rotations (Fig. 2.4).

The extent and severity of the lesions are, of course, in proportion to the severity of the acceleration or deceleration injury. Cerebral lacerations of this type, even in severe injury, are seldom more than 2 cm in depth and, as we know from war experiences of similar superficial penetrating brain wounds, are not in themselves significant as a cause of disturbed consciousness or death. Nevertheless, they are important as a potent source of complication in severe head injury, namely, acute subdural and intracerebral haematomas and contusional brain swelling. Subdural and intracerebral bleeding arise usually from torn veins, and to a lesser extent from tearing of the more robust arteries, at the site of the laceration (Fig. 2.5).

Another potent, although less common, source of subdural bleeding is from the superior cerebral veins which pass from the superomedial border of the cerebrum to drain into the sagittal sinus. In acceleration and deceleration injuries they may be suddenly stretched and torn by rotation of the brain within the dura. **Once venous bleeding begins, irrespective of its source, it is maintained or recommenced, and then hastened, by high intracranial venous pressure due to impairment of the airway, so often seen in the deeply unconscious patient and often**

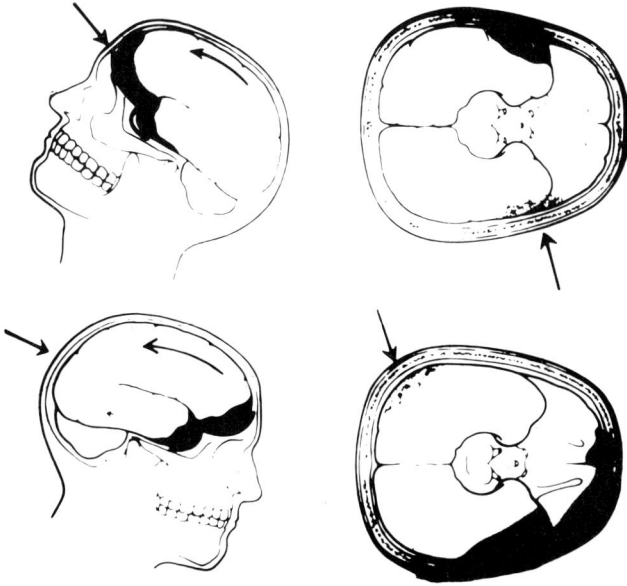

Fig. 2.4.

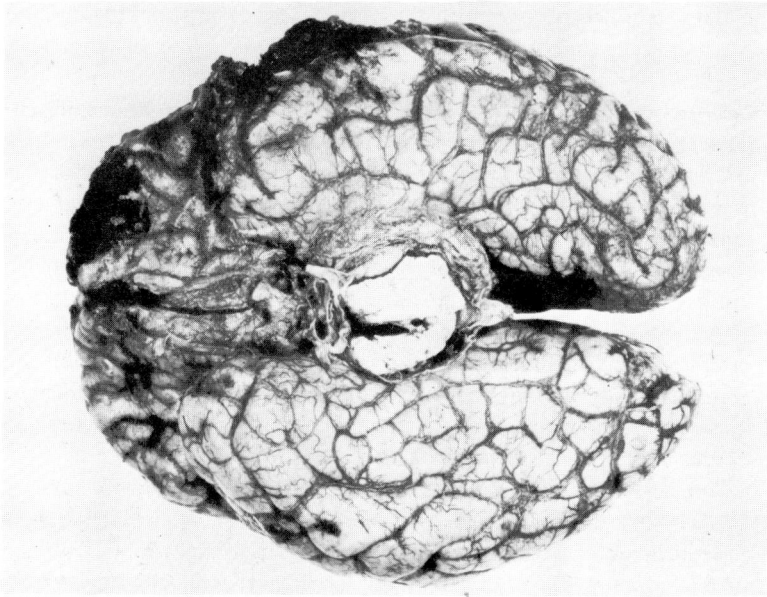

Fig. 2.5.

within seconds of injury. This may occur because the patient is lying on his back or his head is tilted backward, e.g. in a vehicle, so that the tongue obstructs the pharynx. Vomitus, which may occur soon after injury, and blood and secretions are also major causes of respiratory obstruction. Fracture of the facial bones, e.g. floating maxilla or fractures of the mandible call for immediate relief of the obstructed airway.

These acute subdural haematomas (those which show themselves within an hour or two of injury, as opposed to the subacute variety which only show themselves days after injury) are caused by severe acceleration or deceleration injuries and are, in our experience, associated with a very high mortality rate. **Early relief of respiratory obstruction by positioning of the patient, adequate suction and the use of an airway may well reduce the incidence of acute subdural haematoma by lowering of the intracranial venous pressure and prevention of continued bleeding.** Although in many cases operation for evacuation of clot is still performed too late or inadequately, it seems that some other major injury, the primary brain stem lesion, must be responsible for such grave consequences.

It is said that the lesser wing of the sphenoid, by resisting movement of the cerebral hemispheres in this region, largely protects the circle of Willis and its important perforating branches to the basal nuclear region of the brain from injury. However, much clinical and pathological evidence does not support this view. There is a striking similarity between the clinical behaviour, and indeed the EEG changes, of the severely head-injured and those suffering from the severe effects of rupture of an anterior communicating aneurysm. In this latter condition, ischaemic lesions in the territory of supply of the perforating branches of the anterior cerebral arteries have been demonstrated at autopsy; they are the result of spasm following rupture of the aneurysm (Gillingham and Watson, 1953; Gillingham, 1958). It may well be that interference with these important perforating arteries by stretch and subsequent spasm may help to explain the prolonged disorders of consciousness and the autonomic and metabolic dysfunction that follow severe acceleration head injury (Gillingham, 1953) (Fig. 2.6).

Similar lesions of the perforating branches of the posterior cerebral arteries have also been demonstrated in head injury with greater or lesser degrees of haemorrhagic infarction of a primary kind. They are associated with loss of consciousness and increased tone in the limbs and, when severe, with decerebrate rigidity (Fig. 2.7).

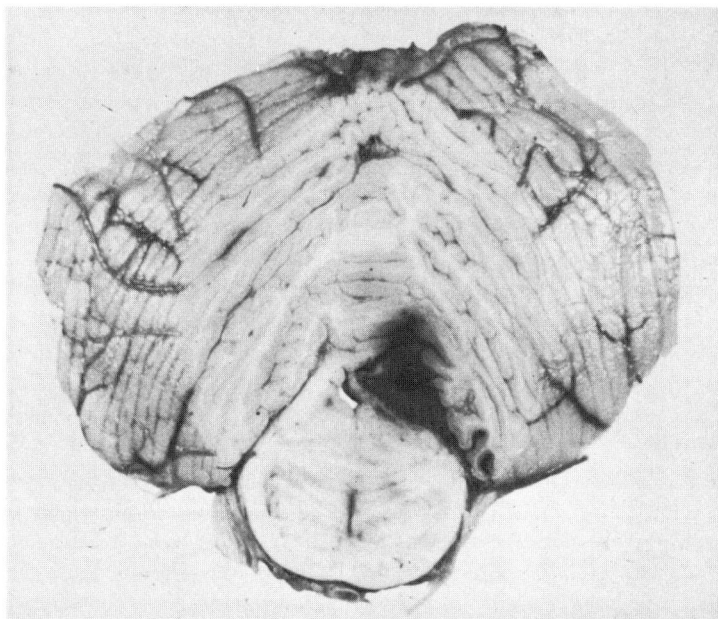

Fig. 2.6.

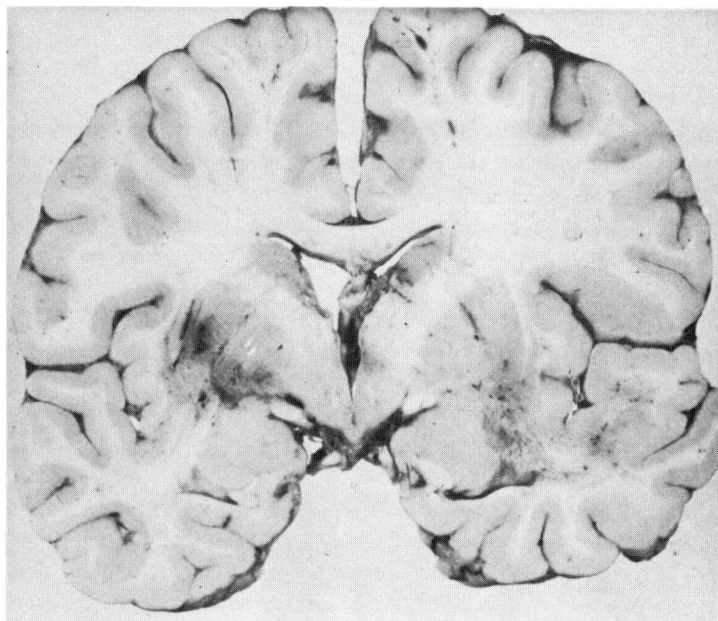

Fig. 2.7.

PREVENTABLE COMPLICATIONS

So much for the immediate pathological changes which follow the sudden cerebral displacements of acceleration injury. Of far greater practical implication are their complications, the haematomas and cerebral swellings, which are preventable or remediable if dealt with promptly. The degree of recovery of a patient with brain injury will depend on the severity of the primary stem lesion, which may be slight, the real problem being the secondary brain stem lesion from late evacuation of clot which might have been prevented in any event. Although expanding lesions are difficult to recognise in the already unconscious patient, where there has been no lucid interval, knowledge of the pathological factors involved in the gradual cerebral displacements which are associated with their development clarifies a somewhat confused clinical picture. **Repeated monitoring of the vital signs in these patients at quarter-hourly intervals is essential as soon as possible after the injury.** Usually they already show a tachycardia and a somewhat raised pulse pressure. Any increase, particularly when associated with a rising respiration rate and increasing restlessness, should make one alert to the possibility of an intracranial expanding lesion.

The explanation of these findings is as follows. When an intracranial clot or swelling occurs, there is progressive lateral displacement of the brain from the clot. Traction upon the striate branches of the anterior and middle cerebral arteries causes further ischaemia of the diencephalon. In the case of a patient already recovered from concussion, these vascular traction displacement effects lead to increasing headache and drowsiness. When there has been no lucid interval and the patient is unconscious, they lead to increasing restlessness (from headache from rising intracranial pressure) with a further lowering of consciousness, culminating in coma. Traction upon the lateral group of perforating vessels from the middle cerebral artery, which supplies the internal capsule, leads to an increasing contralateral hemiparesis.

In addition to lateral displacement, there is an attempt on the part of the brain to make further room for itself in its closed box. At the tentorial hiatus there occurs further displacement. To accommodate the increasing volume within the supratentorial compartment of the skull the mid-brain moves downwards, and at its lateral border the hippocampal gyrus of the temporal lobe herniates downwards between it and the edge of the tentorium. At the same time the midbrain is pushed across and the cerebral peduncle may be pressed against the opposite edge of the tentorium, with consequent hemiparesis on the same side as the clot. Increasing herniation of the hippocampal gyrus stretches the third cranial nerve which lies below it with dilatation of the pupil so characteristically seen in the late stages of increased intracranial pressure from rapidly expanding unilateral supratentorial lesions. **It must be emphasised that dilatation of the pupil is a late sign** (Fig. 2.5).

As the midbrain is displaced downwards, its tiny vessels of supply, which arise from the basilar artery and its short circumferential branches become progressively stretched. The artery is held up by its posterior cerebral branches over the edges of the tentorium and by the posterior communicating arteries, and is unable to follow the downward movement of the midbrain. Resulting ischaemia of the midbrain causes further impairment of consciousness. Finally, as ischaemia progresses, decerebrate rigidity appears and, with infarction of the midbrain, death soon follows.

With the recognition of such displacements from clot or swelling, it can be seen that a good deal depends upon their speed of formation and this dictates the urgency for their relief.

In the past few years some of the less severe primary brain stem lesions seem to have had a better prognosis than we used to believe, especially in children and the young adult. Indeed some of them have completely reversible lesions. There is some evidence that impairment of the airway immediately after injury and/or the intermittent or more continuous straining associated with decerebrate rigidity, may extend smaller lesions as a result of rapid rise of venous, arterial and intracranial tension. **Clearing of the airway at the roadside and the earliest establishment of controlled respiration in the decerebrate would thus seem to be of the greatest importance in the attempt to maintain reversibility of the brain stem lesion. These ideals may be difficult to achieve but considerable effort should be made to establish an efficient organisation and adequate training.**

INITIAL CARE OF THE HEAD-INJURED

The adequate care of the head-injured is dependent, therefore, upon a lively appreciation of the clinical picture which results from the sudden displacements of injury in the first instance and the gradual

PLEASE COMPLETE AS FAR AS POSSIBLE

NAME .... AGE ....

ADDRESS ....

LOCUS OF
ACCIDENT .... TIME ....

CAUSE OF ACCIDENT ....

TIME AND DATE EXAMINED ....

NATURE OF INJURIES ....

HAEMORRHAGE:– (Put a tick √ in appropriate box)

SEVERE ☐   MODERATE ☐   SLIGHT ☐   NONE ☐

STATE OF AIRWAY WHEN EXAMINED:–

CLEAR ☐   OBSTRUCTED ☐   VOMITING ☐

ACTION TAKEN ....

STATE OF CONSCIOUSNESS:–

	When first found	When examined	In Transit
ALERT AND CO-OPERATIVE	☐	☐	☐
DROWSY AND CONFUSED -	☐	☐	☐
UNCONSCIOUS - - - - -	☐	☐	☐
EPILEPTIC FIT - - - - -	☐	☐	☐
"FAINTING ATTACK" - - -	☐	☐	☐

DRUGS GIVEN ....

BY WHOM ....

REMARKS:–

Fig. 2.8.

displacements of its complications in the second. The establishment of first-aid care depending on close cooperation between the accident emergency department of the hospital, fire, police and ambulance services is one of the most important steps in dealing with these problems. Radio communication is essential. Care of the airway and recording of conscious level from the first cannot be stressed too greatly. The introduction of a simple casualty card for this purpose was provided for ambulance crews in 1963 and has been invaluable in estimating trend of level of consciousness which is the key to the earliest recognition of developing haematomas. Prompt assessment and further observation in hospital is the next step (Fig. 2.8).

The main problems at the site of the accident are of

Airway

The first and most urgent problem is hypoxia or anoxia from obstruction which may arise from simple obstruction by the tongue which is more likely to occur in a damaged vehicle with an extended head or when the patient remains on the back immediately after injury or during transportation. A number of deaths have been and are still being recorded following simple concussion and obstruction of this type. Continuing education of ambulance crews and the general public about the correct position of the patient, bearing in mind the strictly maintained neutral position of the neck, is essential if this important lesson is not to be repeatedly forgotten. The correct position is shown in Fig. 2.9.

POSITION OF PATIENT WHEN TRANSPORTED

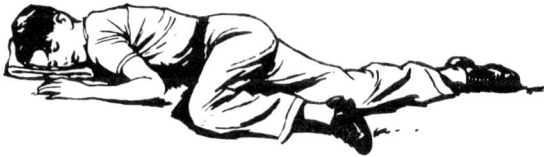

AMBULANCE SERVICE
CASUALTY LABEL

SEMI PRONE — Small, relatively firm pillow.
Neck in neutral position.

AIRWAY CLEAR

Fig. 2.9.

Dentures must be removed, but impacted or broken dentures in the pharynx may cause difficulty and require instruments to dislodge them. Hooking of the tongue forward with the index fingure may be required urgently to relieve obstruction. An oro-pharyngeal tube may help an urgent situation. The causes of obstruction in 27 of a group of 1132 consecutive head injuries (241 moderate and severe, 891 minor) are shown in Table IV.

TABLE IV

Respiratory obstruction before admission to hospital

	Minor head injury	Moderate head injury	Severe head injury	Total
Vomitus	0	3	7	10
Tongue	0	0	1	1
Vomitus and tongue	0	1	2	3
Blood and secretions	0	2	7	9
Blood, secretions and vomitus	0	0	2	2
Blood, secretions, vomitus and tongue	0	1	1	2

There is obviously a major problem when vomitus, blood and secretions obstruct the lower respiratory passages. Efficient suction adequate to deal with semi-solid material, with oro-pharyngeal intubation as a minimum, and the use of the catheter with end and side apertures are basic essentials for any ambulance team. Practical tuition of such ambulance crews in hospital on a continuing basis by anaesthetists should be a matter of routine in all accident/emergency services. Ideally the ambulance crews manning such a service should be specially trained and an intimate part of the hospital team. Only in such a way can rapport and the highest standards of immediate care be maintained, for it is too expensive to staff ambulances with hospital medical personnel. If ambulance facilities are not available, sensible and trained passers-by may save life by positioning the patient as already shown and clearing debris from the mouth and pharynx with a handkerchief. All motorists should carry a first-aid kit comprising a mouth-to-mouth airway tube, two slings and a large newspaper of fairly stiff paper so that it can be folded over to make a 5-inch collar. This can be placed around the neck, overlapped and fixed gently but securely with a handkerchief so that flexion and extension are prevented (Fig. 2.10). This is particularly important during manipulations for control of the airway, extraction from a vehicle, transportation and moving the patient from road to stretcher and

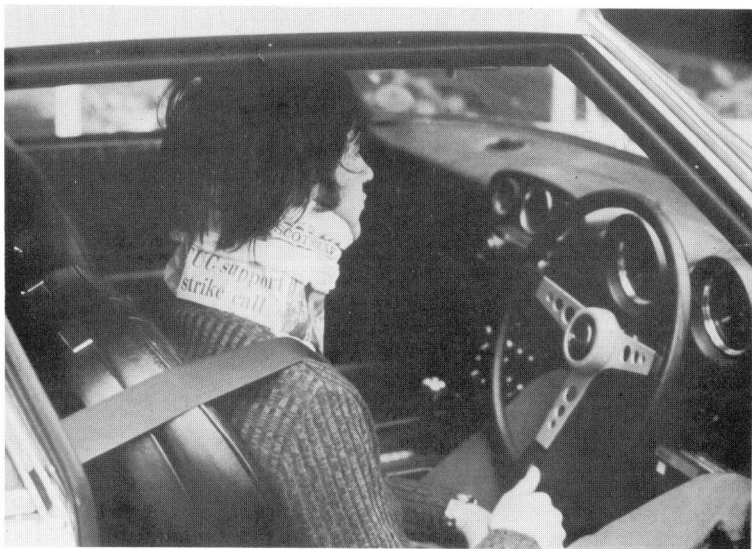

Fig. 2.10.

from stretcher to bed in hospital. Clinicians working in the accident field have seen more than one tragedy of tetraplegia developing for the first time after thoughtless manipulation of this kind; the paralysis, though minimal or not present before, usually remains permanent after such a mishap. **There is much to be said for an examination on the practical elements of first aid for all motorists before a driving licence is granted.**

Apart from hypoxia due to airway obstruction, an equally important problem is that of acute and rapid rise of intracranial venous pressure which occurs at the moment of impact and within the few minutes which follow. Clear cut evidence of the rapid rise of intracranial pressure with respiratory obstruction has been put forward by Hulme and colleagues (1966). Urgent relief of an obstructed airway—with attendant reduction of the increased volume of the intracranial venous bed, cerebral distension and oedema—is obviously essential. Thereby the vicious circle of continuing bleeding into the subdural space and cerebral substance, cerebral distension, venous infarction and oedema can be reduced. A primary brain stem lesion may remain reversible or minimal if the addition of a secondary lesion can be prevented.

Blood loss

Blood loss of significance occurs in only 20 per cent of casualties with head injury alone, but in 50 per cent with multiple injuries (Table V). Nevertheless, death from preventable severe blood loss can occur in two instances:

(1) Bleeding in the older age groups from larger scalp vessels, such as the occipital and superficial temporal arteries, when they are atherosclerotic and remain open. Pressure with the fingers or thumb or by a well-placed and maintained pressure bandage must be applied at once. Pressure bandages are apt to slip, and considerable seepage may have occurred into dressings by the time the patient reaches hospital. When the ambulance arrives at the scene of the accident, artery forceps are usually available and are the best means of controlling such bleeding. Blood or fluid replacement may be necessary during transportation.

(2) From fractures of the skull involving the major venous sinuses. A man of 19 died soon after admission to hospital from exsanguination due to loss of blood from a simple depressed fracture of the vertex involving the outer wall of the superior longitudinal sinus. Subsequent questioning showed an obstructed airway and the loss of a large volume of blood on the road and transportation to hospital. He could easily have been saved by: clearing the airway, the application of an airtight bandage to prevent air embolus, and elevation of the head and upper trunk to lower intracranial venous pressure. Fractures involving the major venous sinuses will cause severe exsanguination if intracranial venous pressure is high. The fact that the bleeding is venous will be apparent from its blue colour and the relationship of the scalp injury to the anatomical sites of the venous sinuses.

The urgent control of haemorrhage from elsewhere in the body is, of course, essential in order to reduce the effects of hypoxia and the ischaemic effects on the brain, particularly the diencephalon which adds to the effects of head injury. Blood or fluid replacement and fast transportation to hospital will occasionally be necessary.

TABLE V

Total head injuries with blood loss = 442
Jan.– Dec. 1967

Grade of blood loss	Total	%
Minor	374	84·6
Moderate	60	13·6
Severe	8	1·8

Total multiple injuries with blood loss = 85
Jan.– Dec. 1967

Grade of blood loss	Total	%
Minor	43	50·5
Moderate	34	40
Severe	8	9·4

Good recording of the history of events and their management is essential if full understanding of the problems involved is to be acquired by the receiving staff of the accident/emergency department. As soon as possible relatives should be contacted so that previous acute and chronic disease or injury suffered by the patient will be known so that action can be taken, e.g. renal disease, atherosclerosis, diabetes and a history of psychiatric disorder.

SPINAL INJURY

The high incidence of minor cervical spinal injury in association with head injury, particularly from vehicular accidents, emphasises the great importance of immobilisation of the cervical spine during extrication. First-aid immobilisation with an improvised newspaper collar has already been described but most ambulances are now

equipped with 'Camp'® collars. The best type of splint is a modification
of the Harrington splint as used by emergency care schemes (MCAP,
1975) (Fig. 2.11).

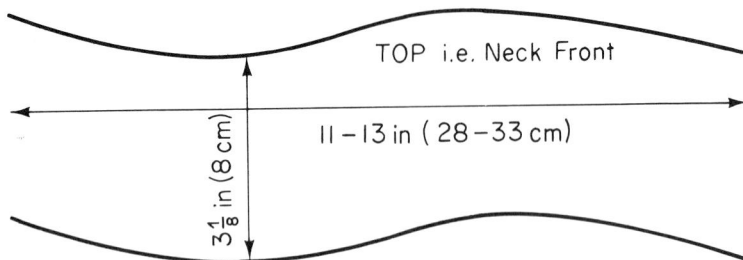

Fig. 2.11. *The cervical collar: for use in suspected cervical or thoracic spinal
fracture in conjunction with the Spinal Board. Materials: Hard
cardboard or, preferably, Vinolay. Cover with 3 in. rib unbleached
stockinette, length being 50–60 in. in order that this will tie around
the back of the neck and can be gently knotted at the front. Pack
the side marked Neck Front with cotton wool in order to make a soft
pad of the collar. The piece of cardboard, which should be long
enough to run under the angle of the jaw to the occiput, will also
prevent hyperextension; this may be particularly useful in elderly
people who sustain an extension type of injury. Moreover, the collar
will serve to hold forward the angle of the jaw, preventing airway
obstruction in an unconscious patient. The collar is applied whilst
the patient is still in the vehicle. It can be fitted in any position and
then rotated into the correct site. The collar does not need to be
pulled tight, and there is no danger of impeding venous return from
the brain.*

The incidence of injuries of the spine at other levels in association
with head injury also occur. They are not so common but care must
be taken to splint the patient as for those in the cervical region though
the situation is rather less hazardous.

Transportation of the splinted patient to hospital should be rapid
particularly if there is evidence of injury to the spinal cord. It is
now known that one of the problems of cord injury is the rapid
development of oedema, usually within four to six hours. If the cervical
spine is subluxated or there is a fracture dislocation the dimensions
of the spinal canal will be reduced to approximately half of normal.

The cord may be contused but not yet compressed and thus there is a partial and potentially recoverable lesion. The development of venous engorgement, hypoxia and oedema will add the factor of compression with rapid ischaemia of the cord within a restricted spinal canal unless the dislocation is reduced by skull traction as soon as possible and in any event within six hours. The use of dexamethasone, 10 mg intravenously, may help to diminish oedema but the evidence is not yet entirely convincing. Reduction of the dislocation is also probably effective in reducing compression of the blood supply of the cord, both arterial and venous, thus reducing the possibility of hypoxia, venous engorgement and oedema of the cord.

This somewhat optimistic approach to spinal cord injury is not entirely without justification from the dynamic pathological standpoint, and there is accumulating clinical evidence to support it. A longer term study of this policy will indicate whether or not there is a reduction of the incidence of permanent tetraplegia and paraplegia. Any means of reduction of this grave disability must obviously be pursued with the greatest vigour.

During transportation conflict may arise over the position of the spinal injured and splinted patient and the management of his airway. In the unconscious patient a mouth or oro-pharyngeal or endotracheal airway may thus be required.

Further improvement in the initial care of the head-injured will depend on many factors. In particular, during the next five years, the most pressing needs are for:

in **education,** continuing education of ambulance crews and the medical and lay public concerning the importance of the avoidance of the second accident if the first cannot be prevented;

in **research,** careful recording and follow-up of patients who have received care at the site of the accident so that the adequacy or otherwise of methods used can be assessed.

REFERENCES

Gillingham (1954), *Proc. Roy. Soc. Med.*, **47**, 10, 869.
Gillingham (1958), *Ann. Roy. Coll. Surg. Eng.*, **23**, 89.
Gillingham (1970), *Med. Sc. and the Law.*, **April**, 104.
Gillingham (1972), *Head Injuries.* Proc. Int. Symp. Edinburgh /Madrid. London: Livingstone.

Gillingham and Watson (1953), Communication to Association of British Neurologists & Society of British Neurological Surgeons.

Hulme and Cooper (1966), Personal Communication.

Medical Commission on Accident Prevention (1967 and 1975), *Broadsheet on Organisation and Equipment.*

3

Chest Injuries

E HOFFMAN

Injuries of the chest are becoming much more frequent. Increasing numbers of road accidents account for about 70 per cent and the remainder are due to falls, crushing injuries, stab wounds, etc.

Although chest injuries account for only 5–10 per cent of injuries in road accidents, they exact a heavy toll in deaths and are found in about half the fatalities (Fig. 3.1). Car occupants and motorcyclists are more likely to sustain serious chest injuries than pedestrians and pedal cyclists. The frequent association of chest trauma with other injuries makes its detection more difficult. The combination of head and chest injury is particularly serious because the anoxia due to chest injury causes cerebral oedema which in turn further depresses respiration. In the author's series (Hoffman, 1976) of 199 fatalities with a fractured skull, 61 also had a haemothorax.

The incidence of penetrating injuries due to stab or gunshot wounds has also been increasing, they were present in 19 of 95 chest injuries admitted to the author's unit over the past three years.

Management has greatly improved in the last two or three decades, mainly due to advances in anaesthesia, appreciation of the role of blood transfusion, the introduction of tracheostomy and positive pressure ventilation, and advances in open heart surgery.

The recognition and management of chest injuries at the site of accidents, during transport, in the accident department and during the first 24 hours will be discussed in this chapter.

PHYSIOLOGICAL DISTURBANCES FOLLOWING CHEST INJURY

The maintenance of respiration and circulation is essential to life,

81

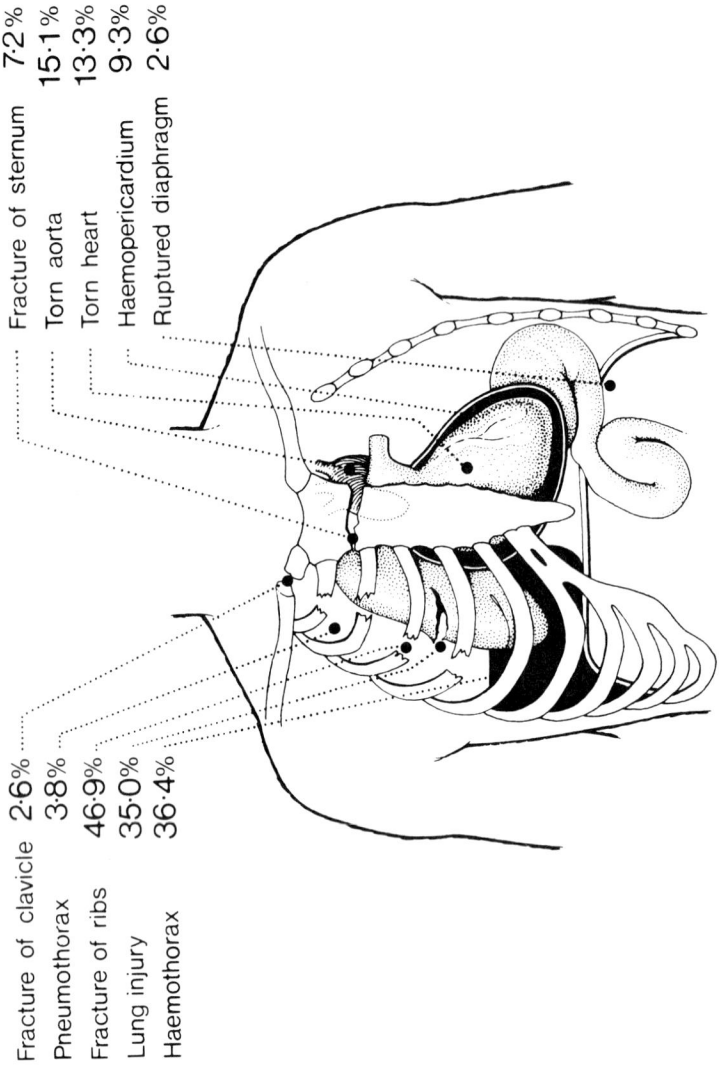

Fracture of clavicle 2·6%
Pneumothorax 3·8%
Fracture of ribs 46·9%
Lung injury 35·0%
Haemothorax 36·4%

Fracture of sternum 7·2%
Torn aorta 15·1%
Torn heart 13·3%
Haemopericardium 9·3%
Ruptured diaphragm 2·6%

Fig. 3.1. Distribution of chest injuries in 344 fatal road accidents. (Hoffman, 1976.)

and a basic knowledge of cardiorespiratory physiology is needed to treat chest injuries effectively.

Two types of respiration take place in the body. External respiration consists of the exchange of oxygen and carbon dioxide in the lungs. Internal respiration deals with the exchange of gases between the blood and tissue cells, and requires an adequate circulation and efficient cardiac function.

In chest injuries, the external respiration is mainly affected. Normal respiration depends on the mechanical function of ventilation and on the exchange of gases within the lungs. Failure of ventilation, i.e. inability to move air in and out of the lungs, is the commonest cause of respiratory failure and is present in practically all severe chest injuries. The reduction of ventilation may be due to depression of the respiratory centre, fractures of the bony thoracic cage, intrapleural compression of the lungs by air or blood or reduction of lung compliance, i.e. of the distensibility of the lung.

The respiratory centre in the brain stem may be depressed by a number of factors, including injuries to the brain, increase of intracranial pressure, a rise of carbon dioxide tension, hypoxaemia and pH changes. It is also depressed by alcohol, sedatives (especially morphine) and general anaesthesia. Central respiratory failure can easily be overlooked because it causes weak respiratory excursions without dyspnoea, in sharp contrast to the acute respiratory distress associated with chest injuries.

Ventilation is greatly diminished in multiple fractures of ribs and sternum, particularly if flail chest with paradoxical respiration is present. This occurs when several ribs are fractured at two or more points and the segment of chest wall in between becomes mobile and moves paradoxically with respiration, being sucked in on inspiration and blown out on expiration. Effective coughing and expectoration of bronchial secretions is greatly reduced or abolished and atelectasis of the underlying lung results. If untreated, these patients drown in their own secretions. Even with a few simple rib fractures pain produces rapid and shallow breathing causing alveolar hypoventilation and retention of secretions.

Compression of the lung by air in the pleural space (pneumothorax) or by a collection of blood (haemothorax) also reduces alveolar ventilation. In tension pneumothorax or in an open pneumothorax due to a penetrating chest injury, dyspnoea may be extreme and, if untreated, rapidly fatal. A large haemothorax may also lead to marked reduction in the circulating blood volume and to hypovolaemic shock.

In patients with a reduced lung distensibility, ventilation–blood flow imbalance is present; in these cases blood flow to the lung is adequate but oxygen is not taken up. This occurs in atelectasis, diffuse lung contusion and post-traumatic lung complications such as 'shock lung', pulmonary embolism or bronchopneumonia. Ventilation–perfusion balance is also affected if the pulmonary artery pressure is reduced, as in haemorrhage, compression of the heart by blood (cardiac tamponade) or diminished venous return. As a result of diminished venous return, cardiac output falls and this is eventually followed by cardiac standstill.

The degree of respiratory impairment and the efficacy of treatment can be assessed by repeated arterial blood gas analyses. The normal range of arterial carbon dioxide tension is 36–44 mm Hg; a rise above 50 mm Hg indicates ventilatory failure; at 80 mm Hg consciousness becomes impaired. The normal arterial oxygen tension is between 80–100 mm Hg; severe hypoxaemia develops if the tension falls to 60–40 mm Hg. The volume of oxygen in the blood also depends on the haemoglobin content, and a patient with severe chest injury is more hypoxaemic if he has lost a lot of blood.

The maintenance of a normal acid-base balance as shown by an arterial pH between 7·34 and 7·45, and a plasma bicarbonate of 23 mmol/l is of great importance. Soon after a chest injury a respiratory alkalosis is often present due to hyperventilation. The lungs however cannot remove sufficient carbon dioxide because of ventilatory impairment, and a respiratory acidosis soon develops. In addition, a metabolic acidosis occurs as the body cannot eliminate some acids particularly lactic acid. The clinical signs of advanced respiratory acidosis are drowsiness, disorientation, hypotension and coma. The myocardium is also affected and a reduction of cardiac output and arrythmias may occur.

There is a close association between lung and heart function, and failure of one system frequently leads to disturbances in the other. The chief causes of acute circulatory failure are severe blood loss, cardiac tamponade, and tissue hypoxia secondary to impaired ventilation.

EARLY ASSESSMENT

In the unconscious patient breathing is best observed by listening for breath sounds with the ear directly over the nose and mouth, while watching for excursions of the chest wall. Respiratory movement of the chest or abdomen without audible air movement in the airway is a sign of total airway obstruction, and unless such a patient is treated within 2–3 minutes, he will die. Fortunately airway obstruction is usually incomplete, with noisy breathing and obvious use of accessory muscles.

Serious oxygen lack, such as occurs in respiratory obstruction, soon leads to cardiac arrest and this may also happen after severe blood loss. Thus as soon as the airway has been cleared the carotid or femoral pulses should be felt; if these are absent, cardiac arrest has occurred. The carotid pulse can be felt if the index and middle fingers are placed on the larynx and then moved laterally pressing gently backward. In the absence of effective circulation, cardiac arrest leads to death within 3–5 minutes.

The recognition of blood loss depends on its amount and on the rapidity with which blood escapes from the circulation. The amount of external haemorrhage from, for example, scalp wounds or compound fractures can be seen and estimated. The amount of concealed blood loss into the chest, abdomen or pelvis can only be assessed from the patient's clinical condition. In a healthy adult signs of hypovolaemic shock do not develop until he has lost about $1\frac{1}{2}$–2 litres, that is about 30–35 per cent of his total blood volume. In the early stages, there is an increase in the pulse rate, sweating, restlessness and thirst; later, the skin becomes cool and pale, perspiration is profuse, the pulse becomes soft, rapid and thready and the respiratory rate rises. **Estimation of blood pressure is an unreliable guide, as in the early stages the pressure may be normal or only slightly lowered even in severe haemorrhage.**

Chest injuries are difficult to detect in fully clothed casualties at the accident site, particularly in the unconscious and in poor lighting conditions. If there is extreme breathlessness or if respiratory distress increases during bag–mask ventilation a tension pneumothorax should be suspected.

Shortness of breath may be present in multiple rib fractures, particularly if there is a flail segment of the chest wall. Paradoxical movements may be seen and confirmed if the flat of the hand is placed on the affected part of the chest and compared with movements on the other side. Respiratory distress in these cases usually develops gradually, but in severe crushing injuries an acute respiratory emergency is present immediately after the accident.

After resuscitation in the accident department, the casualty should be undressed to allow more thorough examination of the chest. Respiratory excursions are first observed; if one hemithorax is prominent and does not move well with respiration, a large pneumothorax or haemothorax may be present. Poor respiratory movements also result from 'splinting' of the chest wall by painful rib fractures. In a flail chest, paradoxical movements may be seen anteriorly or laterally. Posterior paradoxical movement may be missed if the back of the chest is not examined. Physical signs are helpful but should be interpreted with caution. A pneumothorax produces a hyperresonant percussion note, whilst in haemothorax the note is dull; in both cases the breath sounds are diminished.

Examination of the neck should always be carried out. A large pneumothorax and a haemothorax both displace the trachea towards the opposite side. Distended neck veins are present both in tension pneumothorax and in cardiac tamponade. If respiratory distress is absent cardiac tamponade is the more likely diagnosis, particularly in the presence of hypotension, distant heart sounds or a wound in the precordial region.

In patients with multiple injuries all other systems should be examined and **the chest X-rayed only after the patient has been resuscitated.** Upright postero–anterior and lateral chest films should be taken as conditions such as a haemothorax or a ruptured diaphragm may be missed in a supine view. No time should be wasted in taking X-rays if a tension pneumothorax or cardiac tamponade are suspected clinically, as urgent treatment of these conditions is essential.

MANAGEMENT

Chest injuries and their complications can be grouped according the urgency of treatment. Firstly, there are potentially lethal conditions needing immediate treatment, then there are injuries which must be treated within a few hours, and lastly there are cases which can be managed conservatively.

In multiple injuries it is necessary to decide which of the lesions is immediately endangering life. Some of these—such as a subdural or extradural haematoma, an abdominal emergency due to bleeding, perforation of a viscus or an arterial injury—have to be operated on as soon as cardiorespiratory problems are controlled.

When considering the management of chest injuries it is useful to classify the efficiency of the respiratory function into three grades: efficient, impaired and failing. Patients with an efficient respiration can breathe and cough satisfactorily. If the respiratory function is impaired patients cannot breathe properly or cough up their secretions, and will require intubation or tracheostomy. Patients in respiratory failure cannot ventilate efficiently in spite of relief of pain and tracheostomy, and their breathing will have to be assisted by intermittent positive pressure ventilation.

POTENTIALLY LETHAL EMERGENCIES

Potentially lethal injuries and their complications must be recognised immediately and treated urgently. They are: airway obstruction, respiratory failure, tension or open pneumothorax, severe blood loss and cardiac tamponade.

Airway obstruction

Upper airway obstruction is most commonly due to the tongue falling back against the pharyngeal wall in unconscious patients. These patients are also unable to swallow or to cough up saliva, blood, vomit, etc. Upper airway obstruction may also be caused by fractures of the maxilla or mandible, with swelling of adjacent soft tissues, or by an impacted foreign body.

A detailed description of the management of upper airway obstruction has been given in Chapter 1. The subject is of such importance that the basic management of respiratory obstruction will be repeated here. In resuscitation the simplest effective measures should be tried first. In the unconscious patient with respiratory distress, extending the head and lifting the jaw forward is all that need be done in 80 per cent of cases. If the casualty has a good colour and is breathing spontaneously, he should be put into the semiprone position to allow drainage of secretions and to prevent inhalation. The mouth and pharynx are cleared of blood, vomit and foreign material with the finger wrapped in a handkerchief, or preferably with a sucker. All dentures are removed and a large oral airway is inserted. If no respiratory effort is made, mouth-to-mouth ventilation should be started and continued with a bag and mask as soon as it becomes available, using oxygen-enriched air. For ventilation to be effective the chest must be seen to expand. In the unconscious patient who is unable to breathe properly a cuffed endotracheal tube should be inserted to prevent aspiration and allow positive pressure ventilation. Endotracheal intubation should only be carried out by a doctor experienced in this technique, as prolonged attempts at passing a tube may lead to severe hypoxaemia.

Patients with maxillofacial injuries who are unable to sit up should also be placed in the 'coma' position; at necropsy of such cases, inhalation of blood is found in a high proportion.

The increase of spinal injuries following road accidents gives rise to special problems in respiratory first aid and transportation. In the author's series (Hoffman, 1976) 3·1 per cent of surviving hospital admissions and 18·2 per cent of fatalities had fractures or fracture–dislocations of the spine. As a large proportion of these were cervical spine fractures, torsion and flexion of the neck should be avoided during respiratory resuscitation. About 5 per cent of head injuries also have a spinal injury, and a cervical collar should be applied at the accident site in unconscious casualties and in those who complain of pain in the neck. Special care should be taken when freeing such casualties from their cars. The head and trunk should not be twisted and the shoulders and pelvis kept parallel when they are lifted and transported. They are best extricated by means of a spinal board, which should be standard equipment in ambulances. Patients with high spinal injuries should be intubated because of their inability to cough and the danger of aspiration.

Tension pneumothorax

Progressive accumulation of air in the pleural cavity is usually due to a valvular leak from a lacerated lung. As the intrapleural pressure increases the lung on the injured side is compressed, the trachea and mediastinum are displaced to the opposite side and eventually the other lung is also affected. Impairment of the venous return reduces the efficiency of the cardiac pump, and this results in a feeble pulse and hypotension. Extreme breathlessness dominates the clinical picture, and unless promptly relieved the condition is rapidly fatal. Emergency treatment consists of inserting a large bore needle into the pleural cavity in the 2nd or 3rd interspace in the midclavicular line anteriorly, or in the 4th or 5th interspace laterally. An incised finger cot, if available, may be tied to the end of the needle to act as a flutter valve. An intercostal tube should be inserted into the pleural space as soon as possible and attached to a bottle with an underwater seal.

If the lung fails to expand after intercostal intubation and a large quantity of air continues to escape, rupture of a main bronchus should be suspected. Haemoptysis usually occurs and the diagnosis can be confirmed by bronchoscopy. If the pleura remains intact, air from a ruptured bronchus may accumulate in the mediastinum and present as surgical emphysema in the neck. Early thoracotomy and repair of the bronchial tear should be carried out.

An open pneumothorax is caused by a penetrating wound of the chest, and the severity of the clinical picture depends on the size of the opening. In stab wounds little air enters the pleural space, although there may be a tension pneumothorax and severe intrathoracic bleeding. Larger wounds from a gun or an impalement injury are more serious and not compatible with life unless immediately converted into a closed pneumothorax. Penetrating injury of the chest is easily diagnosed because of the typical sucking sound made by air rushing in and out of the wound. First aid consists of covering the wound with a large pad of gauze, until further treatment can be given in hospital where the patient should be intubated and ventilated, and a thoracotomy performed as soon as his general condition allows. Debridement of the contaminated wound is carried out and intra-thoracic complications are dealt with. In a simple stab wound intercostal intubation may be all that is necessary.

Perforation of the lower oesophagus due to blunt trauma or a penetrating injury is rare, and may at first present as a pneumothorax with a persistent air leak. Irritation of the mediastinum and pleural space by leaking gastric contents presents as an acute emergency with circulatory collapse and symptoms similar to peptic perforation. Early repair of the oesophageal tear and drainage of the pleural cavity are indicated.

Technique of intercostal intubation

All medical officers working in an accident unit should know how to introduce a tube into the pleural space (Figs. 3.2 and 3).

A suitable site to decompress a pneumothorax is in the 2nd interspace anteriorly in the midclavicular line. The site should not be too near

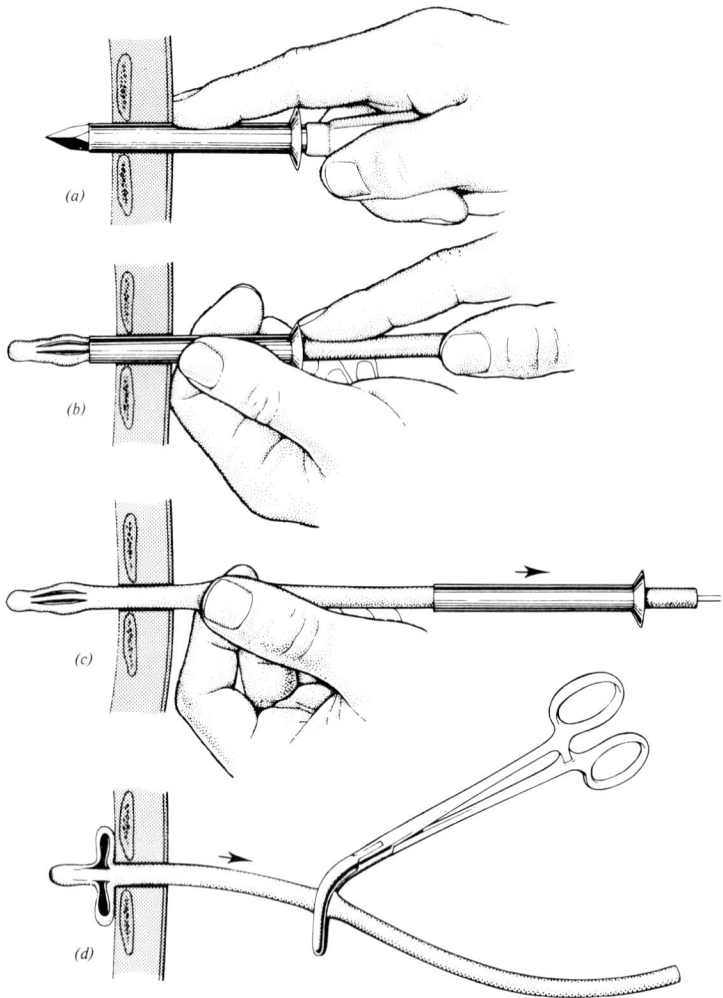

Fig. 3.2. Intercostal intubation:
  (a) Introduction of trocar and cannula into pleural cavity.
  (b) Tube stretched on introducer is passed through cannula.
  (c) Two fingers steady tube while cannula and introducer are
       withdrawn.
  (d) Tube is withdrawn so that flanges touch chest wall. Forceps
       on tube prevent air entry.

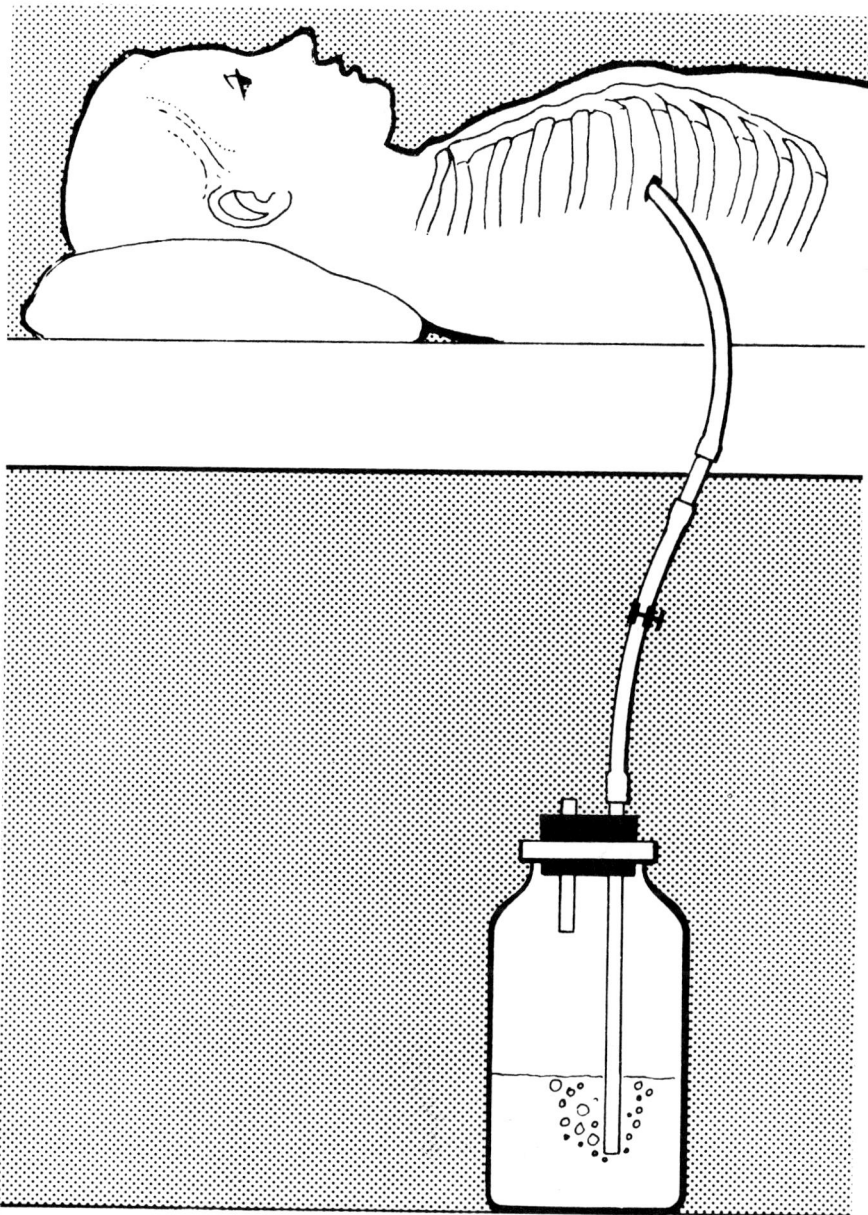

Fig. 3.3. Tube is attached to bottle with underwater seal.

the sternum as the tube could be introduced into the superior vena cava. (In a case known to the author, it had to be extracted at thoracotomy.) Alternatively, the tube may be inserted in the 4th or 5th space in the midaxillary line.

The skin and subcutaneous tissues are infiltrated with local anaesthetic. The needle is introduced until the point touches the lower margin of the rib above the selected interspace; 3 ml of local anaesthetic are then injected deep to the rib. A small skin incision is made and a trocar and cannula large enough to accept the tube introduced into the pleural cavity. A finger is placed on the shaft of the cannula to prevent the trocar penetrating too far into the chest. The catheter stretched on a blunt-ended introducer is then quickly passed through the cannula after the trocar has been withdrawn. A finger on the tube prevents it slipping too far into the chest. The cannula and introducer are then withdrawn while two fingers compress the tube to prevent air entering the pleural space. The catheter is then clamped and partially withdrawn so that its flanges touch the inner surface of the chest wall. It is then attached to a calibrated drainage bottle with an underwater seal. The placing of the finger on the cannula and on the tube is an advisable precaution as, in the author's experience, a tube may later be found to have penetrated the lung when introduced by inexperienced residents.

For drainage of a haemothorax a large-bore tube (e.g. 36–40 FG) should be used, to prevent blockage by blood clots or fibrin, and at times it may be an advantage to insert two tubes. A careful watch should be kept to see that the fluid level in the glass tube leading to the underwater seal moves freely with respiration, as kinking, compression or clotting within the tubing will prevent escape of air and drainage of blood. The amount of blood drained should be recorded so that replacement requirements can be estimated.

Severe blood loss

The clinical signs of severe blood loss have already been described. It is not always appreciated that a patient with a pulse rate of 120 and a systolic pressure below 70 mm Hg, who is pale and sweating may have lost 2–3 litres, i.e. 40–50 per cent of his total blood volume. Table I shows the amount of blood found at necropsy in cases with injuries of the chest or abdomen.

TABLE I

Amount of blood found in 168 fatalities with injuries of the
chest and abdomen (Hoffman, 1976)

Amount of blood (litres)	Haemothorax	Haemoperitoneum
up to 1	48 (50%)	63 (87·5%)
1–2	24 (25%)	6 (8·3%)
2–3	22 (22·9%)	3 (4·2%)
over 3	2 (2·1%)	0

Bleeding into the chest is the commonest cause of concealed haemorrhage. The amount of blood lost is often underestimated in multiple injuries. Head injuries are particularly deceptive, and one should remember that **in an unconscious patient a rapid pulse and a low blood pressure is due to blood loss and not to the head injury.**

The treatment of severe blood loss consists of rapid transfusion of blood or, if none is available, of a salt or dextran solution. If a doctor is present at the accident site and the casualty needs transfusion, he should leave the ambulanceman to attend to the airway once respiratory control has been established, and concentrate on putting up an intravenous drip. When a severely injured casualty arrives in the accident department without a drip, an intravenous lifeline should be established immediately, while another doctor attends to any respiratory difficulties. The infusion should be started with a salt or dextran solution. Rapid crossmatching should make blood available within 20–30 minutes; there is a case for storing group O rhesus negative blood in the accident department for use in exsanguinating haemorrhages.

A common mistake is to let the blood run in too slowly. In hypovolaemic shock, 500 ml of blood should be given every 5–10 minutes until there is clinical improvement, as shown by a stronger pulse and a rising blood pressure. Central venous pressure can be simply monitored by means of a catheter advanced into the superior vena cava. The transfusion should be turned down to a slow drip when the central venous pressure reaches 15 cm water. Distended neck veins are a good clinical sign of overtransfusion. The amount of blood required varies, but in multiple injuries 4–5 litres or more may be needed. In chronic bronchitics and elderly arteriosclerotic casualties, care must be taken to prevent overtransfusion which may give rise to pulmonary oedema and heart failure.

Cardiac arrest

The management of cardiac arrest has been described in Chapter 1. External cardiac massage is at present the accepted method of treatment. It should not be used in some chest injuries, such as multiple rib fractures, or if a large pneumothorax or intrathoracic bleeding are suspected. It should also be avoided in stab or gunshot wounds of the chest, and in cases where damage to the heart or great vessels is a possibility. In these cases, **internal** cardiac massage is the method of choice, and it is also indicated if the carotid or femoral pulses are not palpable after a few minutes of external cardiac massage.

Technique of internal cardiac massage

No time should be wasted on aseptic technique. An incision is made through the skin and muscles in the 5th left intercostal space anteriorly. It starts 2–3 cm lateral to the sternum to avoid the internal mammary artery, and extends up to the midaxillary line. The cartilages of the ribs above and below are divided with a scalpel and this allows an assistant to hold the ribs apart. It is preferable to insert a rib spreader, and an emergency thoracotomy set should be kept in the accident department. The heart is then rhythmically compressed with the flat of the hand against the posterior surface of the sternum. If after a few compressions the heart does not resume its contractions, the pericardium should be opened longitudinally along its entire length in front of the phrenic nerve. To prevent damage to the heart, the pericardium can be picked up with forceps, and a small initial incision is easily extended with a finger protecting the heart.

Cardiac massage is most effective if both hands are used, one in front and the other behind the heart. The heart should be compressed at a rate of about 70 per minute, allowing complete relaxation between compressions. It is essential that pulmonary ventilation should proceed simultaneously using an oxygen-enriched mixture. If cardiac arrest is due to haemorrhage, a rapid blood transfusion should also be given. If blood is not available plasma expanders can be used.

If ventricular fibrillation occurs internal defibrillation is necessary.

The pads of the electrodes are soaked in saline before placing them on the ventricles. With AC the voltage should be set at 110–180 volts for 0·1–0·2 seconds; with DC 20–60 watt/seconds should be used. Electric shocks are repeated until effective; cardiac massage should then be restarted immediately. Supportive therapy with sodium bicarbonate, 1:1000 adrenaline or calcium chloride may be indicated (see Chapter 1).

Cardiac tamponade

Acute cardiac tamponade may be due to a penetrating wound of the heart or to blunt trauma such as may occur in a steering wheel injury. Most cases of cardiac tamponade reaching hospital alive are due to stab wounds. Such injuries lend themselves to surgical repair, as myocardial wounds have a tendency to seal off. The suture of a myocardial wound with two or three interrupted silk sutures is not a difficult procedure. Rupture of the heart due to blunt trauma is usually fatal before arrival at hospital; these cases often have other severe injuries. In the author's series of 344 fatal road casualties, the heart was found to be injured in 46 cases; 24 of these also had a haemopericardium (Hoffman, 1976).

If the pericardial wound is large, blood is rapidly lost into the pleural cavity and the clinical features are those of a massive haemothorax and hypovolaemic shock. If the pericardial wound becomes sealed off, blood and clots compress both atria and ventricles—resulting in a low cardiac output, a fall in arterial pressure and a rise in venous pressure, and eventual cardiac arrest.

Cardiac tamponade should be suspected in patients with penetrating wounds in the precordial region, upper abdomen or back. These patients are typically admitted in circulatory collapse, their neck veins distended and their heart sounds muffled and distant, but with little respiratory distress. At times it may be difficult to differentiate between cardiac tamponade and internal bleeding. In these cases, if the patient's condition permits it, the central venous pressure should be monitored. Cardiac tamponade is likely to be present if the reading is above 15 cm water. Readings should be taken several times as a rise in pressure may only occur after replacement of lost blood. Radiological examination is not helpful, as rapid bleeding of as little as 100 ml can produce tamponade with no evidence of enlargement of the heart shadow.

If the diagnosis of cardiac tamponade is suspected, the pericardium should be aspirated; the removal of even 20–30 ml of blood may be followed by dramatic relief. A long, large-bore, short-bevelled needle is inserted at the junction of the xyphisternum and left costal margin, and advanced at an angle of 45 degrees inward and upward. Constant aspiration while advancing the needle will help to locate the blood and prevent injury to the myocardium. If the condition of the patient allows time for it, a sterile ECG precordial lead attached to the needle will show an elevation of the S–T segment when the needle touches the ventricle.

In cardiac tamponade the present trend in treatment is to proceed to thoracotomy only if the tamponade recurs after aspiration. But the author is in favour of exploring all wounds in the vicinity of the heart, after an unfortunate experience some years ago. A man of 41 was admitted after being stabbed in the precordial region with a pair of scissors some 12 hours earlier. On admission he was dyspnoeic and had a large haemothorax displacing the trachea to the opposite side. His condition improved dramatically after drainage of the haemothorax and blood replacement, and it was decided to watch his progress. A few hours later cardiac tamponade developed and he died before anything further could be done. At postmortem a small amount of blood and clots were found in the pericardium at the back of the heart. The myocardial wound had sealed off.

CONDITIONS REQUIRING EARLY TREATMENT

Chest injuries and their complications which may require early treatment include haemothorax, flail chest, the 'shock lung' syndrome and rupture of the diaphragm. The severity of these injuries may vary; some require immediate treatment and others may be observed for some hours before a decision is made about their management.

Haemothorax

The most frequent source of intrathoracic bleeding is a laceration of the lung caused by the jagged ends of broken ribs. Bleeding into the pleural space from the low pressure lung parenchyma tends to seal off; it may occur immediately following an accident or after an interval. More serious haemorrhage follows injury of the systemic intercostal or internal mammary arteries in the chest wall. The most severe intrathoracic bleeding is due to injuries of the heart or great vessels.

A haemothorax may be difficult to diagnose from physical signs alone, as up to 1 litre of blood may accumulate in the paravertebral gutter and escape attention. Signs of severe blood loss may be obvious long before respiratory distress is apparent. Reports from the literature show that bleeding into the pleural cavity is the most frequently missed site of concealed haemorrhage, and is potentially lethal. In all patients showing signs of blood loss upright anteroposterior and lateral chest X-rays should be taken, a supine view being of little use. In small effusions blunting of the costophrenic or cardiophrenic angles may be seen. In a large haemothorax there will be a basal opacity curving upwards at the periphery or a fluid level.

A small haemothorax needs no treatment as the blood will be absorbed. In small effusions aspiration may at times be preferable (Fig. 3.4). In a large haemothorax immediate blood replacement (see under Blood loss) should be begun, and one or two large bore tubes (such as 36–40 FG) should be inserted into the pleural space and attached to a bottle with an underwater seal. The best place to drain a haemothorax is in the 4th or 5th interspace in the axillary line. Generally most of the blood is drained into the bottle in a short time and then the flow almost stops. If blood continues to escape at a rate of 300 ml or more per hour, immediate thoracotomy should be carried out, to remove blood and clots, and to tie or coagulate bleeding vessels (Fig. 3.5). At times it is necessary to resect a lacerated or infarcted segment or lobe of lung.

The possibility of associated abdominal bleeding should be considered if fractures of the lower ribs are present. In these cases abdominal guarding and tenderness with dullness in both flanks is suggestive. Repeated examinations should be carried out but physical signs are not always easy to interpret. Peritoneal lavage, if the condition of the patient permits it, has proved to be diagnostic in a high proportion of cases. A thoracotomy can then be easily extended into a thoraco-abdominal approach.

Traumatic rupture of the aorta

In a large haemothorax traumatic rupture of the aorta should be

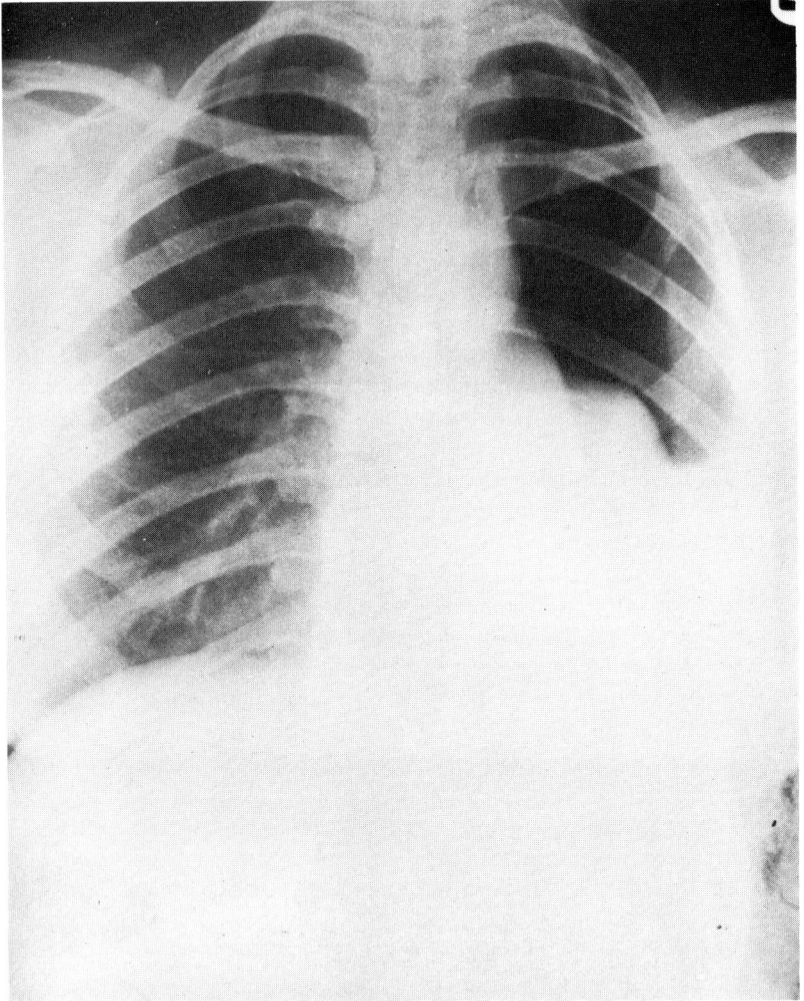

Fig. 3.4. Rib fractures and haemopneumothorax. This woman of 32 was injured while driving her car. X-ray shows collapse of the left lung, a pneumothorax with a fluid level, and fractures of the 7th to 11th left ribs. Following bronchoscopy and aspiration of the haemothorax her lung re-expanded and further convalescence was uneventful.

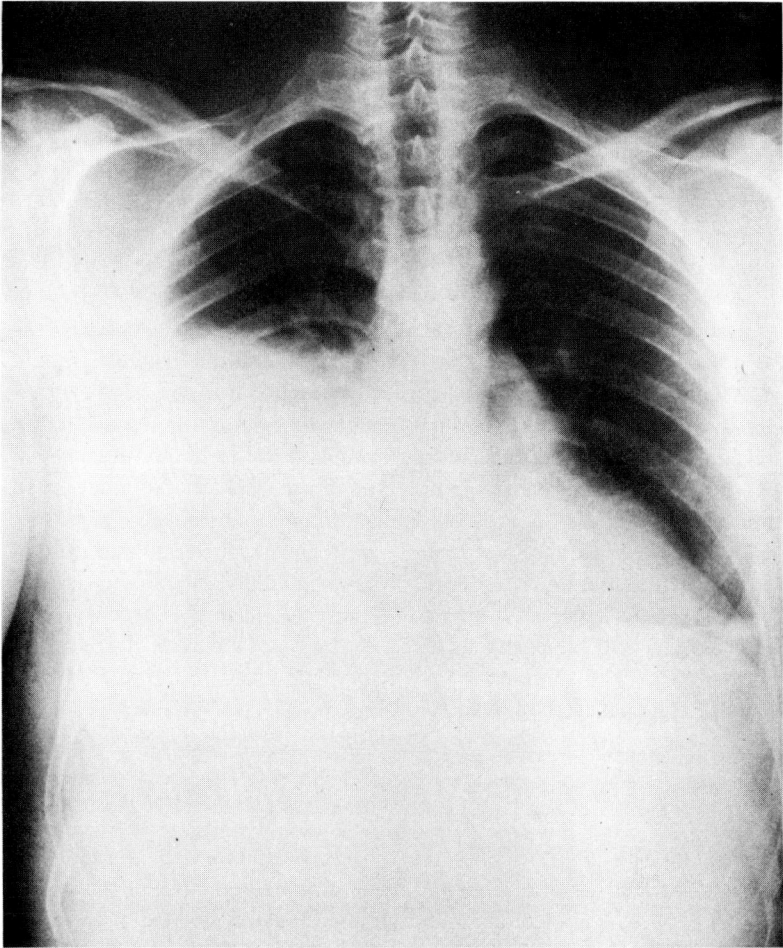

Fig. 3.5. Rib fractures and haemothorax—thoracotomy. A man of 41 was hit by a tanker and admitted 4 days after injury. On admission he was dyspnoeic and showed signs of severe blood loss. X-ray shows a right basal opacity curving upwards laterally. Fractures of the 10th and 11th right ribs are present. At thoracotomy 3 litres of blood and clots were found in the pleural cavity. There was no injury to intrathoracic structures.

suspected, particularly if the sternum or first ribs are fractured. The commonest site of injury is below the origin of the left subclavian artery. Disruption of the aortic wall is thought to be due to a combination of shearing forces and an increase of intraluminal pressure. The tear begins in the intima and proceeds outwards, but if the adventitia remains intact, the patient may be alive on admission. In the author's series, five of the 52 fatalities with aortic injury were admitted alive; three lived for 3–5 hours, one for 11 hours, and one survived for $6\frac{1}{2}$ days.

Aortic injury can be recognised radiologically if progressive widening of the mediastinum is present (Fig. 3.6). Portable X-rays taken in the accident department are not easy to interpret, and the diagnosis should only be considered if good quality chest views are available.

Clinical signs of aortic injury include dyspnoea, chest pain (often posteriorly and not affected by respiration), hoarseness and dysphagia. If the patient's condition permits, an aortogram should be carried out in a centre where cardiopulmonary bypass is available. Increasing numbers of successful operations are being reported under partial by-pass. In desperate cases thoracotomy should be done by the surgeon on the spot, as successful repairs of small tears have also been reported after direct suture in the absence of by-pass facilities. Rarely, the untreated patient survives for a longer period and then presents with a traumatic aneurysm of the aorta.

Flail chest

Crush injury resulting in a mobile segment of chest wall with paradoxical respiration is one of the most serious thoracic injuries. The mobile segment leads to impaired ventilation and collapse of the underlying lung, which then causes shunting of unoxygenated blood, and lowering of the arterial oxygen tension. At first there is little change in the arterial carbon dioxide tension, but when respiratory insufficiency develops, there is both hypoxaemia and carbon dioxide retention. Frequent arterial blood gas analyses together with the clinical findings are a good guide to the degree of respiratory failure and the efficacy of treatment.

Clinical manifestations of a stove-in chest depend on the size of the flail segment. In a large mobile segment with obvious paradoxical respiration extreme breathlessness is present immediately after the accident. First aid at the roadside consists of applying firm but gentle

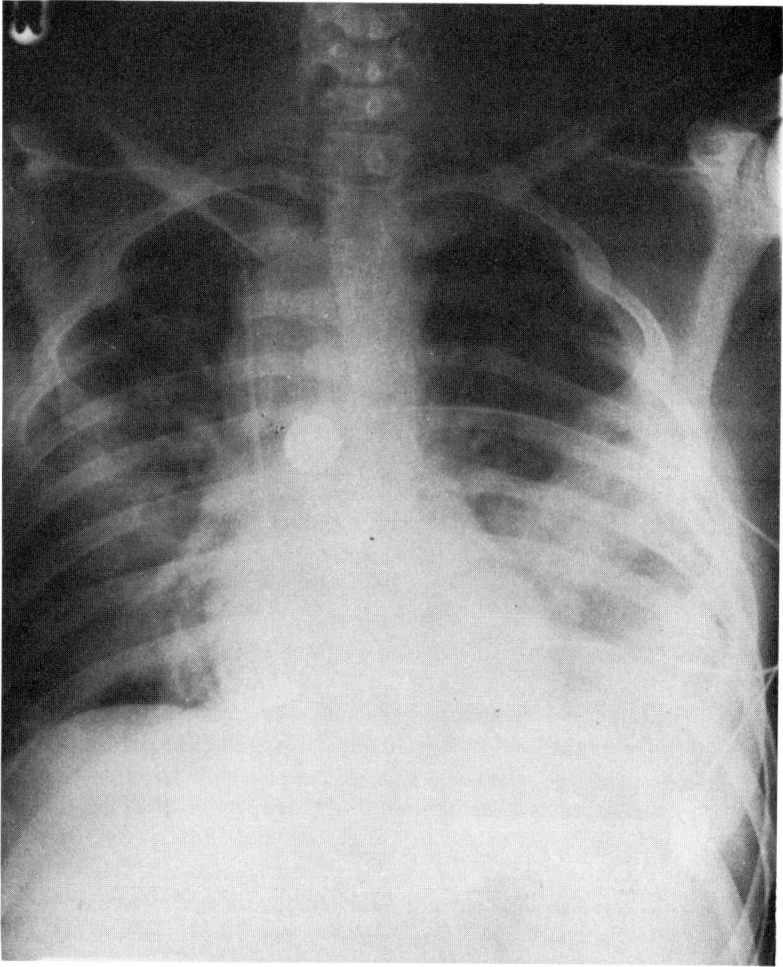

Fig. 3.6. *Aortic rupture. This man of 23 was a passenger in a car involved in a road accident. He was admitted with a compound fracture of the femur and closed fractures of the tibia and pelvis. His fractures were reduced under general anaesthesia and he was admitted to the intensive care unit. He then complained of chest pain and an X-ray showed a widened mediastinum which was correctly interpreted as an aortic rupture. He died in the X-ray department waiting for an aortogram 11 hours after admission. At necropsy, complete division of the thoracic aorta and extensive mediastinal haemorrhage were found.*

pressure over the mobile area to stabilise the chest wall until the patient reaches hospital. In a lateral or posterior paradox, lying on the side or back helps to splint the affected part. As soon as the patient arrives in the accident unit a general anaesthetic should be given, a cuffed endotracheal tube introduced, and controlled respiration begun. If the lung is difficult to inflate, the possibility of a pneumothorax or haemothorax should be kept in mind and the chest intubated if necessary.

More often, if there is only a small mobile segment, the clinical picture of a stove-in chest develops insidiously. Paradoxical respiration may not be obvious at first, and the patient shows no signs of respiratory distress. Within a few hours, however, there is marked deterioration. Cough is suppressed because of pain and sedation, increasing breathlessness develops, and the patient dies drowning in his own secretions. For treatment to be effective early diagnosis is essential. The first signs of hypoxaemia and carbon dioxide retention are a bounding pulse, a raised blood pressure, anxiety, restlessness and confusion. Later the pulse rate increases, breathing becomes rapid, shallow and distressed, and the patient uses his accessory muscles of respiration including the alae nasi.

The introduction of tracheostomy for this purpose has revolutionised the treatment of stove-in chest. It allows aspiration of bronchial secretions, reduces dead space and in the unconscious patient prevents inhalation of saliva, blood, vomit, etc. **It should be carried out in all patients with an unstable chest wall or multiple rib fractures, if they are unable to breathe properly or to cough up their secretions** (Fig. 3.7). In the unconscious and in chronic bronchitics even a minor degree of flail chest is an indication for tracheostomy. It should only be carried out as an elective procedure in the theatre except in acute laryngeal obstruction by a foreign body or oedema, when incision of the cricothyroid membrane may be life-saving.

Modern endotracheal tubes are almost non-irritant and can be used for the first 2–7 days after injury instead of a tracheostomy, and this is preferable in children where tracheostomy should be avoided if possible.

After intubation or tracheostomy the patient's respiratory rate and depth should be carefully watched, and arterial blood gases measured. If paradoxical respiration persists, respiratory excursions remain shallow and ineffective, and the patient is unable to cough up his secretions, intermittent positive pressure ventilation should be begun.

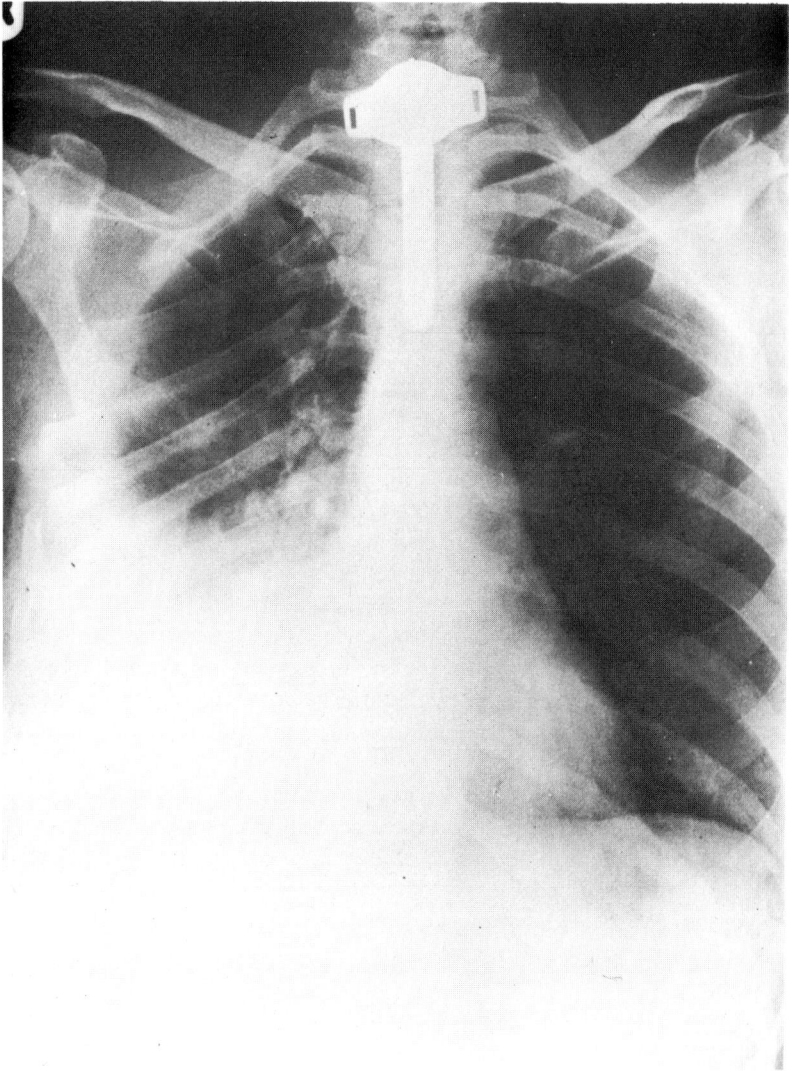

Fig. 3.7. *Rib fractures and haemothorax—tracheostomy. A woman of 37 was knocked down by a car. She had a fracture of the skull and was drowsy and confused on admission. X-ray shows fractures of the 2nd to 9th right ribs. A large mobile chest wall segment and paradoxical respiration was present. Tracheostomy followed by 5 days of mechanical ventilation resulted in uneventful recovery.*

A pneumothorax sometimes develops as a complication of this treatment, and frequent chest X-rays should be taken to facilitate early detection.

Operative fixation of rib fractures has now been largely abandoned except in cases where thoracotomy has to be carried out anyway, as in haemothorax, ruptured diaphragm, etc.

Technique of tracheostomy

Medical officers working in an accident unit should be familiar with the technique of tracheostomy (Fig. 3.8).

It is best done under general anaesthesia with an endotracheal tube *in situ*. A sandbag is placed under the shoulders to extend the neck. A transverse incision gives the best cosmetic result. The incision should be about 4 cm in length and a finger's breadth below the cricoid cartilage, dividing skin, subcutaneous tissue and platysma. The strap muscles are separated in the midline by blunt dissection and an assistant holds the muscles apart till the trachea is reached. A hook under the cricoid cartilage lifts and steadies the trachea. It is usually recommended that the thyroid isthmus should be divided for better access, but it is simpler to retract it downwards. The first tracheal ring should be left intact to prevent stenosis. An incision is made into the trachea between the 2nd and 4th rings, and the opening enlarged to accept a large-bore tracheostomy tube. The endotracheal tube is then withdrawn and a cuffed plastic tracheostomy tube inserted. The introduction of the tracheostomy tube is facilitated if it is guided through the jaws of angled forceps in the tracheal opening. A frequent mistake is to use too small a tracheostomy tube and a large size should be chosen, such as 39–42 FG. Bronchial secretions are then sucked out with a soft catheter. The skin is approximated with two interrupted sutures so that the wound is not closed too tightly. In restless and confused patients it may be advisable to fix the tracheostomy tube to the skin by two stitches to prevent it being pulled out before a track has formed.

In the postoperative period, a strict aseptic technique is essential and this is best carried out if the patient is barrier nursed. The inspired air should be humidified to prevent crust formation. A soft sterile catheter should be used for suction using a non-touch technique or disposable gloves.

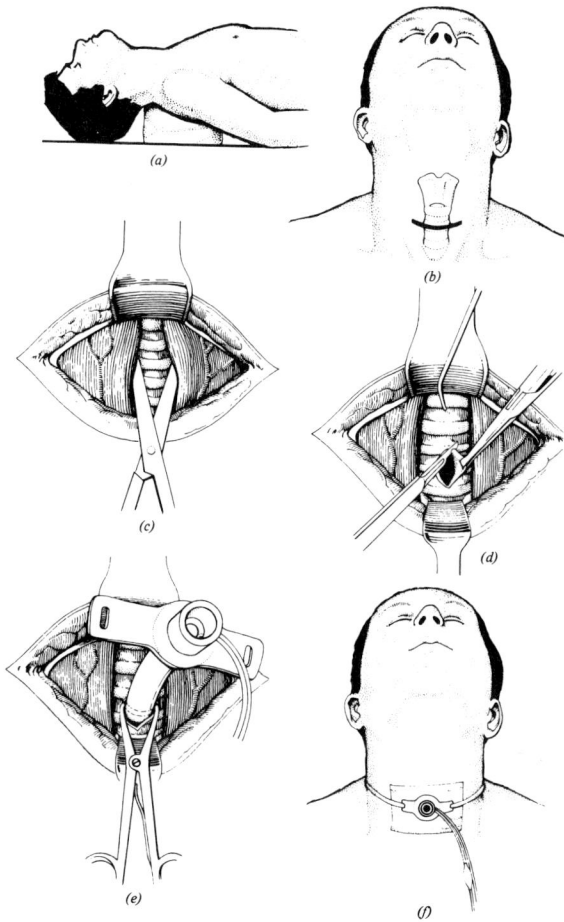

Fig. 3.8. Technique of tracheostomy:
(a) Sandbag under shoulders extends neck.
(b) Transverse incision one finger's breadth below cricoid cartilage.
(c) Separation of strap muscles in midline by blunt dissection.
(d) Hook under cricoid cartilage lifts and steadies trachea. Thyroid isthmus retracted downwards. Opening made in trachea between 2nd and 4th rings.
(e) Introduction of tracheostomy tube facilitated by angled forceps.
(f) Tracheostomy tube in situ.

Shock lung

The shock lung or adult respiratory distress syndrome is a major cause of death following trauma. It was first described in battle casualties during World War II and is now a frequent complication in intensive care units. It has been variously described as the wet lung syndrome, post traumatic pulmonary insufficiency, congestive atelectasis, etc.

Shock lung is a non-specific reaction to a variety of aetiological factors. These include blast injury to the lungs, burns, extensive soft tissue damage associated with serious blood loss, fat embolism, head and chest injuries, aspiration and renal failure. A large proportion of cases are associated with sepsis. Shock lung may also be a complication of treatment in patients who have been overtransfused or given stored blood, excessive volumes of salt solutions, or high concentrations of oxygen or who have been on prolonged mechanical ventilation.

Symptoms usually appear 12–72 hours after injury, with a wet ineffective cough, an increased respiratory rate and progressive shortness of breath. Early blood gas estimations show a hypoxaemia of 60 mm Hg or less which does not respond to treatment with oxygen. There is intrapulmonary right to left shunting which progresses to respiratory failure. Clinical signs may not be obvious at first and serial measurements of arterial blood gases should be done routinely in all seriously injured casualties. Patients should be carefully observed for any changes in the character of their breathing, difficulty with expectoration or moist sounds in the chest. Initially there are no radiological changes; later, fluffy opacities appear in the lung fields.

Early pulmonary oedema may respond to treatment with diuretics, and the author has found frusemide most effective in aborting early and treating established cases. Bronchoscopy is not very helpful as secretions reaccumulate quickly. Medical treatment of pulmonary oedema is well established: oxygen should be given, bronchospasm treated with aminophylline and steroids, and arrythmias with digoxin. If the patient does not respond to medical treatment within a few hours he should be intubated and given assisted ventilation. If despite this symptoms progress, continuous positive pressure ventilation should be started using an end-expiratory pressure of $+5$ to $+10$ cm water. In cases of refractory respiratory failure oxygenation has been maintained for some days by extracorporeal support with a membrane oxygenator but this method is still on trial.

In fatal cases the lungs are found to be congested and oedematous

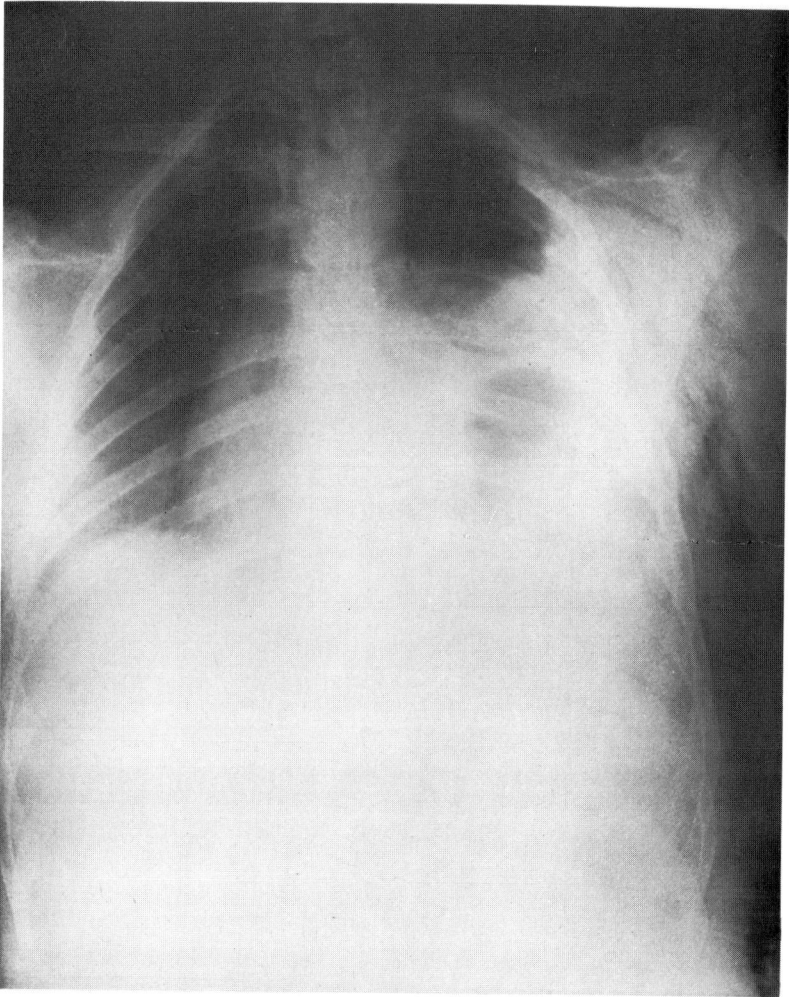

Fig. 3.9. Rupture of the diaphragm. A youth of 18 hit a lamp post whilst driving a car. On admission he was unconscious and dyspnoeic. The upright X-ray shows fractures of the left upper 5 ribs, an air-containing opacity at the left base and surgical emphysema. At thoracotomy most of the stomach, loops of small intestine and the left lobe of the liver were found to have prolapsed into the chest through a diaphragmatic tear. After repair he made a good recovery.

with areas of atelectasis. Microscopically, interstitial oedema and focal haemorrhages predominate at first, later alveolar cell hypertrophy and hyaline membrane deposits are found.

Rupture of the diaphragm

Crushing injuries of the lower chest and upper abdomen may result in rupture of the diaphragm. In the majority of cases the tear is on the left as the right diaphragm is protected by the liver. A small tear may be temporarily plugged by omentum or a viscus, and herniation or even strangulation may occur later. Large tears mostly begin in the central tendon and extend radially, though involvement of the oesophageal hiatus is rare. In these cases herniation of most of the abdominal viscera can occur, and stomach, spleen, liver, colon or small intestine may be found within the chest. In cases of massive herniation severe shortness of breath, pain referred to the shoulder and cardiovascular collapse are often present. Rupture of the diaphragm may be missed if the diagnosis is not kept in mind. Audible peristalsis posteriorly in the chest is diagnostic but not always present. An upright X-ray of the chest is conclusive and shows absence of the diaphragmatic outline, a 'high' diaphragm or radiotranslucent areas in the chest. If a distended stomach fills the hemithorax the appearances can be mistaken for a pneumothorax (Fig. 3.9).

Surgical repair of a ruptured diaphragm should be carried out as soon as possible after initial resuscitation. An abdominal approach is preferable if intra-abdominal injury is suspected. Otherwise it is easier to repair the tear through a thoracic incision which can be extended into the abdomen. In cases with mild symptoms the hernia may be missed in the acute stage and discovered after some time during investigations for vague upper abdominal dyspeptic symptoms.

INJURIES WHICH CAN BE MANAGED CONSERVATIVELY

Some chest injuries can be managed conservatively provided they do not develop complications. They include simple fractures of a few ribs or the sternum, contusion or haematoma of the lung and myocardial contusion.

Fractures of ribs or sternum

Rib fractures are the commonest type of chest injury. A simple fracture of one or more ribs in the young or middle aged is a trivial injury. In the bronchitic or elderly, fracture of even one or two ribs may lead to atelectasis from retained secretions and cardiorespiratory embarrassment.

Rib fractures are the result of direct impact or compression of the chest. In conscious patients the diagnosis is not difficult. They complain of localised pain aggrevated by deep breathing or coughing, and the affected area is tender on palpation. Fractures most frequently occur in the 5th to 9th ribs. If the lower ribs are fractured tears of the liver or spleen should be suspected. The diagnosis of these visceral injuries may be difficult because of reflex upper abdominal rigidity and tenderness which may be due to the fractures. The abdomen should be re-examined frequently to exclude visceral injury.

An upright chest X-ray should always be taken to detect pleural or lung complications, and repeated daily for the first two to three days. The author remembers a patient who was sent home after having been seen in the accident unit with a simple rib fracture. The next day he was brought back having collapsed, his pulse and blood pressure were unrecordable, and at thoracotomy 4 litres of blood and clots were removed from his chest.

Treatment of simple rib fractures consists of relief of pain with analgesics. If this is unsuccessful nerve block of the affected ribs should be carried out and repeated twice or three times daily if necessary.

Sternal fractures are much less common than rib fractures. They occur after steering wheel injuries or direct blows to the sternal region. The majority are transverse fractures of the sternal body, some displacement of the segments may be present but this is rarely severe enough to require surgical correction. The steplike deformity can be felt, and seen on a lateral film. Patients complain of pain in the sternal region aggravated by coughing or deep breathing. The possibility of damage to the heart or great vessels should be kept in mind. Treatment consists of bed rest and analgesics.

Injury to the lung

The extent of damage to lung parenchyma varies with the severity of the chest injury. In multiple rib fractures damage to the underlying lung may be small as the force of the original impact is generally absorbed by the chest wall. Clinical manifestations of lung injury depend on its location.

Peripheral laceration is due to damage by sharp spicules of ribs or to a penetrating injury such as a stab wound. In a lung injury with a pleural tear, air often escapes into the subcutaneous tissues producing surgical emphysema, which may be extensive and alarming to both patient and laymen, but requires no special treatment. Air usually absorbs once the lung laceration has sealed off, or an intercostal tube has been inserted.

If the parenchymal damage is more central, disruption of small blood vessels leads to the formation of a haematoma and this may give rise to chest pain or haemoptyses. Radiologically an opacity with indistinct edges is seen, but later this becomes well defined. At this stage it may be confused with other more serious lesions such as bronchial carcinoma. No treatment is required as the haematoma usually resolves within two to four weeks. If the blood is coughed up a lung cyst appears which is later absorbed.

Myocardial contusion

The diagnosis of myocardial contusion should be considered in steering wheel injuries, fractures of the sternum, compression injuries, or blows to the precordial region. This is the most common heart injury and has a favourable prognosis. Patients complain of precordial pain unaffected by deep breathing. Electrocardiographic changes may be similar to those of myocardial infarct although the pattern is more irregular. Serum transaminase levels are also raised. It is important to make the diagnosis from medicolegal and prognostic viewpoints. Treatment consists of bed rest until electrocardiographic changes have reverted to normal. In a few cases arrythmias and congestive heart failure develop and these should be treated with digoxin and diuretics.

On rare occasions aortic insufficiency results from ruptured cusps or mitral regurgitation from torn papillary muscles of the mitral valve. Both atrial and ventricular septal defects have been described following blunt trauma or penetrating injuries. If heart failure develops surgical correction of these defects after preliminary medical treatment is indicated.

REFERENCES

Barret (1960), Early treatment of stove-in chest, *Lancet*, **i**, 293.

Cleland, Goodwin, McDonald and Ross (1969), *Medical and Surgical Cardiology*. Oxford: Blackwell Scientific Publications.

Frey, Huelke and Gikas (1969), Resuscitation and survival in motor vehicles accidents, *Journal of Trauma*, **9**, 292.

Hoffman (1976), Mortality and morbidity following road accidents, *Annals of the Royal College of Surgeons of England*, **58**.

Hunt (1973), *Pathology of Injury*. Report of a working party of the Royal College of Pathologists. Harvey Miller and Medcalf Ltd.

Illingworth and Jennett (1965), The shocked head injury, *Lancet*, **ii**, 511.

Moore and colleagues (1969), *Posttraumatic pulmonary insufficiency*. Philadelphia: Saunders.

Naclerio (1971), *Chest Injuries*. New York: Grune and Stratton.

Surgical Clinics of North America. Symposium on a physiologic approach to critical care, Vol 55, June 1975.

Sykes, McNicol and Campbell (1974), *Respiratory failure*, 2nd ed. Oxford: Blackwell Scientific Publications.

Symposium on a physiologic approach to critical care (1975), *Surgical Clinics of North America*, **55** (June 1975).

4

Injuries of the Soft Tissues

P S LONDON

A wound is more than just a break in the continuity of the skin. If defined as **a break in the continuity of tissue**, a wound comprehends injuries that occur within intact skin and includes bruises, torn muscles, rupture of the spleen and other visceral damage—which are all examples of closed wounds. If this definition of a wound be accepted, it must also include fractures.When one recognises that with some fractures it is the soft tissues rather than the hard that need to be dealt with, it will be acknowledged that any account of injuries of the soft parts should include fractures that are accompanied by considerable damage to their soft surroundings.

Another noteworthy feature of soft tissue injuries is that they are the ones that can kill a person; fractures, which sometimes seem to be regarded as the be-all and end-all of so-called trauma (which means an open wound, or, more generally, an injury) threaten life only when there is accompanying damage to the soft tissues.

Effects of wounds

In the case of the aptly termed tidy wound the tissues are divided but otherwise undamaged; more widespread force produces untidy wounds with more or less laceration, contusion and destruction of tissue. The principal difference between the behaviour of tidy and untidy wounds lies in the readiness with which they heal. A tidy wound usually needs no more than simple closure for it to heal soundly within about a fortnight but an untidy wound can tax a surgeon's judgement and skill to the utmost and still heal slowly with an associated risk of infection, much scarring and subsequent contracture.

Tidy and untidy wounds are alike, however, in that they cause

112

bleeding, and may cause distal ischaemia, and they interfere with the function of the part. Inasmuch as wounds breach an external or internal surface of the body they carry the risk of infection until the wound has healed soundly. Sound healing does not apply only to the skin or mucous membrane, because this can heal over damaged tissue or even dead tissue in which the seeds of sepsis may remain for a very long time. Nevertheless, the main risk of septic invasion ends when the epithelial barrier is re-established.

THE MANAGEMENT OF WOUNDS

The steps required in an emergency are easily stated as being to provide cover for an open wound, to add tetanus toxoid and perhaps antibiotics in the prevention of infection, to stanch accessible bleeding and to provide comfortable support for the injured part and for the patient as a whole. Each of these essentially simple steps deserves more than passing mention and the conditions vary so much with the circumstances of injury, the number of casualties, the time taken to reach them and effect any necessary rescue, the duration and conditions of transport and the choice of destination that the nature of the wounds themselves deserves detailed attention.

OPEN WOUNDS

Cover

While it is easy to say that wounds should be covered by a sterile and occlusive dressing it does not take much experience of accidental injuries to recognise that this recommendation is, perhaps more often than not, entirely impracticable. The reasons arise from the relative sizes of wounds and dressings, the accessibility of the wound, the complexity of the injury and the skill and experience of those available to use them.

Size of dressing

The first aid kits that can be purchased by the public contain dressings that are large enough for the average domestic or picnic accident but useless for most wounds resulting from accidents on the roads and for many of those inflicted in factories. Some rescue services are provided with pad and bandage dressings up to about 6 in (15 cm) square but even these are not always large enough. The largest dressings in use are usually the result of personal initiative and are based upon a sterilisable and waterproof layer* to which is stitched a sheet of gamgee or comparably substantial and absorbent material. Such a dressing (Fig. 4.1) can be up to 18 in (45 cm) square, and has enough body to provide some support but is not too bulky to go inside an inflatable splint. The waterproof paper is of advantage in the wet but if there is continuing bleeding the blood does not soak through to the surface and comes out at the ends of the dressing. It is important to be aware that by the time this has happened **the dressing may have soaked up as much as one litre of blood.** Such a dressing can be kept on by any of the usual bandages but the crepe or conforming sort are most convenient. Dressings of this nature should be commercially available before long.

A very useful alternative is polyurethane foam, which can be cut up into whatever shapes and sizes are required and sterilised by X-rays after being sealed in plastic bags. As well as being readily absorbent and not sticking to wounds this material fits and supports fractures if it is used as packing or padding or if a strip is rolled several times round a limb.†

Occlusion

Quite apart from the size of dressing it may be impossible to seal the wound from the surface. It requires skill to apply an ordinary cotton bandage in such a way that it will keep a small and relatively thick pad firmly in place. A triangular bandage is unlikely to be better but a crepe or conforming bandage may succeed. Nevertheless, this is not easy as a demonstration and it may be impossible, even for skilled hands, with a wound that is awkwardly situated, on a limb that has been badly broken, with a terrified patient or in darkness, wind or rain.

The lint and bandage dressings of first aid kits are easier to apply

---

* Kimberly Clark, Kleenex® surgical sheet or Vernon Carus, Azowrap®.

† I am indebted to Major G. W. Stanley, MBE, TD, for this account of the practice of the Wellington Free Ambulance Service in New Zealand.

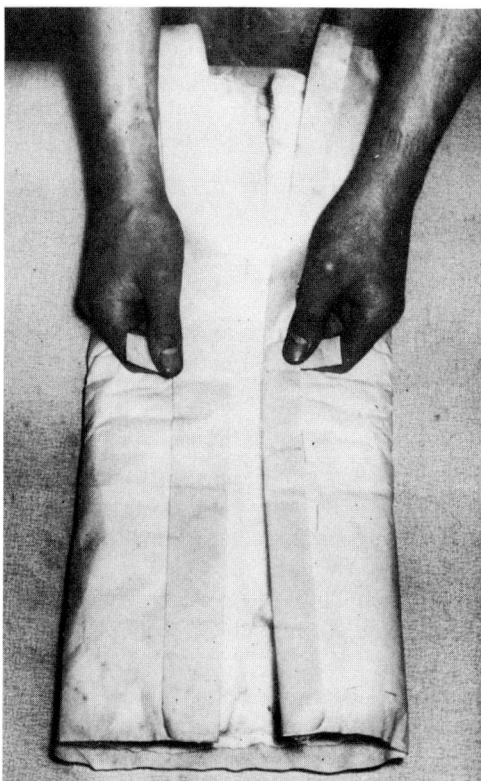

Fig. 4.1. A substantial, waterproof dressing that
can easily be made in hospitals or by
volunteers. The fringe of paper around
the dressing and the tabs of autoclave
tape make it easy to open the dressing
without contaminating it. (Reproduced
by kind permission of John Wright and
Sons, Ltd.)

and they may occlude fairly dry burns, but if there is enough oozing
to soak through to the surface of dressing, it is no longer occlusive.

In practice, a truly occlusive dressing is of doubtful value when
applied to a wound and its surroundings that may be very heavily
contaminated, but it does prevent additional contamination from
without and it hides an unpleasant sight.

In sum, one may say that there is no point in applying a dressing that will cover only part of a wound and be easily dislodged. Whatever the sense of obligation of the rescuers, it is often true that the dressings used could have been left in their wrappings without any disadvantage to the patient.

These comments apply to emergency care at the place of accident; they may not apply in the case of temporary accommodation in a small hospital or other aid post where it may be possible to cleanse thoroughly the skin surrounding the wound and apply an adequately absorbent and well secured occlusive dressing of gauze and cotton wool. Tulle gras may be preferable to dry gauze for the simple reason that it is much less likely to fall off a surface with an awkward contour or position.

Sterility of dressings

What has already been said about the difficulty of applying occlusive dressings applies to a large extent to using sterile dressings. It is not difficult in orderly conditions to extract a dressing from its coverings and apply it to a wound without contaminating the part that will be on the wound but such an action may be impossible in poor light, with inadequate access to the part, a strong wind blowing and fingers made clumsy by haste and anxiety. The ideal might be to have the absorbent part fixed to a sheet of impermeable and sterilisable material that formed one side of a sealed bag. The bag would be opened by tearing off the second side but this would still make contamination very likely in difficult conditions.

For emergency use, it is desirable that a sterile dressing be applied when it is practicable to do so, but it should be remembered that the degree of accidental bacterial contamination of a dressing is likely to be much less than that of the wound to which it will be applied.

Stanching bleeding

Direct pressure

Accessible bleeding can almost always be stopped by direct pressure. Exceptions are bleeding from within the skull and from the lids or eye, which may have suffered a penetrating wound. In these cases a bulky, absorbent dressing kept snugly in place is all that can be offered. Whenever possible the bleeding part should be raised. A first aid dressing that is too small to cover a wound may be large enough to apply the pressure necessary to stop bleeding. Although sterility is always desirable, in the rare case of severe and accessible bleeding, sterility and even cleanliness are much less important than stopping the bleeding and the way in which pressure is applied or maintained is less important than whether it stops the bleeding. If a dressing does not stop bleeding it may be sufficient to add to its bulk and apply a firmer bandage but if practicable, the ineffectual dressing should be removed and an effective one applied.

Indirect pressure

The writer's experience suggests that a supposed tourniquet applied in an emergency is more likely to provoke bleeding by causing venous obstruction than to stop it. If removing the constriction does not stop the bleeding a firm dressing certainly will. The only conditions in which constriction should be used are when it can be applied proximal to inaccessible bleeding from a trapped part and in the rare case of crushing of a limb that is so severe or so prolonged (six hours or more) that the limb will have to be amputated. The constriction must be tight enough to stop the bleeding, and in the case of crushing it should be as close as possible to the crushed part, but because it is painful it should not be applied to a crushed limb until it is about to be released. This prevents the loss of a large part of the circulating blood into the crushed part and may reduce the risk of consequent renal failure. Constriction should be used only by those with the necessary training.

An amputation stump rarely bleeds severely but should be watched carefully after a firm dressing has been applied. In an emergency it may be squeezed in the hands.

The use of pressure points is rarely worth considering and is likely to fail because of collateral circulation.

Assessing bloodshed

Simple practical experiments or illustrations of simulated bloodshed can enable the amount of blood lost externally to be estimated with rough but useful accuracy by merely looking at stains, pools and trickles (Fig. 4.2).

Drugs to prevent infection

Neither tetanus toxoid nor a reinforcing antibiotic such as penicillin need be given at the place of accident and there is no place for applying any antibiotic to the wound, but once the patient is in hospital tetanus toxoid should be given if he is not known to be actively immune.

If the patient is actively immune there is increasing evidence that even a booster dose of toxoid is unnessary within five or even ten years of previous injection (Committee on Trauma, 1972) but it is probably true that a dose of toxoid given unnecessarily is very unlikely to cause harm.

If the wound is heavily contaminated or several hours old and if the patient is not known to have been actively immunized he should be afforded passive immunity as well as receiving tetanus toxoid.

The safest and most reliable substance for inducing passive immunity is human immune globulin (known in Britain by the trade name of 'Humotet®'). The dose is 250 units. Equine antitoxin is still perhaps the most widely available passive immunizing agent but if more than one dose is given the protective effect is much reduced and the risk of anaphylaxis is increased. When there is no alternative, it still has a place in both prophylaxis and treatment, but it must be accompanied by precautions against anaphylaxis. Whether or not penicillin or erythromycin can be regarded as an acceptable alternative to antitoxin depends on the age of the wound. If it is fresh, any contaminating clostridia may be eliminated by an antibiotic before they can produce toxin, but if the wound is more than about 12 hours old and is likely to contain Cl. tetani it is reasonable to suppose that toxin may already have been produced and to administer antitoxin. It must be emphasized, however, that expert opinion is increasingly antagonistic to equine antitoxin.

Comfortable support

Any badly injured limb and the patient as a whole should be made comfortable with suitable support whether or not bones have been

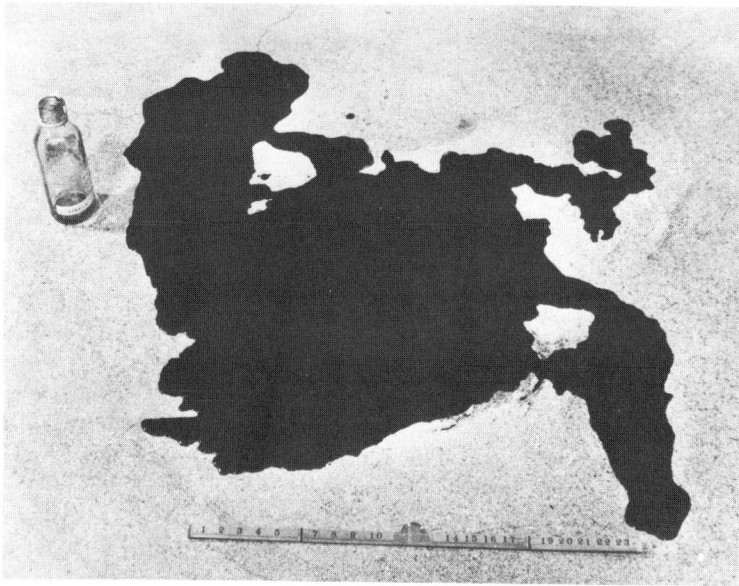

(a)

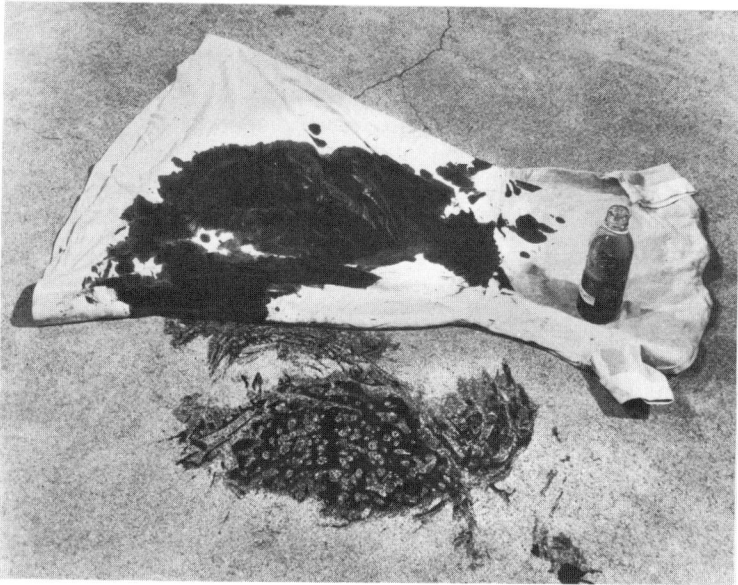

(b)

Fig. 4.2. *Bloodshed: (a) one donation on an unabsorbent surface makes a pool about 2 feet (60 cm) square; (b) half a donation will soak a dress right through and leave a considerable amount of blood on the surface beneath it. (Reproduced by kind permission of Camera Talks Ltd, from the film strip* How much blood?*)*

broken. The term comfortable support is preferred to the word splintage because the concept of splintage customarily entails immobilisation, whereas in fact the application of a splint can be a very painful experience and may do nothing to provide either comfort or support thereafter.

Air splints

Fractures beyond the elbow and at or below the knee can be comfortably and safely supported by air splints. The comfort of a conscious patient is the best guide to the right pressure but if the patient is unconscious the splint should be inflated, then lifted by its further end and then either inflated or deflated until it just buckles. The experienced hand can usually recognise a comfortable supporting pressure.

Air splints can safely be applied over dressings, clothing and footwear, so the latter should not be removed as a matter of course; trousers should not be left crumpled but folded as neatly as possible.

The best splint to use is the cheapest one that has a reliable valve, preferably with an extension tube, and a reliable fastener that is not opaque to X-rays.

Another form of air splint provides comfortable support for the entire body because when it is **deflated** the many plastic balls within it consolidate as a mould for whatever is lying on it (Fig. 4.3).

Reducing deformity

The inflation of an air splint is often the most successful and comfortable means of reducing deformity in a limb but if it is not uncomfortable, is not blanching the skin and has no associated damage to nerves or blood vessels, there is usually no need to interfere with deformity. Only in the case of spinal injury is it dangerous even to attempt to alter the position of the spine in any way. If it is considered necessary to reduce deformity of a limb any attempt to do so may have to be abandoned if it causes more pain. Success is likely to depend upon the manipulator's experience in handling broken limbs and the confidence that he can induce the patient to place in him. Relaxation by the patient may allow deformity to be corrected with little effort or pain. If deformity is corrected there is likely to be rapid swelling afterwards, so whenever possible the firm support of a bandage or an inflatable splint should be provided.

Padding

If an air splint cannot be used it is often best to support the limb by carefully placed pads made from cushions, clothing, blankets or whatever is suitable. This may be more comfortable for the patient than having an upper limb bound to the trunk or the lower limbs bandaged together.

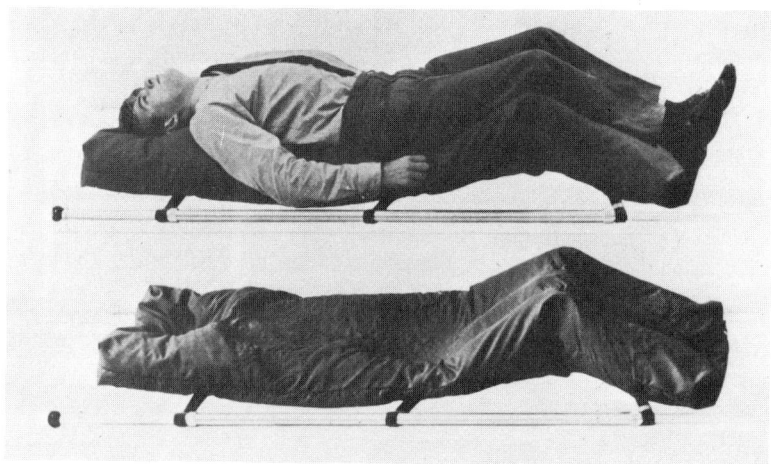

Fig. 4.3. Deflatable or vacuum mattress, which becomes almost rigid when completely emptied of air. (Reproduced by kind permission of Vickers Ltd.)

Splints

Most conventional splints are of doubtful value but emergency packets of plaster of Paris and paper bandages (Fig. 4.4) have proved their worth, while for those that possess and know how to use Thomas's splint there is no more comfortable way of supporting the lower limb (Fig. 4.5) for a possibly painful journey.

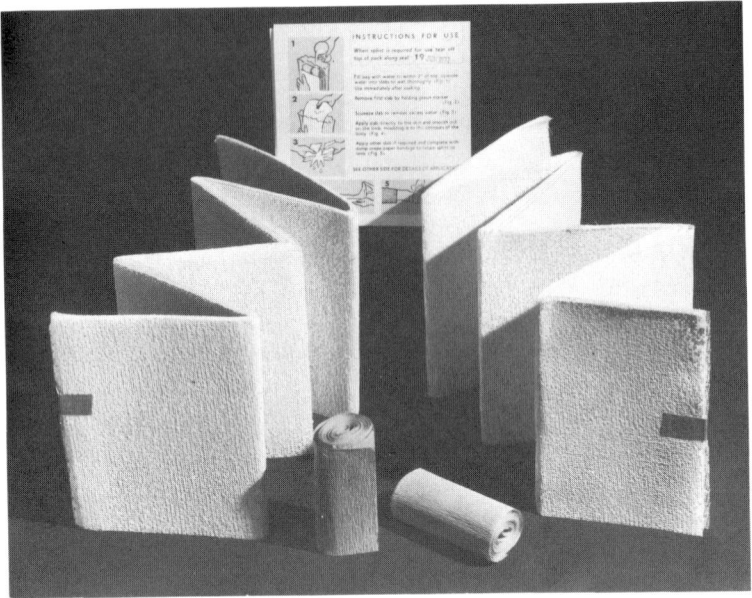

Fig. 4.4. The packet contains plaster slabs and crepe paper bandages for holding them in place. The packet can be filled with water and used for wetting the plaster slabs. (Reproduced by kind permission of Smith and Nephew Ltd.)

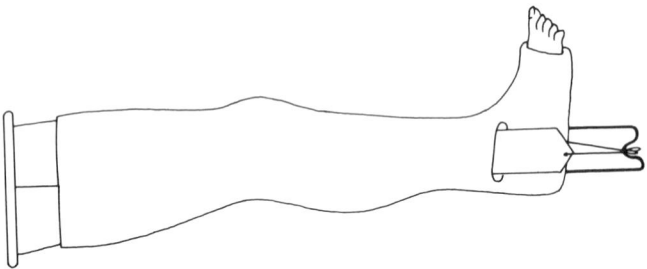

Fig. 4.5. The Tobruk plaster is a Thomas's bed knee splint which is held in place by a plaster of Paris shell over all. Fixed traction is maintained by the strips used for skin traction, which must emerge clear of the plaster.

Some special features of open wounds

Penetration

The circumstances of injury should be considered for evidence that penetrating wounds have resulted. Wounds caused by falls or stabbing, whether accidental or deliberate; wounds inflicted at high speeds and by certain types of machinery, and wounds caused by fine, sharp objects, by injection or by gunshot can all be small, apparently superficial and have few symptoms even when they have in fact penetrated a foot (30 cm) or more. Information of this sort may be of great assistance to whoever becomes responsible for definitive treatment.

Open pneumothorax. If there is any hissing or bubbling at a wound of the chest it should at once be covered by a firm pad fixed in place with strapping. If the patient is then in respiratory distress the largest needle available should be inserted into the pleural space either through the second intercostal space in front, or high up behind the anterior axillary fold. Ready-made valves are on the market but if the finger of a rubber glove, or a finger stall, is tied round the base of the needle and its tip is snipped off it makes an effective valve for releasing a dangerous pneumothorax.

If there is a large hole in the chest wall artificial ventilation, even mouth-to-mouth, is the first need and is much more likely to relieve distress than merely sealing the wound with a suitable dressing. After sealing the wound the pleural space should be drained by the forementioned method.

Foreign bodies. Foreign bodies should be removed only if they can readily be grasped and are not firmly embedded. In the case of impalement it is usually necessary to cut through the impaling object before the patient can be removed. Among the more troublesome foreign bodies are the lead of a copying pencil and the irritant tip of the spike of a blackthorn, which readily snaps off and is left behind. A rare but particularly serious penetrating injury is the injection of oil, grease, paraffin, paint, plastic material or air under pressure from a fine nozzle. The part may be massively distended and in urgent need of wide decompression in an attempt to prevent the death of tightly stretched skin and other tissues.

Penetration outwards. Many open fractures are open from within and in some cases bone is protruding and perhaps tightly gripped by the skin. If this is so, an otherwise desirable attempt to reduce the deformity may have to be abandoned because it would further damage the skin by distortion or pressure. If the bone is not so gripped there is no objection to reducing deformity even though this may take contaminated bone back inside. **The fact of protusion and any obvious contamination should be reported to whoever takes over the care of the patient.**

Fragments of bone found outside the wound are worth saving if they are larger than chips or slivers but any loss of bone should be reported. Any bone that is later put back will be boiled first so that there is no need for any attempt at sterility for fragments sent to hospital.

Bites

These injuries can be classified according to the nature and degree of damage they cause.

Fine punctures. The fine, sharp teeth of cats can easily puncture the joints of the hands and destroy them by infection that is not recognised in time.

Local destruction. Human bites crush the tissues and embed organisms that can make the part a stinking mess within a day or two. If they break the skin they require careful surgical decompression and protection by antibiotics with a wide range of effectiveness. Dogs may bite out tissue but they more often slash with their teeth to produce wounds that may be quite complicated but are almost incised in nature and not destructive so that they will heal well after careful surgical repair.

It should be remembered that in some countries dogs, foxes, wolves and bats can transmit rabies when they bite.

Massive destruction. Large animals, particularly predators, inflict bites in which there is likely to be a risk of death from bleeding as well as massive destruction of tissue. Domestic cattle can inflict severe penetrating wounds and swine have been known to eat unattended infants.

Shark bites are the ultimate in severity and danger (even the crocodile relies on drowning its prey, so that if it can be induced to relax its grip the victim may escape with little final disability). If the victim of shark bite reaches shore alive he should not be taken beyond the water's edge. Aid should be rushed to him there from rescue stations that should be provided where sharks are a known menace. The vital needs are to stop any bleeding and to replenish the circulation as rapidly as possible. Two or even three litres of saline can be given with dramatic benefit and keep the patient alive until blood is available. There is no great advantage in such cases in giving lactated Ringer's solution or- one of the dextrans to start with. When it is decided that the patient can be removed to hospital he should be assured of as comfortable a journey as possible: the need for rushing has passed.

Poisonous bites. The bites of venomous snakes are not necessarily fatal and antivenom should be available in the countries in which they are likely. The doctor's most useful function may be to offer reassurance in an effort to prevent panic. The general rule is that the victim should lie down as and when it is safe to do so and that a venous tourniquet should be applied proximal to the bite, but those bitten by sea snakes may have no alternative to trying to reach help. There may be some benefit from immediate attempts to suck out the venom but there should be no attempt to lay open the wound. Most bitten persons will need tetanus toxoid. If the victim of snake bite elects to cut the bitten part off it is to be hoped that this sacrifice achieves its object.

The bites of scorpions and venomous spiders are less dangerous but should be treated along the above lines.

Severed limbs

Upper limbs that survive reattachment are more likely than lower limbs to become better than an artificial substitute, but whether or not a limb is worth reattaching is for the surgeon concerned to decide. If it appears capable of being reattached the limb should be wrapped in clean or sterile materials and kept as cool as possible. If the wrapped limb is sealed in a plastic bag it can be placed in cold water or packed in ice for the journey to hospital. Washing out the severed part with heparin and antibiotic should be left until it reaches hospital but if there is likely to be much delay in moving the patient to hospital it may be worth sending the limb on ahead for this purpose.

Wounds of the neck

Apart from the possibility of rapidly fatal bleeding from neck injuries, there are the risks of air embolism and suffocation.

Air embolism. This can occur if a large vein is opened and it is more likely if the patient sits up. He should therefore be kept recumbent with a large and firmly retained pad on wounds that carry this risk. If air does enter the circulation it causes failure of circulation and a curious but allegedly characteristic alteration of the heart's sounds. In such cases, it is recommended that the patient be laid on the left side in an attempt to keep the air—or froth—from entering the pulmonary circulation. In theory, froth might be removed by passing either a needle or a catheter into the right ventricle.

Suffocation. If the trachea or larynx is divided it may be necessary to intubate the trachea through either the accidental wound or a surgical one below it.

CLOSED WOUNDS

Diagnosis

Some of these injuries can easily be overlooked unless the patient is examined methodically from head to foot, back and front and not forgetting the perineum, buttocks and urethra, but the extent and duration of initial examination must depend on the conditions.

Inspection

Grazes, bruising and swelling as well as open wounds all deserve attention with the circumstances of injury in mind.

Grazes. If seen on the chest after forcible impact these should prompt a search for evidence of multiple fractures or visceral damage and raise the possibility of rupture of the aorta or diaphragm—or injury of the heart.

On the backs of the shoulders, grazes may be a sign of a flexion injury of the spine, which may be confirmed by a kyphosis, tenderness, bruising and a palpable gap. When examining the back it should be remembered that a posterolateral strip on the under side can remain unseen unless the patient is rolled beyond the lateral position.

Grazes on the knees should direct attention to the hips, and marks of injury on the face and forehead may have been inflicted in the course of hyperextension of the spine. If these signs are present in an unconscious patient it is more important than ever to assume that the spine and spinal cord have been injured.

Bruising. Small bruises over subcutaneous bones may at first be the only sign of fracture; firm pressure on the bone nearby will support this possibility if it causes pain at the bruise.

Bruising over the pubes, in the perineum or by the sacrum suggests fracture of the pelvis, which may be found to be unstable.

Bruising over the spine may be accompanied by a palpable gap between the spinous processes and in the deep fascia. These signs are clear evidence of a dangerous injury such as a fracture–dislocation and evidence of paraplegia should be sought.

Pattern bruising, such as the mark of clothing impressed upon the skin as a bruise, is not to be ignored when it is found on skin not immediately supported by bone. In the neck it may mean that the larynx or trachea has been crushed and ruptured against the spine (Fig. 4.6) and on the anterior abdominal wall it has a similar significance for the viscera (Fig. 4.7).

Massive bruising. Palpation may show that the bruise has a soft centre so that if the skin is indented it yields readily and may be felt to be directly against bone from which it would normally be separated by fat, fascia, muscle, ligament or capsule. In such a case there is the possibility that important blood vessels have been ruptured by the force that has crushed their surroundings (Fig. 4.8). This state of affairs is not to be confused with the crater-like haematoma of the scalp, with which all the layers superficial to the skull are intact (Fig. 4.9).

Massive bruising, which can also follow widespread subcutaneous

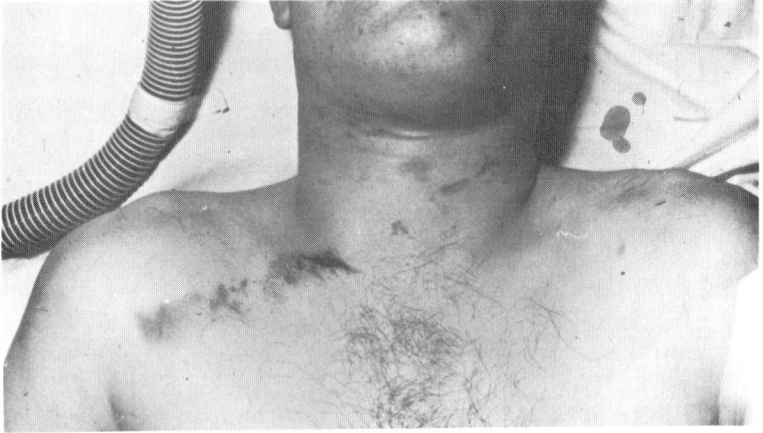

(a)

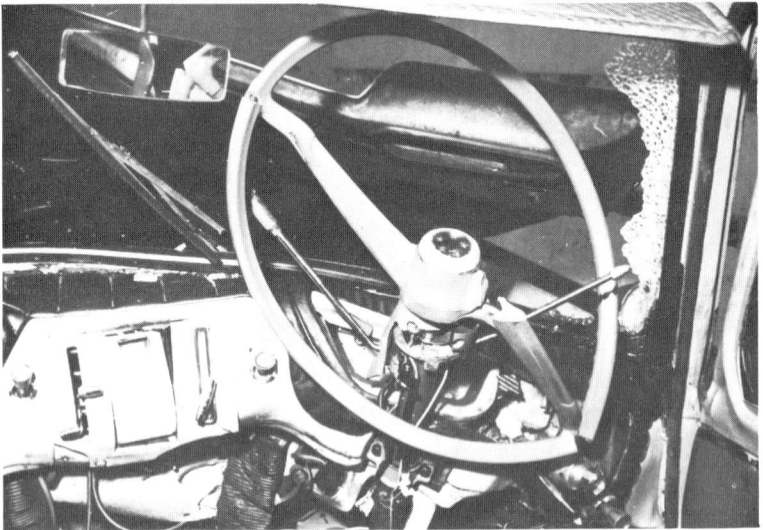

(b)

Fig. 4.6. The force of impact that caused the marks on the patient's throat (a) can be judged from the deformation of the steering wheel (b) which struck it. The surgical emphysema in the neck was more easily felt than seen at the stage illustrated. (Reproduced by kind permission of Mr H Proctor, FRCS (Edin).)

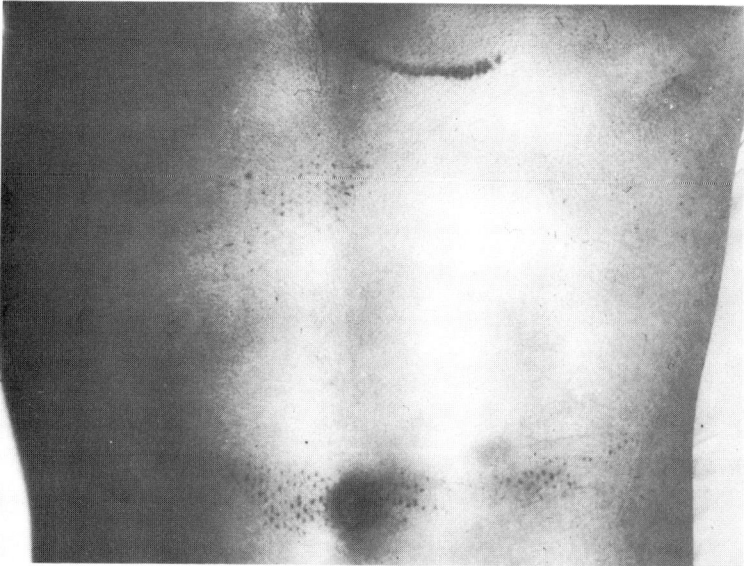

(a)

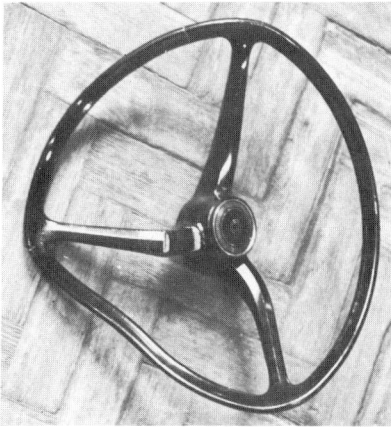

(b)

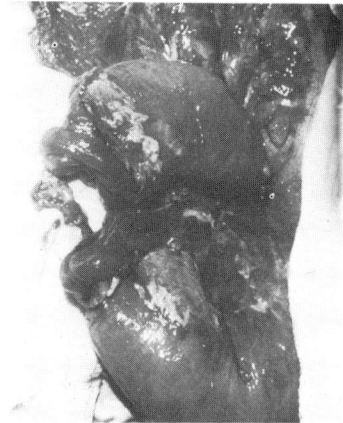

(c)

Fig. 4.7. The pattern of clothing (a) was imprinted on the abdominal wall by the impact of the steering wheel (b) with sufficient force for it to be indented by the lumbar spine and divide the jejunum (c). (Reproduced by kind permission of Mr H Proctor, FRCS (Edin).)

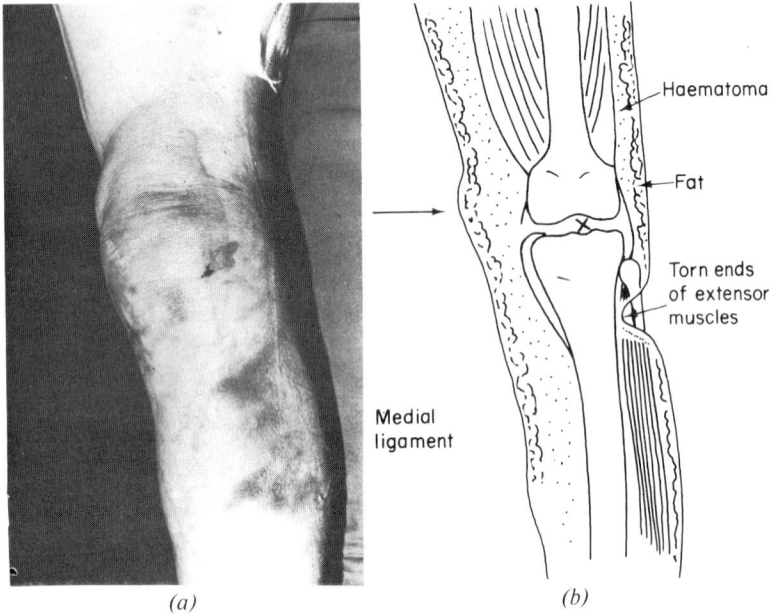

(a)   *(b)*

Fig. 4.8. The effects of violent impact on a limb. (a) Swelling. (b) The arrows show where pressure could press skin against bare bone. The right arrow shows how skin alone separated fingertip from tibia. The anterior tibial artery had suffered the fate of the extensor muscles.

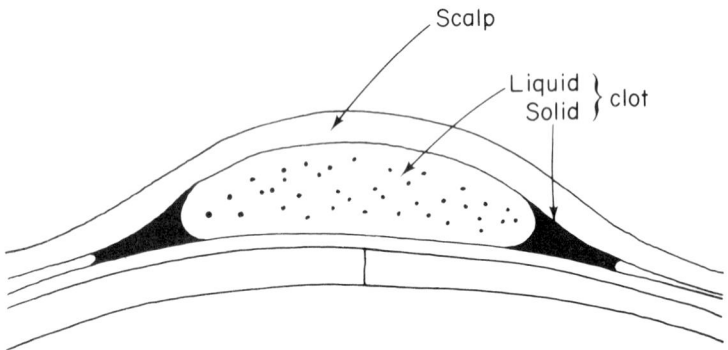

Fig. 4.9. Haematoma of the scalp has a soft centre but all layers of tissue are present.

disruption—a closed form of flaying—can cause so much tension that it kills skin which might otherwise have survived. A warning sign of this danger is the general occurrence of blistering on the summit of a large, tense swelling; it calls urgently for decompression.

Massive swelling. Without visible bruising, this is sometimes a result of surgical emphysema which may appear and spread rapidly from eyebrows to groins (Fig. 4.10).

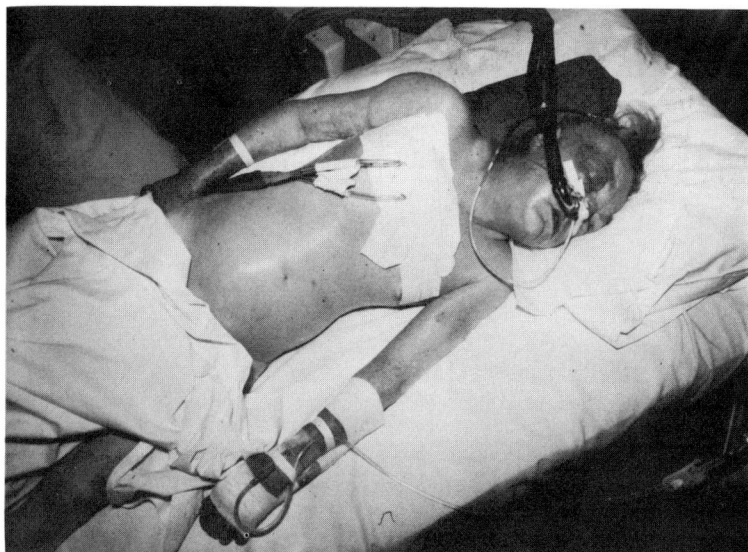

Fig. 4.10. Massive and widespread surgical emphysema. The two tubes emerging from the chest are both pleural drains; there is no need to drain the subcutaneous tissues. Without pleural drainage, artificial ventilation can give rise to fatal compressing pneumothorax, not necessarily with surgical emphysema.

Swelling and bleeding. It is not always possible to distinguish between swelling and deformity, which can coexist, but when a limb is swollen it is swollen by effusion of blood within it. If the swelling of injured limbs be matched by applying putty or felt to normal ones of similar size it is clear just how much swelling can be present but either ignored or misinterpreted. Obvious swelling of an adult's ankle amounts to about half a litre, but this amount of swelling may make no perceptible

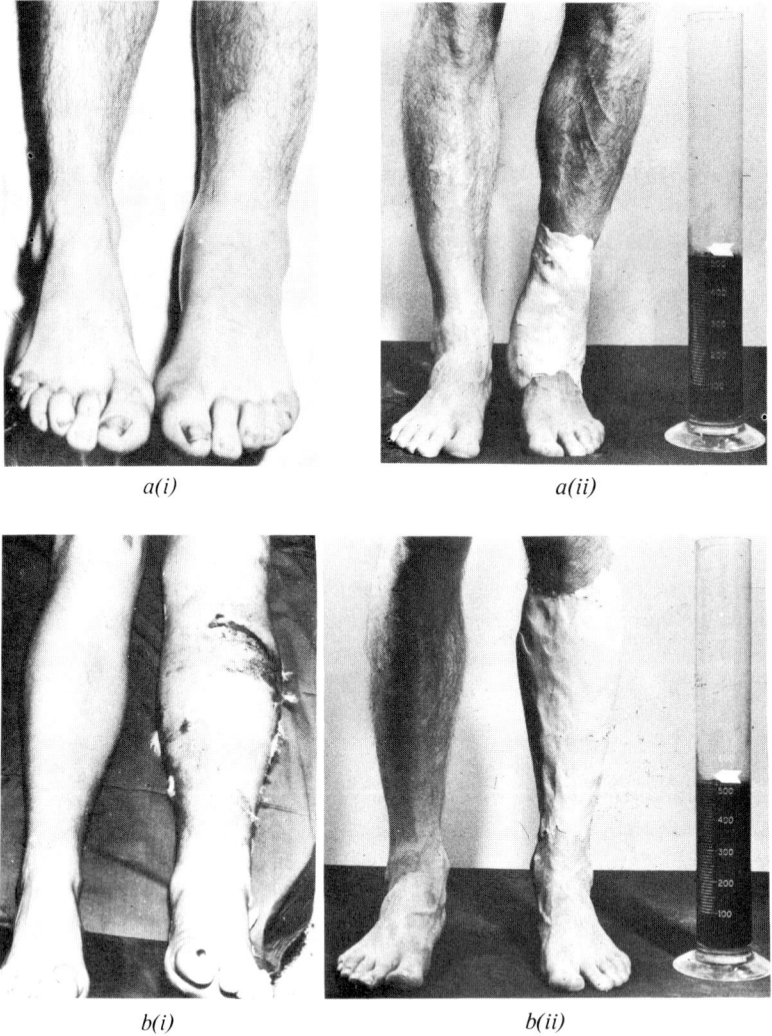

a(i)   a(ii)

b(i)   b(ii)

Fig. 4.11. a(i) The swelling of the left ankle is not remarkable; (ii) shows that
it can be approximately reproduced by applying half a litre of putty
to a normal ankle.
b(i) This amount of swelling obviously much exceeds the increase in
bulk caused by spreading half a litre of putty over the leg (b(ii)).
(Figs. a(ii) and b(ii) reproduced by kind permission of Camera
Talks Ltd, from the film strip How much blood?)

difference to the size of the calf (Fig. 4.11). Here, visible obvious swelling will be not less than about one litre, and in the thigh, twice that.

Although it may take an hour or more for swellings to become massive, it is as well to know the possible significance of those that do. Appreciation of the meaning of swelling may enable a risk of severe but hidden bleeding to be recognised in time for exsanguination to be forestalled.

Deformation. The discerning eye will be able to distinguish between swelling and other causes of deformation of a part. Among them are the stove-in chest with asymmetry of shape and movement, the characteristic shapes and postures of the dislocated hip, shoulder and elbow as well as the more obvious deformities of broken limbs and the more subtle deformities of broken feet (Fig. 4.12) or hands and wrists (Fig. 4.13).

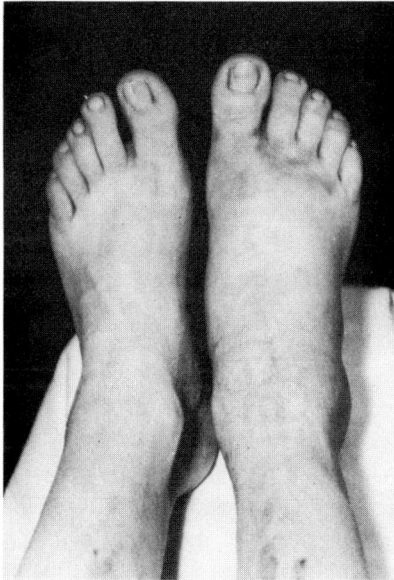

Fig. 4.12. The outward inclination of the right foot near its middle is the result of tarso-metatarsal fracture–subluxation and can easily be overlooked.

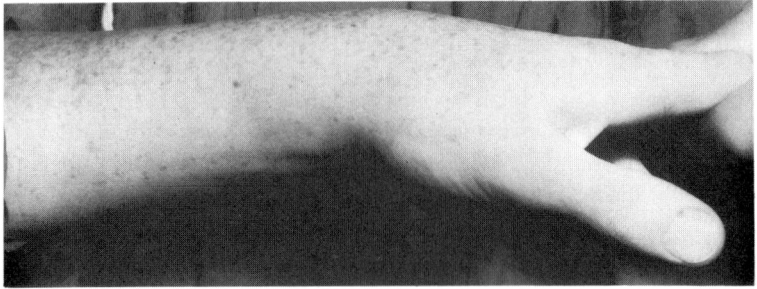

(a)

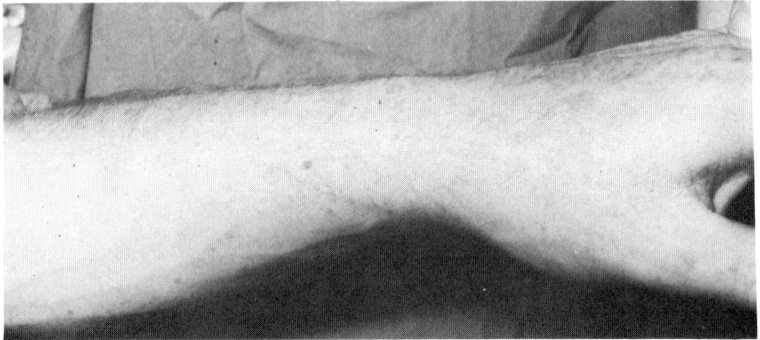

(b)

Fig. 4.13. The right wrist (a) was not much swollen when compared with the left (b) but it was the seat of fracture–dislocation.
Note: the photograph of the right wrist has been reversed to facilitate comparison.

Palpation

As well as the palpation that has already been mentioned in connection with bruises and spinal deformities, it will indicate the position of the trachea, the apex beat of the heart; it may give the first intimation of surgical emphysema and of the inequality of radial pulses that sometimes occurs after rupture of the aorta. Absence of peripheral pulses in a severely injured or chilled patient is of doubtful significance whereas their presence is always reassuring. Absent pulsation in major vessels should be regarded as a sign that the circulation needs to be assisted by compressing the heart.

Percussion and auscultation

These methods of physical examination are not likely to be practicable at the place of accident and may not give much useful information even in hospital.

The value and significance of the foregoing physical signs is not to be judged by the simplicity with which they can be observed in many cases. In the case of injuries of the chest in particular, knowledgeable interpretation of easily notable signs may give all the information necessary to carry out life-saving treatment on the spot and, indeed, can in the early stages be more accurately informative than X-ray appearances (Fig. 4.14).

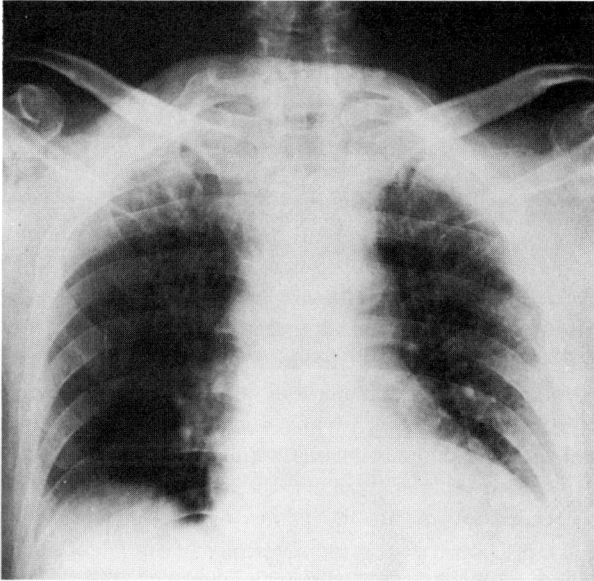

Fig. 4.14. None of the 12 fractures of the left ribs revealed at post mortem can be identified in this X-ray film.

The range of conditions covered by the word emergency is so broad that many sorts of injury need to be considered under this heading and their management needs to be considered from the viewpoints of the doctor on the spot, the doctor summoned urgently to the local cottage hospital and the doctor who has to teach first aiders and other rescuers. Much of the treatment that is practicable in an emergency can be carried out as well by trained assistants as by doctors, but the special contribution that a doctor can sometimes make depends upon his extra skill in recognising and interpreting physical signs and in the use of more elaborate methods of treatment. Both skills are improved by practice and the former can be taught to others to a useful extent.

A LOOK INTO THE THE FUTURE

In spite of the enormous advances in diagnosis and treatment that modern technology has made possible it is difficult to see any striking development that it could bring in the emergency care of injuries of the soft tissues. More widespread use of radio would reduce the delays that occur in taking suitable skill and equipment to the victims of accidents in remote places, but one cannot look for radical alterations in policy for the emergency services. There is a growing interest in and support for the use of doctors at the place of accidents, but even if there were enough doctors in Britain for them to attend all accidents it would waste a great deal of their time. **What can be sought is a national decision to make doctors available when they are likely to reach casualties before an ambulance can, to train and equip them for their tasks, and to insure them against the risks to their lives and limbs. There should also be a review of ambulance services to see to what extent, and in what parts of the country, there is a place for providing advanced training for selected ambulance-men.** Such training might include intubation of the trachea, endo-bronchial suction, venepuncture and the use of apparatus, and perhaps drugs, to record and assist the action of a defective heart. If these practices were to be added to the repertoire of ambulancemen it would be best achieved by service jointly in the intensive care and anaesthetic departments of hospitals and in the ambulance service itself. When necessary for the sake of maintaining the additional skills, the advanced ambulancemen would go back to work in hospital for a month or two.

Another desirable advance would be towards a far greater awareness than the public possess of their capabilities and responsibilities in providing first aid. This would require a determined and persistent campaign of instruction in schools and continuing education, by television in particular, with special incentives for motorists to carry a suitable first aid kit and to know how to use it.

More comfortable journeys in better designed ambulances would be particularly beneficial to those that had suffered extensive injuries and consequent bleeding but the widely held belief that aircraft, particularly helicopters, could usefully play a much larger part than they do in emergency transport gains little support from the facts.

5

Poisoning: (a) in Childhood

ALISON ELLIMAN

The problem of poisoning in childhood is an increasing one. In 1960, approximately 6610 children under 15 were admitted to hospital in England and Wales with poisoning, while this figure had risen to 20 620 in 1967. This rise is partly due to greater awareness by the public and the doctors, but there is almost certainly also a genuine increase in incidence.

The majority of cases of poisoning in childhood are accidental in nature..In toddlers, the most commonly affected age group, this is almost exclusively so, but where the victim is over five years old the possibility of suicidal intent or other disturbed behaviour should be borne in mind. It must also be remembered that poisoning may be a manifestation of child abuse.

Whenever a child presents with signs or symptoms which are not easily explained, the possibility of poisoning should be considered. Often the parents will know or suspect what has happened and will present the doctor with the poison. On the other hand, it may be very difficult to persuade them that the child could be poisoned and to get them to suggest possible causes. It is also possible that excessive therapeutic use, particularly of aspirin, may result in poisoning.

TYPES OF POISON

There are three main groups of ingested poison: drugs, chemicals and plant poisons. There are also poisonous gases. In our urban society, most child poisonings are from the first two groups, but even in the heart of North Kensington, poisoning with laburnum seeds is not unknown. Of the drugs, the commonest is aspirin, and in particular junior aspirins, which look and taste attractive—a toddler can see no reason why he should not eat all of these 'sweeties' when he finds them. Another common drug poison, possibly more dangerous, is iron; it is often present in the homes of toddlers, having been prescribed for the mother in pregnancy. Most parents are wholly unaware of the serious consequences of small overdoses of iron in their children. Again, the tablets are attractive to look at, and a toddler will take several unless he is interrupted.

The commonest chemical poisons are those wholly kept under the kitchen sink. These include bleach, washing-up liquid and furniture polish. Paraffin, often kept under the stairs, is the other common household poison. Weedkillers, and fertilisers, can be consumed in the garden shed, although after the full consequences of paraquat poisoning were appreciated the packaging and presentation of most garden poisons were improved, and if the manufacturer's instructions are followed there should now be little danger.

Another chemical which should not be forgotten is lead. Lead based paint is still available for outdoor use, but it is not infrequently used indoors, and lead is present in old car batteries, which may be found on dumps or abandoned in fields. Lead presents a different problem from most of the poisons discussed here, as the clinical picture is usually subacute, the therapy is more prolonged and epidemiological considerations are important. Poisoning with other heavy metals is occasionally encountered, but is rare.

Plant poisons should always be borne in mind, particularly with unexplained illness in a rural area. The commonest are toadstools, laburnum seeds, foxgloves and deadly nightshade. It is wise in rural practice to have an idea of the local flora and of the poisons growing in the hedgerows.

Poisoning with gases is not common in childhood, but children are often brought to casualty departments after being overcome by fumes from a paraffin heater or rescued from a smoke-filled room. Genuine poisoning is usually due to carbon monoxide, often from town gas in the past, but occasionally from car exhausts. As town gas has disappeared this problem, numerically small to start with, has decreased.

TREATMENT

The aim of treatment is to get rid of or neutralise the poison as

soon as possible. If this can be done efficiently, further treatment
is often unnecessary. Specific advice on the management of a case
of poisoning can be obtained from the nearest Poisons Information
Centre. These centres (listed below) are manned 24 hours a day,
and aim to provide information on all known poisons:

Government sponsored

London	01 407 7600
Edinburgh	031 229 2477
Cardiff	0222 33101
Belfast	1232 40503
Dublin	Dublin 45588

Others

Leeds	0532 32799
Manchester	061 740 2254
Newcastle	0632 25131

Acute poisoning by ingestion

Oral poisons are divided into two groups from the therapeutic point
of view: those where emesis is indicated, and those where it is not.
All drugs belong in the first group, while the second group consists
of caustic substances and hydrocarbons. As a working rule, emesis
should always be employed in the conscious child unless: the substance
taken is caustic, there are burns of the face, neck or mouth, or
the poison is a hydrocarbon (e.g. paraffin, petrol, kerosene).

Controversy continues over whether emetics or gastric lavage
produce the best results. However, most people agree that the
administration of emetics is preferable; this is easy to do, safe, and,
if done correctly, almost always effective. Gastric lavage requires special
equipment, is intensely unpleasant and is not without dangers.

Syrup of ipecac (United States Pharmacapia) is the emetic of choice.
This must be distinguished from ipecac **extract** which is very much
more concentrated and unsuitable for use in childhood. However, **syrup**
of ipecac can safely be administered to toddlers in a dose of 15 ml.
The dose should be followed immediately by 200 ml of water, as
this enhances the emetic action. If vomiting has not occurred in 20
minutes, the dose should be repeated. In 98 per cent of children

this regime will produce vomiting, with very efficient gastric emptying. If vomiting does not occur, gastric aspiration and lavage should be performed.

In the USA most households are equipped with 30 ml of syrup of ipecac, kept in the drug cupboard. Even if a toddler drinks the whole lot, no serious side effects will accrue, but its presence in the house means that poisoning can be treated very quickly, before medical assistance is available. In this country syrup of ipecac is seldom available in the house, **but it is certainly something which should be in every doctor's bag.**

If emesis is not indicated, copious quantities of fluid should be administered to dilute the poison. In the case of a known caustic substance, the antidote may be administered, e.g. dilute vinegar or other weak acid if caustic soda or other strong alkali has been ingested, or sodium bicarbonate if the poison is an acid. This treatment may be valuable in severe burning of the mouth, pharynx or oesophagus, but the most important thing is that fluid should be administered promptly. For this reason, water or milk are commonly used as they are usually immediately available. The protein in milk gives it some buffering action, and both these substances will wash the burnt areas and dilute the remaining poison. There is some evidence that hydrocortisone is beneficial in caustic burns of the oesophagus, and this should be administered as soon as possible in such cases. Admission to hospital is wise in all but the mildest cases, as perforation of the oesophagus is a real possibility. The late consequence of this type of poisoning is stricture of the oesophagus due to scarring, and this may require surgical correction.

Gaseous poisoning

Obviously the most important thing here is to remove the child from the poison. Usually, with a child, the easiest way of doing this is to pick him up and carry him out of the poisoned atmosphere. If this is impossible, for instance if the child is trapped or there are serious injuries, every effort should be made to bring fresh air to the child and discontinue the flow of poisonous gas. It should be remembered that there may be legal action following such an incident, and before the child is removed, careful note should be taken of his position, etc.

SPECIFIC POISONS

Drugs

As has already been stated, in all cases of drug poisoning, the stomach should be emptied. With aspirin it is never too late to do this, but with other drugs the procedure is pointless more than four hours after ingestion. In the following discussion it is assumed that syrup of ipecac has already been employed, and the stomach emptied, as first aid treatment.

Aspirin

Aspirin is not dangerous up to a dose of 100 mg/kg body weight. If the total dose is known with confidence to be less than this, no action need be taken, but above this dose the child should be carefully observed.

The effects of aspirin poisoning are, initially, stimulation of the respiratory centre causing overbreathing and respiratory alkalosis. This is followed by metabolic acidosis, which also produces overbreathing as a compensating mechanism. If a child is overbreathing following ingestion of aspirin, this should be taken as a sign of significant poisoning, and he should be admitted to hospital. The excretion of aspirin is significantly improved by forcing alkaline diuresis, and this should be undertaken in any child who has symptoms of mild or moderate poisoning. The serum salicylate level can easily be estimated, and the significance of the result interpreted by reference to Fig. 5.1. Hypoglycaemia may occur in salicylate poisoning, and a high sugar intake should be ensured to prevent this. If the poisoning is very severe, haemodialysis may be employed.

Iron

Iron is a very dangerous poison, as little as 300 mg elemental iron/kg body weight being sufficient to kill a child. This is equivalent to 900 mg ferrous sulphate/kg. The immediate effect, within one to two hours, is profound gastrointestinal upset with copious vomiting and diarrhoea, the fluid thus lost containing blood. This fluid loss may lead to shock at once, or there may be a latent period when the child appears well, followed at 24 to 48 hours by collapse. This stage is followed by convulsions, coma and death.

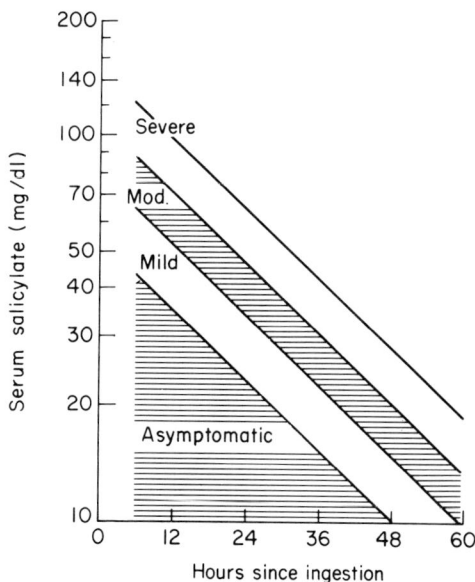

Fig. 5.1. Nomogram relating serum salicylate concentration and expected severity of intoxication at varying levels following ingestion of a single dose of salicylate.

It is important in iron poisoning to keep up with loss of fluid into the gut, and also to administer chelating agents. Plasma or blood may be needed to combat shock and blood loss. Desferrioxamine causes chelation of the iron, and should be administered orally (5 g) and intramuscularly (2 g) at once in all cases. If the child is symptomatic, intravenous treatment should be started.

Sedatives

Of the sedatives, nitrazepam is the safest. Deep sleep follows an overdose but death has not yet been reported. Whenever possible, therefore, nitrazepam should be prescribed for night sedation. At the other extreme is methaqualone (Mandrax), where a relatively small overdose can cause serious harm. The clinical features are unconsciousness with muscular hypertonia and convulsions. There may be papilloedema and pulmonary oedema. Treatment is supportive: forced diuresis and dialysis do not increase the rate of disappearance of the drug.

The commonest problems with overdose of sedative are with the barbiturates. Again, relatively small doses may cause problems, these being respiratory and circulatory depression, hypotension and hypothermia. Plasma barbiturate levels have to be interpreted in the knowledge of whether a barbiturate with a long, medium or short action has been taken, as the tissue-bound proportion varies. Forced alkaline diuresis increases the rate of elimination of long-acting barbiturates from the body, as do peritoneal and haemodialysis. With short- and medium-acting barbiturates these measures are of limited use and treatment is supportive. In severe poisoning it may be necessary to give artificial ventilation, and to sustain the blood pressure with meteraminol. Exchange transfusion has been employed in an attempt to hasten the elimination of barbiturates.

Atropine-like substances

This group includes all the atropine derivatives, e.g. Eumydrin (methylatropine), some of the drugs used in Parkinsonism, e.g. Artane (trihexyphenidyl), and some of the psychoactive drugs, e.g. orphenadrine. The effects are delirium, hot dry skin and mouth, hyperpyrexia, tachycardia and dilated pupils. In severe cases this progresses to convulsions and coma. Again, forced diuresis should be employed with dialysis if necessary. Neostigmine may help, but it is debatable whether it is of any value. Diazepam has been used to good effect in the control of the delirium and convulsions.

Phenothiazines

Overdose of phenothiazines gives rise to ataxia and extrapyramidal signs, and this should be suspected in a child who develops such signs unexpectedly. Again, treatment by forced diuresis is helpful.

Alcohol

Alcohol is a potentially serious poison in childhood, causing gastric irritation, hypoglycaemia and cerebral depression. It is fairly common following weddings, Christenings or other family celebrations, when several toddlers may go round draining all the half-empty glasses, and be found either staggering or unconscious at the end of the party. It may be very difficult to estimate how much has been consumed in this situation, and if the child is unconscious the blood alcohol level should be estimated without delay. Severe intoxication is present if this is 300 mg/100 ml or above. Intravenous glucose or sucrose should be used to maintain the blood sugar, and the rate of elimination is increased by forced diuresis and peritoneal dialysis.

Household products

There is a continuous supply of new products for use in the house or garden, and it is with these products that the poisons information centres play a very useful part in identifying poisons. If the trade name of the offending product is known, the poisons centre will supply a list of toxic contents, some idea of the harmful dose, and advice on treatment. A few of the commoner household poisons are:

Bleach

This is a very common cause of poisoning. The child may be burnt on the face or chest, or in the mouth, in a severe case. Treatment is directed at diluting the poison with copious fluids. Ipecac and gastric lavage are contraindicated.

Disinfectants

These also may cause local burning, and again no attempt should be made to empty the stomach. Water or milk should be given, and if there is evidence of burning, the child should be observed in hospital.

Petroleum products

As a rule the hazard with these products is aspiration pneumonia. For this reason every effort should be made to prevent the child from vomiting, as this increases the risks considerably. Following the ingestion of paraffin most children will develop a cough and mild X-ray changes, although fortunately more serious aspiration problems are rare. The systemic toxicity of these products must also be borne in mind, although luckily it is rare to encounter it. Severe poisoning may lead to a state resembling alcoholic intoxication, and this may proceed to coma and cardiovascular and respiratory collapse.

Turpentine substitute falls into this category, being a distillate of petroleum.

Benzene derivatives

This group includes naphthalene (found in mothballs) and turpentine. The effects include gastrointestinal upset, haemolysis, renal failure, liver necrosis and central nervous system depression. Although aspiration is dangerous, the systemic effects of these poisons are severe enough to outweigh its danger. Gastric lavage is probably preferable to the induction emesis, as the risks of inhalation are reduced. In the unconscious patient a cuffed endotracheal tube should be inserted before lavage is undertaken. In severe intoxication exchange transfusion should be considered.

Paraquat®

This weedkiller is an extremely dangerous poison. It causes early problems, due to caustic effects on the upper gastrointestinal tract. Late problems include hepatic and renal damage, but death is usually after 6–10 days, and is due to a proliferative alveolitis leading to respiratory failure. In one case where this was treated by lung transplant, the graft also developed proliferative alveolitis. Treatment is a matter of urgency, and should be by forced diuresis initially, followed by haemodialysis. In spite of rapid treatment death may follow.

Paraquat is contained in the industrial weedkiller Gramoxone®, and one mouthful of this may be fatal. There is also some in the garden products Weedol® and Pathclear®, but if these are properly prepared it is probable that a large volume would have to be taken to be toxic.

Lead poisoning

There is usually a subacute or chronic history of ill health, irritability, pica (habitually eating paint, paper, clothes, soil, etc.) and symptoms of anaemia in a child with lead poisoning. The late case may present with coma, convulsions or other symptoms of encephalitis. The diagnosis should be suspected in a child with glycosuria, particularly if he is also anaemic; blood film shows basophilic stippling in the red blood cells. The definitive test is the blood lead, and the paediatric upper limit of normal usually accepted as 36 mg/dl. If the level is over 80 mg/dl treatment should be undertaken urgently, as encephalitis may occur. As a first stage in treatment the child should be removed to a lead-free environment and the bowel should be emptied using enemas and laxatives. If chelating agents are administered parenterally before this is done, further absorption of lead from the gut may occur.

Chelating agents commonly used are penicillamine (orally) and dimercaprol or calcium edetate systemically. The lead is chelated by them and excreted through the kidneys. The blood lead may not fall rapidly, or may fall and rise again; this is due to the resorption of lead from the bones, which continues for a considerable time. Because of this the chelating agents should be given for six weeks to two months, and the blood lead should be monitored after treatment is discontinued. For long term therapy, oral penicillamine is the drug of choice.

It should be remembered that chelating agents also bind iron, and that the compound formed by dimercaprol and iron is toxic. Iron should therefore not be administered during this phase of treatment, in spite of the anaemia which may be profound. If necessary this will need to be corrected by transfusion. Oral iron and oral penicillamine will also neutralise each other before exerting a therapeutic effect. It is therefore a good general rule not to give iron while a child is being actively treated for lead poisoning.

If a case of lead poisoning occurs a careful search should be made for the source. The District Community Physician should be notified, and samples of paint, etc. analysed. Other children in the house should be checked as they may also be affected, and such places as the play-school, or the baby-minder's house should be remembered as possible sources. When sampling suspected areas, care must be taken that all layers of paint are examined, as successive generations of painters may simply have applied non-toxic paint over lead-based paint. It should also be remembered that there are other sources of lead, for example old car batteries.

Plant poisons

The treatment of poisoning by plants is the treatment of the individual poisons involved. For instance with laburnum seeds and deadly nightshade berries treatment is as for atropine poisoning. Digitalis is contained in the leaves of the foxglove, and is also found in several other plants.

In the toadstool family, *Amanita muscaria* gives rise to muscarine poisoning, characterised by gastrointestinal disturbance, sweating, salivation, meiosis, delirium, convulsions and coma. Treatment should include subcutaneous atropine. *Amanita phalloides* (the Death Cap toadstool) is an extremely toxic fungus, containing poisons as yet incompletely identified; 60–100 per cent of human consumers die. The onset of symptoms is usually 6–15 hours after ingestion and at first these are limited to the gastrointestinal tract, with pain, vomiting and mucous and bloody diarrhoea. This is followed by degenerative changes in the liver and severe jaundice. There are also toxic effects on kidney and heart, and death is usually from cardiac failure about a week after the ingestion. Treatment should initially be directed towards emptying the gut, and thereafter dehydration and shock must be promptly treated. The degree of toxic change may be lessened by intravenous glucose, plasma or blood.

Carbon monoxide poisoning

Carbon monoxide is toxic because of its high affinity for the oxygen-binding sites on the haemoglobin molecule. This results in the formation of carboxyhaemoglobin, which is much more stable than oxyhaemoglobin. Thus the tissues become deprived of oxygen and the patient dies of asphyxia. He does not become cyanosed, as the carboxyhaemoglobin molecule does not produce cyanosis, and blood containing this compound has a bright red colour similar to arterial blood. Treatment consists of administration of oxygen in as high a concentration as possible, and this is a situation where hyperbaric oxygen has an important role if it is available. The higher the partial pressure of oxygen reaching the lungs, the greater will be the chance of driving off the carbon monoxide.

WHY CHILDREN BECOME POISONED

It is difficult to define the reasons why some children become poisoned.

Obviously there is an element of carelessness in childhood poisoning, as it is much less likely to occur if poisons are inaccessible. Nevertheless it remains true that certain children are more likely to become poisoned than others in the same environment. A retrospective study of a small group of poisoned children and matched controls was, however, unable to define any difference between the two groups (Baltimore and Meyer, 1969). The parents in both groups felt that the most important preventive measure was the method of storage of drugs and other potential poisons, but there was no significant difference in methods of storage between the two groups. Personality studies on the two groups of children showed no significant difference between them, except for a slightly increased incidence of daredevil behaviour in the poisoned group. There was no significant difference in the number of accidents requiring medical attention between poisoned children and the control group. This is perhaps surprising, as one might have expected accidental poisoning to have been one manifestation of accident-proneness. However, it was felt that a study of a larger group of children might reveal a significantly greater number of accidents in the poisoned group. It may be that in the future accidental poisoning will be seen as one manifestation of disturbed behaviour in childhood. This would certainly help explain why repeated poisoning is so common, and why it may be limited to one child in a family.

One definite behavioural difference between the poisoned and non-poisoned children was reflected in the incidence of pica, or exaggerated oral tendencies, manifested in eating paint, clothes, paper, soil, etc. About half the poisoned children exhibited pica, while only a quarter of the control children habitually ate inappropriate things. Pica may be a primary behaviour problem, or may reflect an underlying iron-deficiency anaemia. If the latter is true the pica may resolve when the anaemia is treated. Pica and anaemia are usually both present in lead poisoning. In these cases it may be very difficult to decide whether the pica antedated the poisoning, and thus was a contributory factor, or followed the poisoning and was a manifestation of it.

PREVENTION

It will be appreciated that the problem of prevention is complex. A great deal can be done by encouraging better storage habits in parents, perhaps to the extent of providing free locking medicine cabinets to all homes, and by pleading with manufacturers for better packaging. A toddler-proof container is probably a near impossibility, and greater emphasis should perhaps be laid on packaging products in non-toxic quantities. This is particularly relevant in the case of iron and aspirin. Some of the more toxic gardening products are supplied in sublethal quantities, but as yet this is not a commonplace occurrence.

It is very helpful to parents to have paediatric medicines dispensed in a palatable form, and great emphasis is placed on this by the drug companies nowadays. However, it must be borne in mind that any child will drink a bottle of raspberry syrup or eat all the little orange sweets in the bottle, without appreciating the danger. It is therefore extremely important to exercise care in the storage of these medicines. The chief offender is junior aspirin, a product which is quite unnecessary. Aspirin need never be used in a dose of less than 75 mg and this dose can be obtained by crushing a quarter of an adult soluble aspirin tablet, and dissolving it. The abolition of junior aspirin preparations might well reduce the incidence and severity of aspirin poisoning in children.

If a child exhibits pica, the possible existence of iron deficiency anaemia or lead poisoning must be explored. When these have been excluded, this child and the child who suffers repeated episodes of poisoning should be regarded as exhibiting disturbed behaviour. They are probably seeking attention and should be managed accordingly. It may be necessary to invoke the help of a child psychiatrist.

All in all, prevention of poisoning in children is not easy. Psychological studies may produce a clearer understanding of the aetiology and therefore of preventive or therapeutic avenues to explore. In the meantime we must fall back on obsessional attention to the education of parents, packaging, and storage methods if we are to reduce the seriousness of this problem.

REFERENCE

Baltimore, Jr. and Meyer (1969), A Study of Storage, Child Behavioural Traits and Mother's Knowledge of Toxicology in 52 Poisoned Families and 52 Controls, *Pediatrics*, **44**, 816.

FURTHER READING

Barltrop (1968), Lead Poisoning in Childhood, *Postgrad. med. J.*, **44**, 537.

Matthew (1971), Acute Poisoning—Some Myths and Misconceptions, *Brit. med. J.*, **1**, 519.

Poisoning and Drug-Induced Disease (1970), *Medicine*, **4**.

Poisoning in Childhood (1970), *Pediatric Clinics of North America*, **17**, 1970.

Reid (1970), Treatment of the Poisoned Child, *Arch. Dis. Childh.*, **45**, 428.

Poisoning: (b) Self-Poisoning

(Reprinted from *Medicine*)

MANAGEMENT
(HENRY MATTHEW)

Taking an overdose of a drug is now so common that it fully warrants the description of the modern epidemic. In Britain at least 15 per cent of acute adult medical admissions to hospital have taken an overdose. This must be a conservative figure for there is evidence, at least in Edinburgh, that GPs treat 30 per cent of their patients who have taken an overdose at home. Figure 5.2 shows the steady rise in admissions to the Edinburgh Royal Infirmary's unit for the treatment of acute poisoning in adults. Acute poisoning in children is also increasing, though the toddler is more likely to swallow household items such as bleach rather than medicine.

Classification

Suicide

In Britain the main drugs taken with the clear motive of self-destruction are barbiturates. Carbon monoxide poisoning, still popular as a method of suicide, is likely to decline further with the more widespread domestic use of natural gas. However, most suicides take steps to avoid being found alive.

Accidental poisoning

Since the myth of barbiturate automatism has been exploded, it is unacceptable to certify an adult as dying from accidental barbiturate or other drug poisoning. Accidental drug poisoning is still common

152

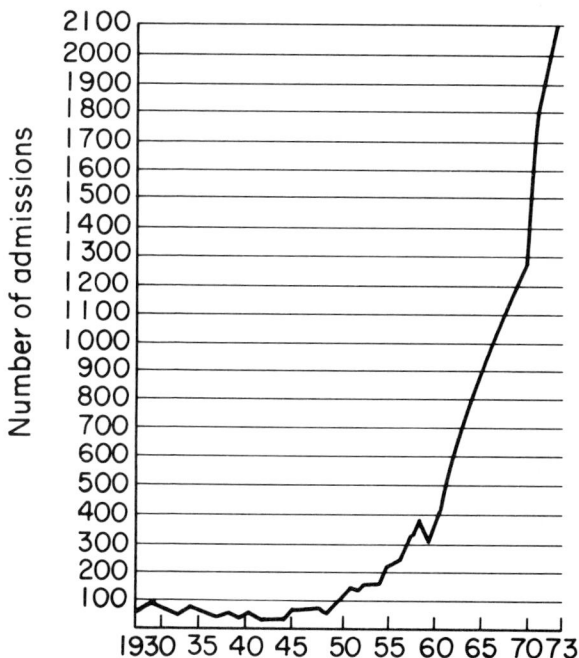

Fig. 5.2. Yearly admission of poisoned patients to the Royal Infirmary, Edinburgh (1928–1973).

in toddlers, who most often swallow aspirin, iron or the contraceptive pill. In recent years teenagers in Britain have been increasingly experimenting with drugs and also with various glues, solvents and aerosols, and being unaware of the potency of the agents concerned, or of their own intolerance to them, may suffer the effects of overdosage.

Manipulative self-poisoning

Most patients who take an overdose are not attempting suicide, they are indulging in an impulsive, manipulative act undertaken to escape from an intolerable situation. Thoughts of self-destruction do not occupy a large or often, indeed, even a small part of their minds at the time of taking the overdose.

Self-poisoning is not limited to any one social class but is most common in social classes IV and V. It is definitely associated with poverty, unemployment, alcoholism, a broken marriage or divorce, and above all with a broken home in childhood. It is more common in urban than in rural practice. In a marriage it may often be the spouse and not the victim of the overdose who requires the greater help.

Some children, because they have taken tablets, are identified as being accident-prone. They are not in fact accident-prone so much as indulging in manipulative self-poisoning. This must be understood if they are to be correctly treated.

Drugs involved

Not surprisingly, fashions in prescribing are reflected in the different drugs taken in conscious impulsive acts. This change is illustrated in Fig. 5.3, which can only reflect prescribing habits in and around Edinburgh; however similar trends are evident elsewhere. Paradoxically it is in some ways a favourable trend. Although one can only deplore the increasing numbers taking overdoses to exhibit their distress, if an overdose must be taken it is clearly better that it be a benzodiazepine, such as chlordiazepoxide (Librium®, Tropium®), diazepam (Atensine®, Valium®), lorazepam (Ativan®), or nitrazepam (Mogadon®), since even 100 tablets or more are unlikely to produce severe effects. For example, there is no authenticated death from a nitrazepam overdose.

Mixtures

Figure 5.3 refers to the chief drug which patients claim to have ingested, but they tend increasingly to take more than one drug at a time. This occurs in about 30 per cent of episodes and alcohol is drunk at the same time in a further 30 per cent. Any such mixture inevitably produces a confused clinical picture.

Patients' statements

These are likely to be nearly 50 per cent wrong about the type of tablets taken, despite the name of the drug now being on the bottle. Patients will exaggerate the number of tablets if they feel the doctor is insufficiently impressed by their plight or they will play it down

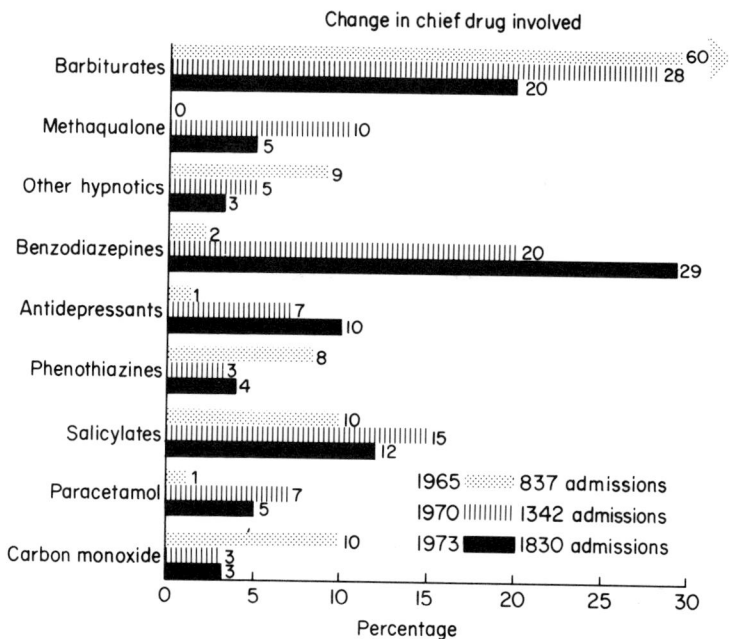

Fig. 5.3. *Admissions for self-poisoning to the Royal Infirmary, Edinburgh (1965, 1970, 1973).*

if they feel guilty. Many patients simply measure the quantity in handsful.

Diagnosis

Since overdosage is so common there should be no difficulty in diagnosis. If a person between 15 and 55 is drowsy or unconscious and there is no evidence of head injury, then he has taken an overdose until proved otherwise; similarly with children when there is some unusual presentation with excitability, drowsiness, convulsions or vomiting.

With adults the diagnosis of acute poisoning is best arrived at by the history and the circumstantial evidence. It should not be necessary to resort to skull radiographs, echoencephalography and lumbar punctures in more than about 1 per cent of unconscious poisoned patients. Few drugs in overdose produce specific diagnostic features; those which do are listed below.

Skin blisters. In unconscious patients, often on an area of erythema and contiguous skin surfaces where pressure has been applied, these strongly suggest an overdose. This is most often seen in barbiturate poisoning, but is also recorded in overdosage with methaqualone (4 proprietary brands), meprobamate (4 proprietary brands), glutethimide (Doriden ®), opiates and tricyclic antidepressants.

Venepuncture marks. In young people who may have been taking intravenous drugs (mainlining), one should inspect the veins on the backs of the hands, the cubital fossae, forearms and inner aspects of the calves for puncture marks. The rectal, vaginal and sublingual plexus of veins may also be injection sites.

Identification

Only rarely is there a specific antidote available to counteract the effects of the poison taken. This means that one should not spend valuable time, either in the home or immediately after admission to hospital, trying to find out the drugs involved. Nevertheless one should attempt, when the time is opportune, to identify the drug taken. This can often be done from the shape and markings of the tablets or capsules. If the identity of the suspect drug is not clear it should be sent to the hospital with the patient.

Laboratory investigation. Qualitative identification of the drug in gastric aspirate, blood or urine will confirm the diagnosis and the drug involved. However, doctors tend to seek laboratory support too often: there are few methods which will provide the answer accurately and rapidly, so that laboratory reports seldom influence the management to any great extent. Furthermore, laboratory data must always be related to a specific patient; the outstanding example of the misleading interpretation of laboratory data is seen in epileptics, who because of their high tissue tolerance and ability to metabolise phenobarbitone (Gardenal®, Luminal®) rapidly, may well be conscious at a barbiturate blood level which might be lethal to anyone unaccustomed to barbiturates.

If laboratory help is needed for severely poisoned patients and is in short supply, the most helpful tests are blood gas analysis and electrolyte estimations. Laboratory help may also be needed for medico-legal reasons.

Poisoned patients who have been unconscious for more than 30 hours have increased levels of certain enzymes, especially serum creatine kinase, which are consistent with skeletal muscle injury. It is important not to ascribe the elevated enzyme levels to heart or liver damage. Prolonged coma is also associated with an increase in fibrin degradation products and in other indices of coagulation and fibrinolysis.

Hospital or not?

Children. A family doctor may be uncertain whether to send a poisoned child to hospital. Some countries have Poisons Information Centres which will provide information about toxicity and the likely clinical features, as well as a guide to treatment.

Adults. For adults who have taken an overdose my advice would be that of the Hill Report (1968): 'all cases of deliberate self-poisoning should be referred to a designated poisoning treatment centre'. The report goes on to state that 'all cases of deliberate self-poisoning should receive psychiatric evaluation and social help'.

Psychiatric help. With poisoning patterns changing to drugs which merely render patients drowsy instead of producing serious physical changes there is a danger that doctors may feel it is not necessary to send such patients to hospital. These patients are then treated at home, perhaps with little or no attempt made to find out the underlying psychiatric or social distress which drove them to take an overdose. It is important to remember that the type of drug and the size of overdose bear no relation to the severity of the underlying psychiatric and /or social upset.

Treatment

Antidotes are available for less than 2 per cent of drug poisonings. Therefore the aim is to manage the effects of the poison, and intensive supportive therapy is vital. One must rapidly assess the severity of the poisoning according to four criteria: grade of coma, respiratory failure, shock and hypothermia.

The grade of coma. This is readily assessed by testing the patient's response to painful stimuli. Four grades are acceptable:

(1) Drowsy but responding to vocal command.
(2) Unconscious but responding to minimal stimuli.
(3) Unconscious and responding only to maximal painful stimuli.
(4) Unconscious and no response whatsoever.

Little valuable information is to be gained from assessing pupil size or their reaction to light, or testing limb reflexes.

Respiratory failure. This is the most common immediate cause of death from overdose, and all those concerned with the management of a poisoned patient must ensure that he has a clear airway and good ventilation, by removing debris from the throat, positioning the patient on his side, inserting an oro-pharyngeal airway and, if necessary, starting artificial ventilation.

The Wright's spirometer can provide a useful measure of respiratory function. A minute volume of over 4 litres in the absence of marked tachypnoea indicates adequate respiration; one below 4 litres suggests significant respiratory depression and a need for blood gas analysis. Oxygen therapy with a Ventimask, hand ventilation or a mechanical respirator may be required.

The drugs used to stimulate drug-induced respiratory depression have been disappointing. However, I have found doxapram hydrochloride (Dopram®) useful in some cases, but the response is very short-lived. Tracheostomy is seldom needed. There is debate as to how long cuffed endotracheal intubation can be continued, but the increasing use of Portex® tubes has lengthened the time, and 72 hours and longer is now acceptable.

Shock. What really matters is tissue perfusion, especially of the brain, heart, lungs, liver and kidneys; however, tissue perfusion is difficult to measure and the blood pressure in the arm is a reasonable guide.

If the systolic pressure falls below 80 mm Hg then steps should be taken to improve the circulation. This is easily done by raising the foot of the stretcher or of the bed, failing which 5 mg metaraminol (Aramine®) should be given iv: the dose can be repeated twice at 20-minute intervals. If these injections are of no avail, low molecular weight dextran or plasma should be given, preferably with monitoring of the central venous pressure.

The best way of reversing shock is to improve the oxygenation and so correct the acid-base state. If acidaemia is contributing to shock and this is confirmed by blood gas anaysis an infusion of bicarbonate is required.

Hypothermia. Significant when the rectal temperature is below 35°C. Avoid reheating with shock cages and warm blankets. Wrapping in a foil space blanket is usually effective, but in severe hypothermia heating the inspired air is helpful.

Preventing further absorption

After attending to patients' ventilation, shock and hypothermia, one must try to evacuate the stomach, whatever the drug taken. If a patient is conscious then with his head dependent, or with a child in the spanking position, irritate the pharynx with the fingers or, better still, the handle of a spoon. If this does not induce vomiting it should be tried again after the patient has swallowed some warm water.

Emetic drugs. Syrup of ipecacuanha has its advocates and I would support its use in a dose of 15 ml, even in a toddler who is conscious, provided its limitations are understood. It requires, on average, 18 minutes to take effect, also one can never be sure that most of the poison has been eliminated, so if the drug ingested is especially dangerous further measures are indicated.

Sodium chloride is often used as an emetic in treating conscious poisoned patients. A dose of 50 g salt in 200 ml water is employed but the effect is unpredictable and may precipitate hypernatraemia, hyperpyrexia and pulmonary oedema.

Gastric aspiration and lavage. I would not advocate these measures outside hospital. If an adult has swallowed less than 10 tablets or capsules they are unnecessary. They should be undertaken if the drug was taken within the previous 4 hours, the exceptions being salicylate when it is never too late, and tricyclic antidepressants, when the period is 12 hours.

The danger of aspiration and lavage—the fact that patients inhale material from the stomach into their lungs—is often exaggerated. In fact, the conscious patient's protective cough reflex prevents this, and in the unconscious patient one forestalls the possibility by inserting a cuffed endotracheal tube. In the severely ill patient with a cuffed endotracheal tube in place the time of ingestion may not be known, but nothing is lost and much may be gained by aspiration and lavage.

Technique. The correct size of tube must be used; I recommend a 30 English gauge Jacques tube. As a rule no special lavage fluid is needed apart from warm water, except in babies when saline should be used. After the procedure all lavage fluid should be removed, although 10 g desferrioxamine in iron poisoning, and 50 ml castor oil in glutethimide poisoning, should be left in the stomach. In acute salicylate poisoning there is good evidence that activated charcoal given within 30 minutes of the aspirin effectively reduces the severity of poisoning.

Fluid and electrolyte balance. There need be no great urgency in setting up a drip infusion but for the severely poisoned patient it is helpful to have an infusion going in case of cardiac arrest. An infusion of 1500 ml/24 hours in the form of a rotation of 1000 ml 5 per cent dextrose and 500 ml normal saline is usually adequate to maintain hydration. In severely poisoned patients one must also attend to electrolyte imbalance and acidaemia.

In my experience the chances of recovery from a severe overdose are greatly dependent on the standard of nursing. Bladder catherisation is done too frequently. It carries risks of infection and good nurses can secure bladder emptying by fundal pressure. Catheterisation is, however, mandatory in certain situations (see below).

A raised temperature. This frequently occurs during recovery of consciousness, the rise often being proportionate to the degree of initial hypothermia and/or the duration of unconsciousness. This rise in temperature should not be regarded as an indication of infection and prophylactic antibiotics should not be given. It is probably caused by generalised tissue injury, particularly of skeletal muscle.

Attempts at enhancing elimination

Because of their training to be activists in therapy, too many doctors rush into methods which purport to increase elimination of a drug and so shorten the period of unconsciousness. These include forced diuresis, peritoneal and renal dialysis, exchange transfusion and passage of blood over charcoal or ion exchange resins, and are appropriate only for a few drugs:

(1) Barbitone (Hypnogen ®), which is now very seldom prescribed.
(2) Phenobarbitone which is to some extent excreted by the kidney; dialysis is of value in severe poisoning.
(3) Salicylate, which responds to forced diuresis.
(4) Amphetamines, which respond to forced acid diuresis, although it is very difficult to achieve acidification of the urine owing to the respiratory stimulant effect of these drugs and the consequent respiratory alkalosis.
(5) Ethchlorvynol (Arvynol ®, Serenesil ®) which, despite its high lipid solubility, is dialysable.
(6) Carbamates such as meprobamate—severe overdosage can be treated by forced diuresis.
(7) Lithium salts (Camcolit ®, Lithium Phasal ®, Priadel ®), which are eliminated by the kidney and can be dialysed.

Intensive supportive therapy is thus clearly the only rational treatment in the vast majority of patients suffering from drug poisoning.

Specific features of overdosage

I have already described the main features and management of poisoning with the majority of hypnotic drugs. The drugs listed below have features in overdose which help in diagnosing the particular drug involved and may be important for deciding the treatment needed in addition to intensive supportive therapy.

Methaqualone. Even with severely depressed consciousness there may be hypertonia with increased limb reflexes, myoclonia and convulsions. The plantar responses are often extensor and there may be papilloedema. There may also be acute pulmonary oedema although respiratory depression is rare.

Glutethimide. Papilloedema may occur with this drug, associated with sudden episodes of apnoea, the pupils being dilated and unresponsive to light. It is important to keep watch on the optic discs; on the slightest suggestion of papilloedema infuse 500 ml 20 per cent mannitol iv over 20 minutes followed by 500 ml 5 per cent dextrose over the next 4 hours.

Chloral hydrate (Noctec ®). Patients may report a burning retrosternal pain and vomiting, both very uncommon in the usual drug overdosages.

Ethchlorvynol. This drug can usually be diagnosed from the characteristic smell of the gastric aspirate. The effects of overdose are often prolonged, severe respiratory depression being common.

Phenothiazines. In phenothiazine poisoning the unconscious patient may have signs of Parkinsonism, dyskinesia (especially torticollis) and convulsions. Hypotension, cardiac dysrhythmias and hypothermia are common. The dyskinesia and convulsions respond to benztropine (Cogentin ®) 2 mg iv and the dysrhythmias to conventional measures, provided hypothermia has been corrected.

Carbamates. The carbamates are rapidly absorbed and, more importantly, rapidly metabolised. However, they may produce profound effects with marked hypothermia and hypotension, and since a reasonable amount of active drug is excreted in the urine, forced osmotic diuresis is indicated in severely poisoned patients.

Tricyclic antidepressants. The important features, apart from depressed consciousness and respiration, are hyperreflexia leading to convulsions, hypotension and cardiac dysrhythmias. Other features are dry mouth, dilated pupils, lack of bowel sounds and urinary retention. Hallucinations may be prominent on recovering consciousness.

It is important to realise that the toxic effects wear off in about 18–24 hours, so if resuscitative measures are required they must not be abandoned too soon. Avoid the pitfall of applying the usual grave prognosis to unconscious patients with fixed dilated pupils.

Physostigmine salicylate iv will temporarily restore consciousness and reverse many of the other features, but the life-threatening cardiac dysrhythmias do not respond to this antidote, which should only be

used on the very rare occasions when the dangers of continuing unconsciousness outweigh those of the powerful antidote.

Monoamine oxidase inhibitors. The effects of overdosage resemble
those of the more common reaction to tyramine-containing foods
such as cheese, and include agitation, hallucinations, tachycardia,
hyperreflexia, convulsions, sweating and hyperthermia. There may
be hypo- or hypertension. Management is the same as for the cheese
reaction.

Opiates. These are one of the rare situations for which an antidote
is available. The depressed consciousness and breathing as well as
the pinpoint pupils respond as if miraculously to intravenous nalorphine
(Lethidrone®), which should be given even when an opiate is merely
suspected. Nalorphine itself, without an opiate to counteract, will
depress respiration further but this is easily dealt with in hospital.
The newer antidote, naloxone (Narcan®), has the important advantages
of having no central respiratory depressant effect, and of antagonising
synthetic opiate derivatives such as pethidine (Pamergan®) and
pentazocine (Fortral®). The initial dose of nalorphine is 15 mg iv and
it is important to continue the injections for some hours because
of the frequency of relapse. When dealing with opiate addicts remember
that the antidote may provoke an acute withdrawal reaction.

Salicylate. Fortunately people remain conscious after swallowing an
overdose of salicylate and usually vomit, thereby lessening the severity
of the restlessness, roaring in the ears, deafness, hyperventilation, perspiration and pyrexia which soon follow. Associated with these features
is a raised serum salicylate level, a lowered serum potassium and
initially a respiratory alkalosis. A metabolic acidosis supervenes after
about 12 hours, but sooner in children and at lower serum salicylate
levels.

Management. In salicylate poisoning it is never too late to start gastric
aspiration and lavage. A serum salicylate level over 50 mg per cent
within 12 hours of ingestion in an adult, or over 30 mg per cent
in a child, warrants forced alkaline diuresis. This cocktail infusion
is effective and requires no laboratory monitoring:
    Saline 0·9%—0·5 litre
    Dextrose 5%—1 litre

Sodium bicarbonate 1·26%——0·5 litre

Potassium chloride——3 g

This mixture is given at a rate of 2 litres/hour for 3 hours and thereafter 1 litre/hour until the serum salicylate level is less than 35 mg per cent. In children the infusion rate should be 30 ml/kg/hour and the serum potassium measured frequently.

In severe salicylate poisoning, if an adult is drowsy and has not taken a second drug, correction of the underlying acidaemia is urgently needed.

Paracetamol. In contrast to salicylate, this drug can produce profound effects with as few as 20 tablets or 10 g. Fortunately vomiting often occurs shortly after ingestion but even this may not prevent hepatic, renal and cardiac damage. Diagnosis is usually simple since the patients remain conscious. Plotting the plasma paracetamol level against the time since ingestion will determine whether treatment is indicated, with penicillamine or dimercaprol if cysteamine is not available.

Digitalis. In general the effects of digitalis poisoning depend on the state of the patient's heart. In a child or healthy adult digitalis chiefly affects the conducting mechanism causing a bradycardia with a prolonged P–R interval and dropped beats leading to asystole. In an already damaged heart ventricular ectopic beats, coupled rhythm and ventricular tachycardia are more common. Maintaining a normal potassium level is all-important. Bradycardia is treated with atropine sulphate, 0·6 mg intramuscularly repeated as necessary, ventricular dysrhythmias being managed conventionally. Poisoning of any severity requires insertion of a cardiac pacemaker if only as a prophylactic measure. Toxic effects are generally over in 48 hours if renal function is adequate.

Iron. The initial feature is a haemorrhagic gastroenteritis which if severe may lead to shock. After an interval, usually hours, patients may pass frequent black offensive stools and suffer severe headaches, confusion, convulsions and coma which may be associated with shock. Acute liver necrosis may then ensue. The chelating agent desferrioxamine (Desferal®) is no substitute for intensive supportive therapy; for adults gastric lavage should be done with a solution containing 2 g desferrioxamine/litre warm water, at the end of which 10 g desferrioxamine in 50 ml water should be left in the stomach. At the same time inject 2 g desferrioxamine in 10 ml water intramuscularly in adults. If the plasma iron is above 500 μg/litre in a toddler and 800 μg/litre in an adult, then desferrioxamine is given by iv infusion at a rate of no more than 15 mg/kg/hour. The maximum infusion dose is 80 mg/kg/24 hours; larger amounts tend to increase shock.

Psychiatric assessment

I have already stressed the importance of all self-poisoners having a psychiatric and social assessment; hospital admission is an important factor in preventing repetition. Psychiatrists differ in their assessment but over a large series it is likely that a quarter of patients will fall into each of the following categories:

(1) depressive illness
(2) personality disorder
(3) alcoholic problems and/or drug addiction
(4) no psychiatric disorder (this group comprises the adolescent behavioural upsets)

Prevention

In children. Prevention amounts to educating parents to store drugs in locked or inaccessible cupboards, to regard medicines as medicines and not as sweets, and to avoid being seen by children when either taking or hiding tablets. The profession should urge the safety packaging of drugs with the utmost vigour and discourage manufacturers from making tablets which resemble sweets.

Preventing adults from taking overdoses is a much more complex problem, which is discussed in preventive aspects.

FURTHER READING

Central Health Services Council and Scottish Health Services Council (1968), *Hospital treatment of acute poisoning.* London: HMSO.
Dreisbach (1974), *Handbook of poisoning: diagnosis and treatment,* 8th edn. Los Altos: Lange Medical.

Gleason, Gosselin, Hodge and Smith (1969), *Clinical toxicology of commercial products*, 3rd edn. Baltimore: Williams and Wilkins.

Goodman and Gilman (eds) (1970), *The pharmacological basis of therapeutics*, 4th edn. London and Toronto: Collier-Macmillan.

Matthew, Proudfoot, Brown and Aitken (1969), Acute poisoning: organisation and work-load of a treatment centre. *Br. med. J.*, **3**, 489.

Matthew (1971), Acute poisoning: some myths and misconceptions. *Br. med. J.*, **1**, 519.

Matthew and Lawson (1975), *Treatment of common acute poisonings*, 3rd edn. Edinburgh: Churchill Livingstone.

PREVENTIVE ASPECTS
(HAMISH BARBER)

The history of the adult self-poisoner has usually been one of long-standing emotional and social instability, as outlined in Matthew's classification; the factor triggering the self-poisoning episode is often relatively trivial in itself, perhaps no more than another domestic row or additional expense that cannot be met. Self-poisoning is an escape from the seemingly insoluble problems of reality and the means are either sedatives prescribed earlier for the patient (for good reasons), or those of some other member of the family.

Incidence of self-poisoning in general practice. In an average practice of 2500 patients, 12·6 per cent of the population at risk (age range 18–80 years), or 315 patients, will be on treatment with psychotropic drugs, with women outnumbering men two to one, in the UK.

Diseases classified as mental disorders (International Classification of Diseases 290–315) account for 8–10 per cent of the family doctor's workload and thus in a practice of 2500 patients for 1200 consultations each year, involving about 300 patients. Furthermore, many other patients will have important psychological or social adjuncts to their main organic illness. In this average practice there will be between 5 and 9 instances of self-poisoning each year—a small number in view of the number of patients at risk.

Patients at risk

Despite this relative rarity of self-poisoning, it should be possible to identify those patients particularly at risk. 'Frequent attenders' (more than 15 consultations per year) who have no single organic condition justifying high attendance are at risk particularly if their doctor diagnoses anxiety or depression and is tempted to prescribe a sedative or antidepressant. Women between 18 and 40 are particularly likely to fall into this category. Other vulnerable groups are families receiving social security benefits who have a history of instability or deprivation, and patients who are apparently dependent on sedative drugs or seem to require repeated courses of antidepressants. Identification of the patient's basic problems, and intervention by a health visitor or social worker at an early stage, may help to alleviate social or psychological situations which might otherwise lead to self-poisoning.

A minimum of sedatives, tranquillisers and antidepressant drugs should be prescribed, and then only for patients where treatment is likely to be successful over a short period. A sedative is not a justifiable alternative to a consultation; time spent in listening to the patient and providing explanation and support, particularly when the support is continued by a social worker, is the first line in management. If drugs are prescribed, it is impracticable to give less than a week's supply; a reasonable compromise is to arrange to see the patient once a week or fortnight, when the prescription may be repeated if necessary. For those who are dependent on hypnotics, it is sufficient to prescribe 4 weeks' treatment at a time, unless there is evidence to suggest that the patient is likely to poison himself. If repeat prescription cards are used, safeguards must be built in to ensure that prescriptions are not issued more often than intended, and the prescription should never be repeated for longer than 3 months without the doctor seeing the patient and reassessing both the diagnosis and his treatment. It is important to try to ensure that the patient does not hoard drugs at home: this is frequently impossible, but careful monitoring of prescriptions can minimise the risk.

Aftercare

In the short term

Following an episode of self-poisoning there is little to be gained by returning the patient to the same environment which precipitated the incident. Hospital discharge information should not be relegated to a letter which might take time to reach the family doctor: details of the patient's state and the psychiatrists' and hospital social workers' reports should be telephoned to him, and he should then take immediate and positive steps to continue his patient's aftercare. The patient may return home to recrimination from relatives, and with feelings of guilt and despair magnified by the continuance of the problems he sought to escape. Repeated visits from the family doctor and the health visitor can do much to help and the social work department should be asked to intervene urgently in the family's domestic affairs.

In the long term

After this initial support the doctor should monitor the patient's future consultations and ensure regular communication between all the agencies involved with the patient. The case notes should have the self-poisoning incident noted in such a way that it is always obvious to the doctor at each consultation, so that he can not only be more careful in prescribing, but also keep a check on the factors which led to the self-poisoning.

FURTHER READING

Parrish (1971), The prescribing of psychotropic drugs in general practice, *J.R. Coll. Gen. Practitioners*, **21**, 92, suppl. 4.

EMERGENCY MANAGEMENT
(DAVID GIBBONS and ARIEL LANT)

Immediate action

If poison has been inhaled, remove patient immediately into fresh air; if poison has been absorbed through skin, remove contaminated clothing and wash skin thoroughly with water.

Safeguard vital functions

Airway

Ensure patency. Clear obstructing tongue, teeth, vomit or bronchial secretions. Lie the patient in semi-prone position and ensure this position is maintained during transportation to hospital. If an unconscious patient fails to respond to painful stimuli insert an oropharyngeal tube. If the gag reflex is absent insert a cuffed endotracheal tube.

Heart

If heart is not beating, ventilate and begin external cardiac massage.

Ventilation

Assess by measurement, not clinical judgement. With a Wright's flowmeter, a minute volume over 4 litres in the absence of marked tachypnoea usually indicates adequate respiration. In an adult, a minute volume below 4 litres, or central cyanosis, signifies respiratory depression and an arterial blood sample should be taken for measuring pO_2, pCO_2, pH and bicarbonate. Give oxygen and ventilate if necessary. If there is significant CO_2 retention, controlled O_2 should be given, e.g. by Ventimask. Titrate the concentration of inspired oxygen given to maintain an arterial pO_2 of 70–90 mm Hg. Hyperbaric oxygen at two atmospheres pressure, if available, is the treatment of choice for CO poisoning.

Circulation

Elevation of the lower limbs may be all that is required to cope with vascular shock. If the systolic blood pressure cannot be maintained above 90 mm Hg in a patient over 50, or above 80 mm Hg in a younger person, give iv metaraminol (Aramine ®) 1–2 mg and repeat if necessary after 20 minutes. Aim at a systolic level of 90–100 mm Hg. If these two injections fail then infuse low molecular weight dextran or plasma, preferably monitoring central venous pressure. Severe metabolic acidosis may require infusion of 8·4 per cent sodium bicarbonate. In resistant shock give iv cortisol 300–500 mg every 6 hours.

Convulsions

Control with iv diazepam (Atensine, Valium) 5–10 mg.

Diagnosis

History and circumstantial evidence

Examine the unconscious patient carefully for venepuncture sites and unusual routes of drug administration. Check the presence of skin blisters, suggesting barbiturate, glutethimide or tricyclic antidepressant overdosage.

Samples for identification

Retain any tablets, capsules or empty containers, vomit and an aliquot of gastric aspirate.

Urine sample. Take 50 ml without preservative. Mention lignocaine to the laboratory if it was used when obtaining a catheter specimen.

Blood sample. Take 10 ml in lithium heparin (in a plain tube if lithium poisoning is suspected). These samples may assist further management and also.be of medico-legal importance.

Supportive management

Antidotes

Unfortunately there are few specific antidotes. Some useful general examples are listed in Table I.

Emetics

Never induce vomiting in the patient who is unconscious or has swallowed a caustic corrosive poison, paraffin or other petroleum distillates. Remove any dentures. Place children in the spanking position, adults on their side, head down. Irritate the pharynx with fingers or a blunt spoon handle, or give 15 ml syrup (not tincture) of ipecacuanha. Allow 15–20 minutes for this to act, but remember that the patient may lose consciousness in the meantime. Note that vomiting may not empty the stomach completely; this is important if a serious poison has been taken. **Avoid apomorphine**—protracted vomiting and shock may result. **Avoid saline emetics**—dangerous hypernatraemia can occur.

TABLE I

Some poisons with specific antidotes

Corrosives: Acids—give alkali (e.g. milk of magnesia)

Alkalis—give acid (e.g. dilute vinegar or citric acid)

Bleach—Sodium thiosulphate 5 g in 200 ml water orally **plus** calcium gluconate 10% 10 ml iv, repeated as necessary, if bleach contains oxalic acid

Cyanide—**give immediately** cobalt edetate (Kelocyanor $^{®}$) 1·5% 20 ml iv over 1 minute, then 50 ml dextrose 50% iv immediately **or** sodium nitrate 3% 10 ml iv over 3 minutes, then sodium thiosulphate 50% 25 ml iv

Iron salts— **1.** desferrioxamine 2 g in 10 ml sterile water intramuscularly, followed by iv infusion; rate not exceeding 15 mg/kg/hour (maximum 80 mg/kg/day) **2.** leave desferrioxamine 10 g/50 ml in stomach after lavage (1 g chelates approx 85 mg Fe^{3+})

Lead—give calcium disodium edetate (Ca Na$_2$ EDTA) 15–25 mg/kg by slow iv injection twice daily; maximum dose 75 mg/kg/day. The injection is given as a 0·5–3% solution in 5% dextrose or normal saline

Mercury and other heavy metals—give D-penicillamine up to 1·5 g/day orally **or** dimercaprol (BAL) 2·5 mg/kg every 4–6 hours by deep intramuscular injection, reducing to 2 injections/day over the next 3 days and then 1 injection/day until recovery

Organophosphate anticholinesterase insecticides—give pralidoxime 30 mg/kg in 5 ml sterile water by slow iv injection, repeated in 1 hour **plus** atropine 2 mg iv followed by 1 mg every 10 minutes until bradycardia and miosis are corrected; **large doses of atropine may be required to save life**

Opiates—give nalorphine 5–10 mg iv or intramuscularly, **or** naloxone (Narcan) 0·4 mg iv or intramuscularly (naloxone also antagonises synthetic opiate analogues); **acute withdrawal may be precipitated in opiate addicts**

Gastric lavage

Note contraindications as for emetics. Gastric lavage should be performed only in hospital, and within 4—6 hours of the drug ingestion (with salicylates it is never too late). Remove any dentures. Place the patient head down on his left side—or prone with his head projecting and supported—with an inflated cuffed endotracheal tube in position if he is unconscious. For adults use a 30 English gauge Jacques tube lubricated and passed through the mouth (Fig. 5.4). Aspirate the stomach using 300 ml warm water (38°C, 100·4°F) for each lavage. For children use a narrower tube, e.g. 17 English gauge, and use isotonic saline for babies. Repeat until the washings are clear (5—10 litres). In general leave nothing in the stomach afterwards, but see p. 164. Keep the aspirate and first washings for drug indentification.

Hypothermia

Use a low-reading rectal thermometer. 35°C (95°F) or less indicates

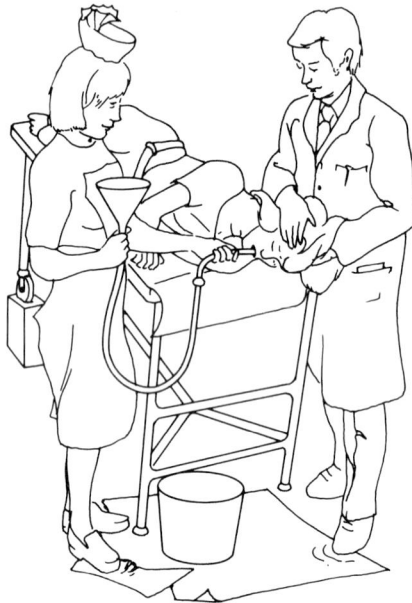

Fig. 5.4. Gastric lavage with a Jacques tube.

significant hypothermia. If patient is hypothermic use only arterial blood for investigations.

Hydration

In the absence of overt dehydration there is no urgency for intravenous fluid and electrolyte replacement within the first 12 hours. Aim at maintaining hydration with 1500 ml in 24 hours, alternating 0·9 per cent saline with 5 per cent dextrose. With severe poisoning, attend to electrolyte imbalance and acidaemia.

Physiotherapy

Turn the patient regularly, with special care to skin. Forget about respiratory stimulants and prophylactic antibiotics, but treat diagnosed infections appropriately.

Catheterisation

Perform in the unconscious patient only if bladder fails to empty with fundal pressure or if forced diuresis is being undertaken.

Enhancing elimination

Methods for increasing removal may be successful with a few drugs (see p. 161).

Psychiatric assessment. See p. 167.

6

Immediate Care

KEN EASTON

That the application of prompt, trained, medical care saves lives and prevents unnecessary disabilities, is now generally accepted. 'Immediate Care' schemes in which doctors voluntarily join with the statutory rescue services to give such aid are now established throughout the United Kingdom and are evolving rapidly in many other countries, notably West Germany and New Zealand.

While most progress has been made within the last decade, the origins date from the late 1940s when traffic was increasing following World War II, and road accidents were accounting for more deaths and disabilities than had resulted from the previous armed conflict.

Personal involvement has been continuous since 1949 when as Medical Officer to the RAF Regiment depot Catterick, Yorkshire, I was allowed to organise on the spot medical care for victims of accidents on a 15 mile stretch of the narrow A1, on which serious mishaps occurred with monotonous regularity. The base was at station sick-quarters, and many of the injured were our own airmen, soldiers, or their dependants. By comparison, airfield accidents were few and minor. Some still remember with gratitude the attentions of the young RAF nursing attendants who were somewhat disconcerted to be referred to in newspaper headlines as 'the angels of the A1'.

Experience gained then, and subsequently in general practice in the same area, and from working with both military and civil rescue services, formed a basis for the introduction of the pioneer Road Accident After Care Scheme of the North Riding of Yorkshire in 1967. By 1965 over 2000 accidents had been attended personally in the locality, and the need for giving organised care was being recognised nationally by those directly involved. At that time contact was made with Professor Eberhard Gögler of Heidelberg, who had just published the results of a highly organised and funded rescue scheme based on his university surgical clinic (Gögler, 1965). I felt that eventually a similar high degree of medical skill could be allied with rescue services in the UK, but covering all rural areas remote from hospitals, and involving the general practitioners in the immediate vicinities.

Catterick is a village astride the main road from London to Scotland and has retained its associations with the armed forces since Roman times, when it was an important military staging post. It is midway between London and Edinburgh, and at the crossroads for east-west traffic of tourists from the Lake District and heavy goods vehicles from industrial Teeside. Until the A1 was widened to a dual carriageway and the by-pass completed in 1960, serious accidents were a daily and nightly occurrence. Villagers let their houses be used as first aid stations, and the proprietor of the transport café would send hot soup and food to accident scenes via his own network of lorry drivers. No payment for this was asked or expected. In those early days of the National Health Service the nearest provincial hospitals, at least 15 miles distant, were offering devoted and advanced immediate care despite the usual lack of staff and facilities. The ambulance service was in an embryo stage, our own being an extension of the local voluntary St John Ambulance Brigade. Vehicles were outmoded and often singly manned. Training was given by local doctors on a voluntary basis and only to the standards of simple first aid. When laymen were extending themselves in such humanitarian acts, it was inevitable that doctors should join in the communal effort even though the National Health Service pays nothing for such work. This kind of voluntary service has been a vital factor for the success of Immediate Care schemes and it should be considered carefully in any future administration. An international correspondence developed with individuals encountering similar problems, and in the North East of England the College of General Practitioners arranged talks to interested doctors.

In 1965 there was an historic accident near Catterick. The cab of one heavy lorry which had run into the back of another was so deformed that normal cutting gear was ineffective. Rescuers had to stand by for an hour while more powerful equipment was brought from a private garage nearby. During that time the badly injured driver suffered unnecessary pain, and his passenger bled quietly to death from an amputated leg. An immediate approach to Parliament, asking both for improved integration of the rescue services and for better equipment for the fire services, met with a surprising reply. We were told that not only were fire services not obliged to attend persons trapped in road accidents but that any improvements in rescue procedures would necessarily depend upon local voluntary action. This advice was acted upon. Our two fire services bought the most modern equipment available, and the ground was prepared for starting the Road Accident After Care Scheme (RAAC).

By 1966 the annual toll of the roads in UK was 8000 killed and 400 000 injured, 100 000 seriously, and road accidents were recognised as the pandemic of society. Home Office figures showed that deaths and injuries in industry, in homes and at sport equalled those on the roads. At this time the improvements recommended in hospital casualty departments, and in the ambulance services (Platt, 1962) had not been implemented; a doctor rarely travelled from hospital to accident scenes, and the plight of those seriously injured was sad indeed.

A resolve was made to try and improve local rescue services and to encourage others to follow suit; to remind Parliament repeatedly of its responsibility towards the injured and of the obvious gap in medical care; and, with this aim in view, to accept any invitations to address influential lay or professional audiences, or to serve on relevant committees if invited.

The first to join me in this venture was the late Dr E L R McCallum who died tragically in 1971. We addressed the BMA Annual Scientific Meeting at Bristol in July 1967, calling upon the profession to study the needs in their own localities. The Annual Representative Meeting supported unanimously a motion that Parliament be asked to improve rescue services nationwide and assist their integration. In that same month we called the initial meeting of what was to become the RAAC scheme (Easton, 1969 and 1972).

THE ROAD ACCIDENT AFTER CARE SCHEME, NORTH RIDING OF YORKSHIRE

The meeting was held at the Richmond Police Headquarters, and a talk was given stressing that life saving and rehabilitation began at the roadside. Although there should be no unavoidable delay in transferring the injured to hospital it was essential that the most skilled medical care available should be given on site and in transit. The main aim of such care during the 'therapeutic vacuum' (Gögler, 1965) should be the maintenance of a clear airway to prevent hypoxic brain damage, and the restoration of lost blood volume. Attention should be paid to the controlled extrication of trapped persons, analgesia and splintage being applied where necessary. In this, doctors would act as colleagues of ambulancemen and personnel of other services.

Those present, doctors from hospitals and general practice, officers of police, ambulance and fire services, a pathologist, Medical Officer of Health, County Councillors, and a Member of Parliament, readily agreed to set up a pilot scheme. By a combination of resources this would give the injured benefits similar to those provided by teams based on hospitals, but would cover a vastly greater area. There were to be no financial, administrative or professional barriers to impede integration. A steering committee was elected and the scheme registered as a charity. Members of the general public requested that they should be allowed to associate themselves by providing money from individual donations or from organised fund raising. This was gratefully accepted, and the funds raised covered the initial cost of special equipment and part-time secretarial help.

It was agreed that complete records would be kept of every accident attended thus providing an overall picture of the effects of the teamwork upon survival and rehabilitation of the injured. These records would be for the use of the steering committee only, and not for litigation. Postmortem reports might point to the needs for improvement of rescue techniques. If possible, photographs would also be taken at accident scenes for training purposes.

Members offered their services to help start similar schemes elsewhere. After six months of detailed planning the Scheme was put into operation in December 1967. It speaks well for the care taken in the planning stage that the practical running of the Scheme has remained efficient and unchanged since then. The cooperation of our Ambulance Officer in personally coordinating all records over so many years is particularly appreciated.

The ambulancemen and their trade unions have supported the Scheme's efforts from the first, but at one time ambulancemen were worried because some newspapers suggested that emergency care doctors were ousting them from their primary role of giving immediate care to the public. It was possible through talks to the ambulancemen's annual conference in Torquay, and through press and television, to make it very clear that doctors were voluntarily joining teams in order to help in a most onerous task.

The Scheme area covers over 1000 square miles (259 000 hectares) of sparsely populated countryside through which run the trunk roads A1, A66, A19, and, since 1960, the motorway A1(M). It takes in the moorlands of Swaledale and Wensleydale, with its War Department Training areas, and farmlands, rivers, railways and aerodromes. **Any sudden illness or accident from whatever cause is attended, although the main work has proven to be with road accidents.**

Those involved are the hospitals at Darlington, Northallerton and Catterick Garrison; the ambulance services of Northallerton, Richmond, Thirsk, Bainbridge, and Darlington; the York and North East Yorkshire police; the fire services of Northallerton, Richmond and Darlington; and 34 volunteer general practitioners. Within each practice at least one doctor is always available to attend accidents in his own or a neighbour's area. In addition a consultant anaesthetist and an orthopaedic surgeon have joined in an advisory capacity, and local ministers of religion of all denominations have offered their help if called upon.

Call out is from Northallerton Police Control (Fig. 6.1) and is simultaneous for police, ambulance, doctors, and if necessary, the

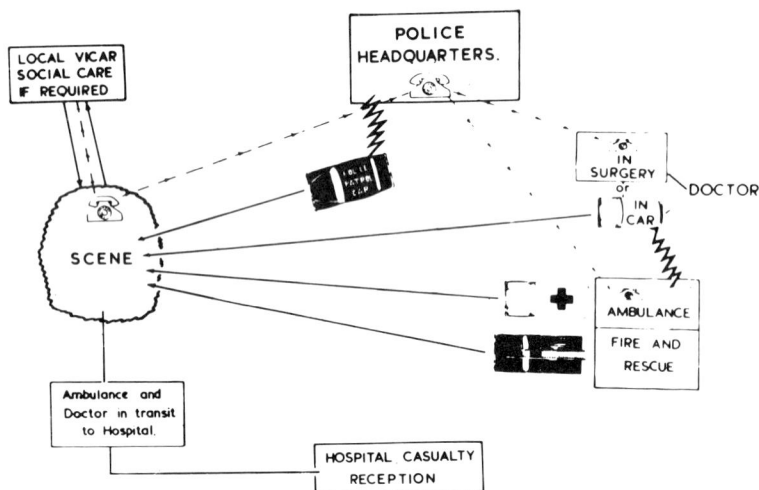

Fig. 6.1. Call out plan RAAC.

fire service. On the wall of the police control room is a map delineating practice areas, with an index of practice or home telephone numbers. Remote practices, and those in the worst situations for accidents are equipped with radiotelephones (eight), linked with the ambulance network and having 'Delta' call signs. Such communication is essential for the efficient working of an immediate care scheme. The doctors are willing to be called to every accident even though their special skills may be required at perhaps one in every five, but at this their speedy presence is vital. In practice the police have become selective in assessing incoming 999 calls and seldom ask for help unnecessarily. Our busiest doctor is singlehanded and attends about 50 calls each year. Depending upon weather and the seasons, calls tend to come in quick succession followed by periods of relative inactivity.

It has been understood from the start that in the absence of a doctor the senior ambulanceman is responsible for medical care and will take the critically injured to hospital without delay. If it is necessary for the doctor to accompany patients to hospital the police take charge of his car and deliver it to him wherever is most convenient.

Our equipment has formed the basis of that recommended by the Medical Commission on Accident Prevention in the Immediate Care Broadsheet 1975 (see below). The doctors and emergency ambulances carry specially designed large wooden boxes which open at the roadside to form a working platform. This is in addition to the Laerdal Modulaide kit. The largest dressings at present commercially available are not always adequate, and we make our own from gamgee tissue, 18 in × 12 in and 14 in × 8 in (46 cm × 30 cm and 36 cm × 20 cm), each with safety pins and 2 in (5 cm) bandages attached. Dr Snook's carefully designed 'Mediflash' doctor's beacon available on loan from the British Medical Association is sometimes inadequate for situations in which we are involved. We favour the Parkinson beacon which is also attached magnetically, with green to the fore and red to the rear, but has a more effective light and a revolving interior reflector. It must be noted that this can be used only with the permission of one's own Chief Constable.

The police cars all carry the basic Laerdal 'Resusciaide' kit, ventilation bags and airways, neck splints, spinal boards, large dressings and suction apparatus, in addition to their normal first aid equipment.

The Tauranga–Thomas traction splint for fractures of the femur is carried on ambulances. It can be applied quickly and ensures comfortable journeys over rough terrain to hospitals sometimes as much as 40 miles (64 km) distant.

With such adequate equipment on all vehicles attending accidents multiple casualties can be treated, and passing doctors can also participate.

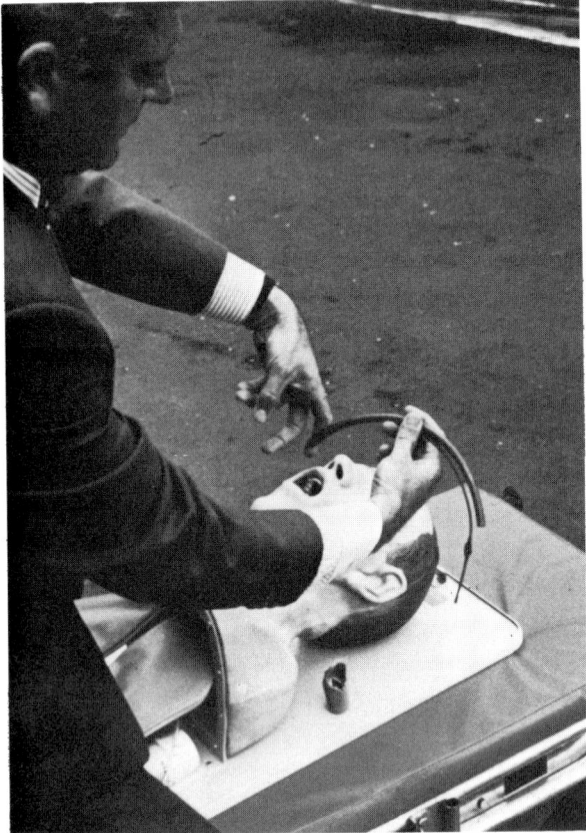

Fig. 6.2. Laerdal Manikin for blind oral intubation.

Training

The scheme doctors receive instruction from their specialist colleagues at hospitals, correlated by the postgraduate tutor. The specialists and certain of the general practitioners also instruct participant ambulance, police and firemen. Mutual instruction can always be given and received at the scenes of accidents (Documenta Geigy, 1969).

Wherever possible photographs are taken for record purposes and for future training instruction. The lifesize Laerdal manikins are used for teaching intubation, infusion, and cardio-respiratory resuscitation in the classroom (Fig. 6.2).

A colour film (16 mm, 20 min) of the RAAC rescue teams, 'Road Crash', is available on videotape for professional audiences, from Roche Products Ltd, 15 Manchester Square, London.

A number of slide/tape presentations suitable for professional and lay audiences can be loaned from the Medical Recording Service Foundation, RCGP, Kitts Croft, Writtle, Chelmsford CM1 3HH:

68–16 Roadsmash: Rescue is Your Concern (Updated 1976)
69–41 Roadside First Aid
71–72 Accident
71–90 Every Doctor's Roadsmash Drill
71–97 Equipment for Use at Road Accidents
73–70 Roadsmash Rescue (Fire and Ambulance)

Suggested equipment for doctors' cars (See Table I)

TABLE I

	Approximate price £.p	Supplier
Rear bumper: red reflective strip	1.07	Halfords
Windscreen: yellow reflective triangle		
Rear window: red reflective triangle		
'DOCTOR' Beacon: flashes red to rear, green to front; magnetic base	19.80	Parkinson Radio-telecommunications 141 High Street Blackpool
(Car radiotelephone if financially feasible)		

TABLE I—cont.

	Approximate price £.p	Supplier
Personal Equipment		
Protective reflective jacket ('DOCTOR' front and back)	3.25	Cowling Signs & Displays Ltd Fircroft Way Four Elms Road Edenbridge, Kent (073-271 3601)
Torch with flashing beacon: e.g. MOTORMATE— complete	2.66	Halfords etc.
Warning triangle	0.57	Halfords etc.
Large scissors: e.g. 10 in (25 cm) shears	1.65	Halfords etc.
Fybriter skirt pencil	0.10	Woolworths etc.
Space blanket (Aluminium / polyester foil blanket: adult size)	0.90	F W Equipment Co Ltd Whitehall Props Town Gare, Wyke Bradford, Yorks
Frac-straps (set of 5)	7.50	F W Equipment Co Ltd
Fire extinguisher: KP 2, light-weight 2 kilo dry powder. £10.80 less 15% + VAT	10.10	Chubb Fire Security Foundry Lane Horsham, Sussex (0403-60161)
Short spinal board	1.50	Home made
2 × 8 ft (2·6 m) Britax spinal board straps (DSB 779) @ £1.85 each + VAT	4.07	Britax Ltd Byfleet, Surrey
Report forms		

TABLE I—cont.

	Approximate price £.p	Supplier
Resuscitation equipment and dressings,		
Modulaide 'Doctor' Bag— basic version	71.72	Vickers Ltd Med. Engineering
Suction—Jet suction Unit		Priestly Road
Add 2 spare cartridges	2.20	Basingstoke, Hants
Inhalation /Ventilation— Resuscitation bag, adult & child's mask, 4 airways		RG24 9NP
Intubation—Laerdal Laryngoscope, 2 blades, 8 right-angle adaptors		
Set of inflatable splints (femur, leg, arm)	10.66	Vickers Ltd
Suction Catheters FG 10, FG 12	0.38	
Endotracheal tubes—Magill's cuffed $1 \times 5 \cdot 5$, 1×7, 2×9	2.16	
IV cannulae—Medicut: 2×14 g, 2×18 g	0.75	
Dressings		
Large: $6 \times$ Surgipads 8 in $\times$ 8 in (20 cm $\times$ 20 cm)	0.26	
$4 \times$ Melolin 8 in $\times$ 12 in (20 cm $\times$ 30 cm)	0.28	
Small: $6 \times$ Melolin 4 in $\times$ 8 in (10 cm $\times$ 20 cm)	0.24	
10 packets $\times$ 5 filamented gauze swabs	0.22	
Adhesive tape: 1 in $\times$ 5 yards (2·5 cm $\times$ 4·5 cm)	0.28	
Dressing scissors: 7 in (18 cm)	0.70	

TABLE I—cont.

	Approximate price £.p	*Supplier*
Giving set: 2 × Baxter BR 1 @ 36p each	0.72	
Dextran 40: 2 @ 94p ⎫ Normal Saline: 1 @ 30p ⎭	2.18	
Haemaccel, (in plastic bottle) has many advantages as an infusion fluid for on-site treatment		Hoechst Ltd (now imported into UK)
Cut down set	7.70	
Crepe bandages: 3 × 3 in, (7·5 cm), 2 × 4 in (10 cm)	0.57	
Triangular bandages × 4	0.60	
Spencer Wells Forceps size 7	1.32	
Elbow immobiliser	2.75	Medical Supply
K Y Jelly 1 × 24 g	0·13	Association Ltd Bourne Road Bexley, Kent
Empty large Modulaide Bag in 'disaster orange'	7.45	Vickers Medical
Mediprep swabs × 5	0.04	Pharmax Ltd
Medisache × 2	0.03	Ethical Pharmaceut Bourne Road Bexley, Kent DA5 1NX
Tauranga—Thomas portable traction splint	20.00	Simonsen & Weel Hatherley House Hatherley Road Sidcup, Kent DA14 4BR (01-300 1128/9)

TABLE I—cont.

Alternative	Approximate price £.p	Supplier
Vitalograph Emergency Resuscitation Outfit E 24–A3 Complete with all instruments for emergency intubation and suction in carrying case.	56.38	Vitalograph Ltd Maids Moreton House Buckingham (02-802 3691)

Supplied by doctors

'DOCTOR' sign on passenger sun visor (available from Pulse)
Safety belts
Reflective number-plates
Four-way flasher unit
Plastic water-carrier
Waterproof kneeling-sheet
Surgical or disposable gloves
Cervical collar
Blood-grouping bottles
IV Analgesic: Fortral/Pethidine
Disposable syringes: 2×2 ml, 2×10 ml, and needles
Tourniquet
(Stethoscope)
Pen

The records of attendance of RAAC members from 1967 to 1975 are shown on p. 187 (Table II).

The nine people who died in transit to hospital were all receiving advanced care by doctors. The postmortem reports stated that the injuries were so severe as to be incompatible with life. But for the quick arrival of the rescue teams these people would have been classed as 'dead on arrival at scene'.

The time for ambulances and doctors to arrive at the scene varies between 9 and 20 minutes from call out, depending on the location. Being nearer to the accidents the doctors are often the first of the services present, closely followed by the police.

While the statutory services are meticulous in sending in reports the doctors tend to be forgetful at times. After an exhausting experience, a shower and change of clothes, and before facing a full day's work such lapses are readily understood. Thus the published figures for doctors' attendances should be taken as the minimum.

First aid teaching

However quickly the rescuers are alerted the first on the scene is usually a layperson, and it is an accepted duty of many of the scheme's doctors to instruct for the first aid societies of St John, Red Cross, and St Andrew. Much of our teaching is incorporated in the joint first aid manual of these societies (third edition 1972).

In addition the following advice is given, and some petrol companies and garages have accepted the invitation to use it as a free handout to motorists.

ROAD ACCIDENT AFTER CARE SCHEME —INSTRUCTIONS TO THE PUBLIC*

First on the scene of an accident

What do you do if you are first at the scene of an accident? The first instinct is to run to the car and start pulling people out. **Don't!!** The men whose job it is to sort out the bloody chaos after road crashes say, 'A high percentage of the people hurt in cars and pulled out by frantic rescuers are made worse, even killed'—and this is fact.

Every crash is different, so there are no rules. But here is some basic advice gleaned from experience of accidents in several busy traffic areas.

What to do first

Park your car far enough away from the scene to protect it. Stop for a second to think. What are the conditions at the scene? If the crashed car is upside-down people may be trapped inside—so hail

---

* Compiled by the late Dr Alexander Mather, MBE, Institute of Advanced Motorists (with permission of the Institute).

TABLE II

RAAC SCHEME

Scheme commenced 23.12.67

Year	Accidents attended	D.O.A.	Casualties attended					Present at scene		
			Died at scene	Died en route	Seriously injured	Slightly injured		Police	Doctors	Fire service
1967	9	3	—	—	5	6		7	7	1
1968	267	16	—	—	157	261		130	166	13
1969	321	18	—	1	165	284		159	171	20
1970	380	23	3	4	164	367		221	216	28
1971	335	26	3	1	193	369		211	208	22
1972	360	27	—	1	199	355		249	172	29
1973	361	16	1	—	196	359		251	190	30
1974	334	16	—	—	187	254		222	147	9
1975	290	19	—	2	169	233		179	136	3
Totals	2657	164	7	9	1435	2488		1629	1413	155

D.O.A. = Dead on arrival at accident scene

passing cars and send them in opposite directions to find telephones and ring the **Police**. Give the extent of the crash, exact location, the number of injured, and services required. It is wise to send one car and then another in each direction with this information. The Police will inform Fire Brigade, Ambulance, Doctor, and breakdown vehicle if necessary. What else can happen? More cars can crash into the already crashed car.

It is often more important to **'protect the scene'** than go at once to the injured. Flag down the first cars, get the drivers to pull off the road, send them as flagmen with some white object to wave, **both ways**, and not just 50–100 feet but 500–1000 where they can give adequate warning.

Dealing with victims

As soon as you get to the wreck turn off the ignition and lights to prevent fire. If the victims of the crash are hurt but not bleeding profusely leave them in the car(s) until trained help comes. Ensure that the injured can breathe. **Don't twist, turn, or move them**. If they are lying in the road (cover them with a blanket or coat), leave them there, and take steps to guard them from the traffic. A doctor says: 'We often see people die who could have been saved if they had not been moved by inexperienced volunteers.' Even a victim with a broken back can usually be saved if allowed to lie unmoved. But well-meaning people *lift* them out of wrecks, *stuff* them into the back seats of cars, and rush them to hospital—with serious results.

If people are pinned

Often accident victims otherwise unhurt appear to be trapped, when they are merely held by a foot twisted under a seat. If so crawl in and gently release the foot. *Make sure the car will not roll while you do this.*

Lifting cars

People sometimes get injuries or further injuries because motorists try to lift cars, find they cannot, and let the car fall back. Four men can sometimes lift one side of a car—but if you try this, be sure that you are not pushing the other side down onto someone (this has been done).

Fire

If fire does not start right away you can relax a bit, for it rarely starts afterwards unless a thoughtless motorist lights a cigarette. Fire in the wiring usually begins as smouldering under the bonnet or dashboard. **Don't** let this panic you into immediately moving the injured. *Do three things:* (1) disconnect the battery; (2) locate the fire; (3) attack it with fire extinguisher, blanket, or earth.

While waiting for the ambulance

If you are a skilled first aider you may or may not have plenty to do. If you *have* you will be convinced of the importance of your training. If you are not a first aider you will have time to think, and *wish* you had attended instruction classes. It might have been *your* wife or child that needed your help.

We advise motorists to carry a small first aid kit at all times even though this is not compulsory as in some other countries. The most comprehensive is that marketed by Laerdal (Fig. 6.3). The contents are all essential and include a lucid instruction manual, and protection for both rescuer and rescued. When not in use the pack can be used as a pillow.

THE ROLE OF THE MEDICAL COMMISSION ON ACCIDENT PREVENTION (MCAP)

The chairman of the BMA scientific programme in 1967, the late Mr Norman Capener, was also chairman of the Medical Commission, and he invited representation of RAAC on that Commission, the aims being mutual. This avuncular relationship has given access to the far ranging associations of the parent body under the auspices of the Royal Colleges.

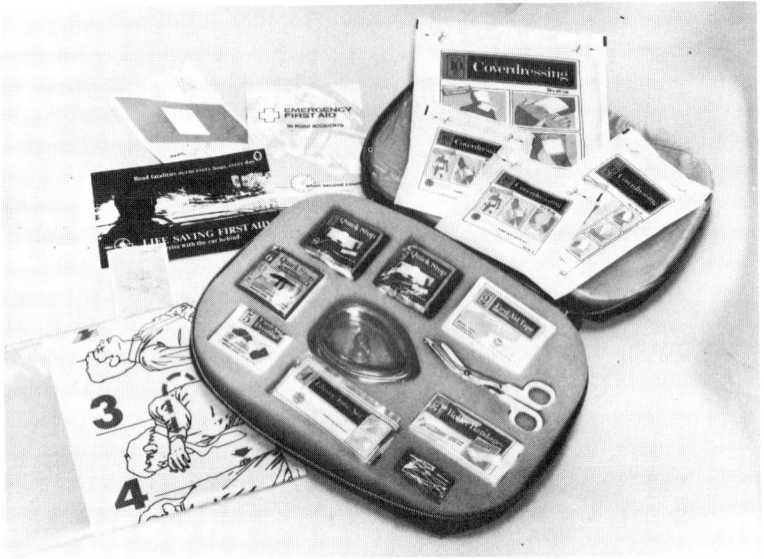

Fig. 6.3: Laerdal motorist's kit.

As new schemes have come into existence in the UK it has been important to have national cohesion, a centre for exchange of information, and a source of help and encouragement to others if requested. The Immediate Care Subcommittee (ICS) of the Commission's Rescue and Resuscitation Committee fulfils this role. Over 50 schemes and 1100 volunteer doctors are now operational (Fig. 6.4). Wherever a new scheme is mooted it is suggested that a simultaneous approach be made to the Commission and to neighbouring schemes (see Table III).

The address of the Medical Commission is 50 Old Brompton Road, London SW7 3EA (Tel 01-584 9240).

The subcommittee meets quarterly in London, and has an elected representative from each of the new regions. Observers or deputies are invited from other schemes to all meetings, and observers or representatives from the police, fire, and ambulance services, and relevant ministries are always present in advisory capacities. A token contribution is asked from registered schemes, related to the numbers of participating doctors, to cover secretarial expenses.

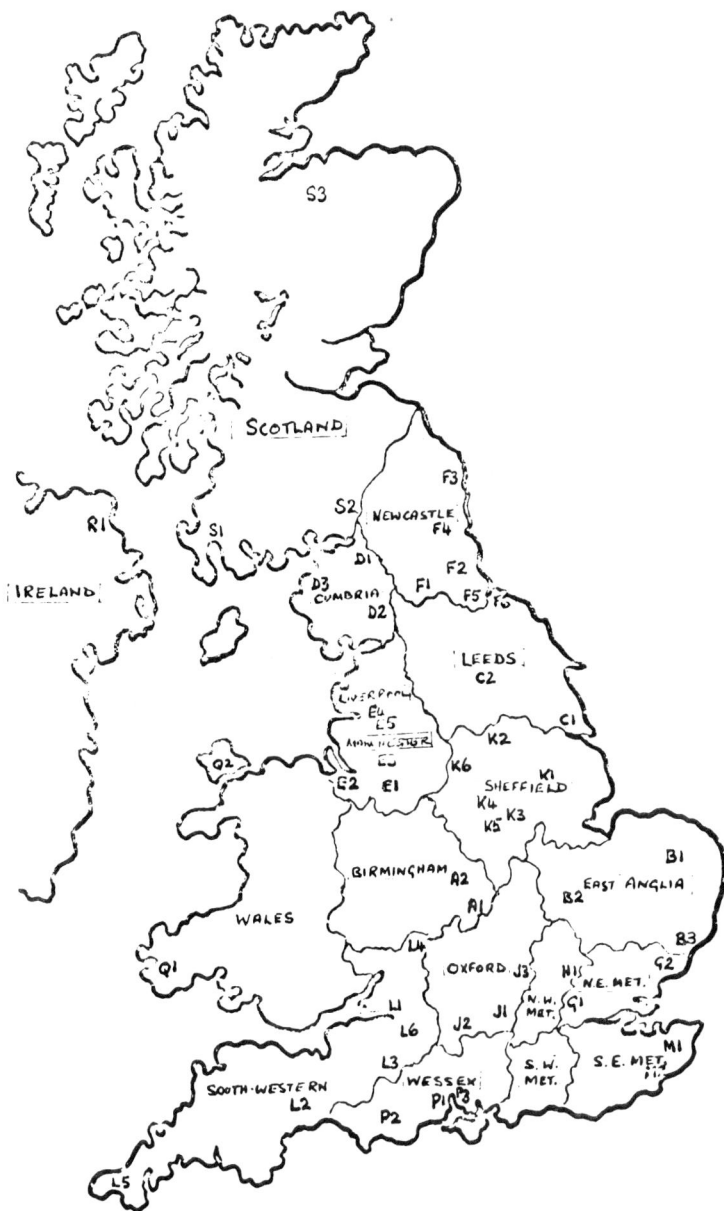

Fig. 6.4. Plan of immediate care schemes operational 1975.

TABLE III

Immediate care schemes known to be operational at 1 October 1975

(R) indicates area representative and member of ICS Sub-committee.
The figures in parentheses indicate the number of doctors participating
in a scheme

Birmingham

A1 (R) Rugby Doctors Accident & Emergency Service
        38 Clifton Road, Rugby, Warwickshire   (21)
A2   Coventry & District Accident Rescue Service
        28/32 Stoney Staton Road, Coventry CV1 4FJ   (9)

East Anglia

B1 (R) Norfolk Accident Rescue Service
        Eynsford House, Reepham, Norwich   (132)
B2   Mid-Anglia GP Accident Service (MAGPAS)
        The Surgery, 84 High Street, Huntingdon   (86)
B3   Suffolk Accident Rescue Service
        c/o Health Dept., Elm Street, Ipswich, E. Suffolk   (90)

Leeds

C1 (R) Yorks E. Riding Voluntary Acc. & Emerg. Serv.
        The Grange, Newport, Brough, E. Yorkshire   (26)
C2   Harrogate Area Accident After Care Scheme
        22 Hollins Close, Hampsthwaite, Yorkshire   (12)

Cumbria

D1 (R) Penrith & Dist. Accident & Emergency Scheme
        36 Wordsworth Street, Penrith, Cumberland   (30)
D2   South of Westmorland Accident Scheme
        The Surgery, Capt. French Lane, Kendal, W'land   (26)
D3   Maryport Emergency Unit
        c/o Midland Bank Limited, Maryport, Cumberland   (4)

Liverpool & Manchester

E1 (R) Cheshire Road Accident Service
        Birchfield, Bunbury, Nr. Tarporley, Cheshire   (12)
E2 (h) Chester Royal Infirmary
        St Martin's Way, Chester   (hospital scheme)

TABLE III—cont.

E3 (h)   Warrington Infirmary
         Kendrick Street, Warrington, Lancashire   (hospital scheme)
E4   Lives in Danger Organisation (LIDO)
         Withy House, Station Road, Bamber Bridge, Nr. Preston   (3)
E5 (h)   Preston Royal Infirmary
         Deepdale Road, Preston, Lancashire   (hospital scheme)

Newcastle
F1 (R)   Yorks N. Riding Road Accident After Care Scheme
         Stepping Stones, 32 Low Green, Catterick Village, Richmond,
         Yorkshire   (32)
F2   Darlington & District Accident Scheme
         147 Coniscliffe Rd., Darlington, Co. Durham   (10)
F3   Northumbria Accident Service
         1 Thirlmere Ave., Marden, N. Shields, Tyne & Wear   (20)
F4   Durham Accident After Care Service
         6 Blind Lane, Chester-le-Street, Co. Durham   (47)
F5   Stokesley Dist. Road Accident After Care Scheme
         Health Centre, Stokesley, Middlesbrough, Yorks   (4)
F6   Whitby Accident Care Service
         Cherry Garth, Stakesby Vale, Whitby, Yorks   (7)

North-East Metropolitan
G1 (R)   Chingford Major Accident Scheme (N. E. Met. London)
         122 The Ridgeway, London E4   (6)
G2   North-East Essex Doctors Emerg. Serv. (NEEDES)
         43 Lexden Road, Colchester, Essex   (50)

North-West Metropolitan
H1 (R)   N. W. Metropolitan Area Accident Unit
         Benington Old House, Benington, Herts   (4)

Oxford
J1 (R)   Road Accident Emergency Care Scheme (Oxon)
         The Surgery, Nettlebed, Henley-on-Thames, Oxon   (50)
J2   Road Accident Emergency Care Scheme (Berks)
         High Street, Chieveley, Newbury, Berkshire   (50)
J3   Road Accident Emergency Care Scheme (Bucks)
         Nashville House, Brill, Aylesbury, Bucks   (50)

TABLE III—cont.

Sheffield

K1   Lincolnshire Integrated Vol. Emerg. Serv. (LIVES)
        The Old Mill House, Tetford, Lincs.   (100)

K2 (R) Doctors Accident Rescue Team (DART)
        54 Thorne Road, Doncaster, Yorkshire   (11)

K3 (h) Nottingham General Hospital
        Accident & Emergency Dept. Nottingham
        (hospital scheme)

K4 (h) Royal Hospital
        Accident & Emergency Dept., Chesterfield
        (hospital scheme)

K5 (h) Derbyshire Royal Infirmary
        London Road, Derby   (hospital scheme)

K6   Ashenfell, Baslow, Bakewell, Derbyshire   (1)

South-Western

L1 (R) Frenchay Hospital Mobile Resuscitation Unit
        Dept. of Anaesthetics, Frenchay Hosp. Bristol
        (hospital scheme)

L2   Cullompton Accident & Emergency Service
        Health Centre, Cullompton, Devon   (3)

L3   Somerset Acc. Voluntary Emerg. Service (SAVES)
        Bilbao House, Mells, Frome, Somerset   (60)

L4   North Gloucestershire Accident Scheme
        The Surgery, Barton Road, Tewkesbury, Glos   (6)

L5   2 Morrab Road, Penzance, Cornwall   (6)

L6 (h) Accident & Ambulance Research
        Crossways Farmhouse, Dunkerton, Bath   (hospital scheme)

South-East Metropolitan

M1 (R) Wye Accident After Care Scheme
        Wye Surgery, Wye, Ashford, Kent   (2)

M2   Kent Accident Rescue & Emerg. Service (KARES)
        16 Hillcrest Road, Hythe, Kent CT21 5EU   (4)

TABLE III — cont.

Wessex

P1 (R) Hythe Road Accident & Emergency Cover Scheme
        Hythe Medical Centre, Hythe, Southampton SO4 5ZB   (15)
P2   Dorset Immediate Care Scheme For Accidents
        The Surgery, White Cliff Mill Street, Blandford,
        Dorset   (26)
P3 (h) Southampton General Hospital
        Department of Anaesthetics, Southampton, Hampshire
        (hospital scheme)

Wales

Q1 (R) Pembrokeshire GP Accident Scheme
        Eryl Mor, St Davids, Haverfordwest, Pembs   (10)
Q2 (R) Gwynedd Acc. Prevention Rescue & After Care
        The Surgery, Nevah Wen, Bennlech, Angelsey   (12)

Ireland

R1 (R) Ballyclare Accident Unit
        Health Centre, George Avenue, Ballyclare, Co. Antrim,
        Northern Ireland   (5)

Scotland

S1 (R) West Galloway Voluntary Accident Scheme
        Four Winds, Glenluce, Wigtownshire DG8 0PU   (20)
S2   Emergency After Care Scheme
        Achnacarry, Glasgow Road, Lockerbie, Dumfries   (12)
S3   Riverdale, Aviemore, Invernesshire   (9)

Insurance

Rescue work is dangerous, and general practitioners are classed as independent contractors. It is therefore essential that participants are insured adequately in case of injury or death when on voluntary service. The Commission recommends the following cover provided by the Medical Insurance Agency Ltd, and is negotiating for improved terms as our numbers increase.

TABLE IV

INSURANCE COVER	COST	INSURER
Insurance cover: Benefits £20 000 death and capital sums. Temporary total disablement at £20 per week for 8 weeks. All Risks cover on the Doctors Bag for an amount of £200. All Risks cover on personal effects for £100. The cover operates from the time the doctor receives advice from central headquarters of an accident, until his return to his surgery or home.	£1.25	Medical Insurance Agency Ltd 53 West Street Brighton, Sussex (0273 21633/4)

The premium is £1.25 per doctor and the Insurer requires a quarterly declaration of the number of doctors participating in the scheme. There is no liability if a doctor, during the normal course of his duties, sees an accident and attends.

The immediate care schemes' symbol

This symbol has been adopted nationally to identify fully trained and equipped doctors who have volunteered to serve at all accidents if called upon (Fig 6.5).

Police and rescue services throughout the country now recognise the plastic disc displayed notch uppermost in the windscreen of a doctor's car. It must be removed if the doctor is not travelling in the car.

A similar badge, in cloth, can be sewn to protective clothing as a means of identification at accident sites. At scenes of major accidents a doctor should also carry an identification card, preferably with an attached photograph of himself, and signed by a police official. In some places these are already being supplied by area ambulance officers.

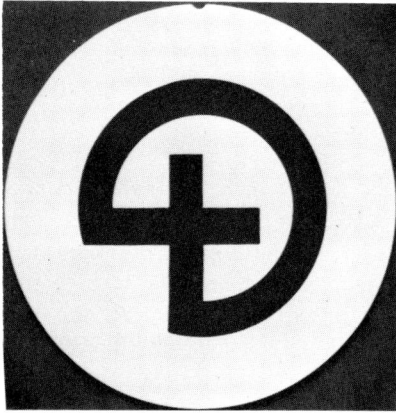

*Fig. 6.5. Immediate care schemes doctors'
symbol.*

SURVEY OF IMMEDIATE CARE SCHEMES

There are now so many Immediate Care schemes that it would be impossible to attempt to describe each in detail. Dr R A A Johnson of the Wye Scheme conducted a survey of ten, each unique in its way (Johnson, 1974). I would like to quote some of his observations:

"Initial organisation

Most of the general practitioner schemes have been organised after a meeting of interested practitioners with representatives from the emergency services, hospital administrators, accident surgeons, and county and regional medical officers, thus ensuring cooperation in resolving local problems. A committee formed from this meeting has then started the organisation. Success is dependent on willing and enthusiastic cooperation of all concerned.

Often suspicion of the organiser's motives, or even opposition, may be met from several quarters. A good example of this is the natural reluctance shown by some ambulancemen to interference from practitioners, and the fear that ambulancemen will become drivers and porters if doctors attend accidents. Once schemes have started, almost without exception these fears have been allayed, and all concerned now value the close working relationship that has been established . . .

Records and evaluation

The doctor records details of all incidents attended. Some schemes have devised a simple form of reporting, largely completed by ticking appropriate boxes on standardised forms. Somerset had managed to persuade one of the pharmaceutical firms to produce their forms in triplicate; one copy for the hospital one for the doctor, and the other for the records officer. Most schemes have a records officer . . .

Finance

Five of the schemes visited are registered charities, and fund raising is organised by a separate committee or public relations officer. Public support everywhere was enthusiastic, and money was raised in a variety of ways. These included gifts from organisations such as Rotary, Lions, Round Table; personal donations, deeds of covenant, Urban and District Council support, and from local industry . . .

Finance is required for equipment, insurance, and administrative costs. The Scottish scheme(s) are the only general practitioner schemes financed by a hospital board.

Conclusions

It is apparent that standardisation of schemes in size, organisation, communications and call out would be impractical, as local demands must be considered. Hospital-based schemes are better suited to towns, whereas general practitioner schemes can be made to function equally well in town or country.

Doctors participating should do so only if they are keen, and not because they have been persuaded or embarrassed into doing so by their colleagues. The existence of an efficient scheme is likely to be of considerable value in the event of a major disaster.

Participants in a scheme have the advantage of additional equipment for use in their day-to-day work, and may have the facility of efficient radiotelecommunications. The success is totally dependent upon the closest teamwork among the services concerned, and upon an efficient call out and communications system."

MAJOR ACCIDENTS

In the United Kingdom, in the years 1965 to 1975, the average annual toll from *major* accidents was 290 killed and injured. By contrast, in 1974/75, the annual toll from accidents of an everyday nature accounted for 5 million hurt, 300 000 seriously injured, and 20 000 killed. One third of this total was from road traffic accidents.

The immediate care schemes which are now geared to attend the daily disasters could well be integrated into regional plans for major accident procedures.

It is notable that during the Moorgate tube train disaster, in which 42 were killed and 60 injured, the North East and the West Metropolitan Schemes (G1, 2; H1) were in attendance (Winch, Hines, Booker and Ferrar, 1975).

The Harrogate after care scheme (C2) was involved in initial care to casualties of the Grassington coach crash on the remote Yorkshire moors, when 32 were killed and 14 injured.

Political considerations

In their fourth report to the House of Commons in January 1974 the Expenditure and Social Services Committee recommended that 'finance should be provided by the Government to immediate care schemes to cover the purchase of equipment and radiotelephones. The Government should also examine the feasibility of establishing a national scheme for the insurance of medical personnel attending the scene of accidents'.

'. . . one Minister should take overall responsibility for the organisation of rescue services, and for procedures for dealing with all types of accidents.'

In their reply (January 1975, recommendation 13), the Government indicated that the new Area Health Authorities were required to have plans for dealing with major accidents, these to be coordinated with the police (under the Home Office). The Government could not agree to making the organisation of rescue services the responsibility of one department, but they were willing to consider suggestions for improvements to the present arrangements for coordinating the various accident and emergency services. In Scotland the Secretary of State already had responsibility for the major services of health, police, and fire.

The advantage of having one person ultimately responsible has been shown by the rapid spread of immediate care schemes in Scotland. Official help has been given in order to meet specific problems, and all efforts have been integrated for the common weal. A model example of this coordination is given in the final Report of the Tayside Health Board—Perth and Kinross—District Working Party on Road Accidents, September 1975.

The Medical Commission on Accident Prevention is conducting an independent national survey of the value of the voluntary work done by immediate care schemes to fill obvious gaps in medical care over the eight year period from 1968.

Perhaps the results of this survey might enable Parliament to give official recognition to such schemes and thus ease many of the present administrative problems.

AIDS TO RESCUE

(Some of the following were published originally as letters by the author to the British Medical Journal, and these are reproduced by kind permission of the Editor.)

Improvised stretcher, blanket lift

When dealing with road accidents it is essential to lift the injured from a vehicle with the utmost gentleness, and, if at all possible, in the position in which they are found. Within the confines of a saloon car this may be extremely difficult, using the normal points of access and relying upon gripping clothing without dragging or twisting the body, to say nothing of the contortions required on the part of the rescuer. Matters can be be simplified by using one blanket as shown in Fig. 6.6.

The aim is to put a cradle under the patient with minimal disturbance, and to produce handholds at a distance.

One end of the blanket is rolled up twice, and the remainder infolded upon itself like a Venetian blind until a narrow strip is produced

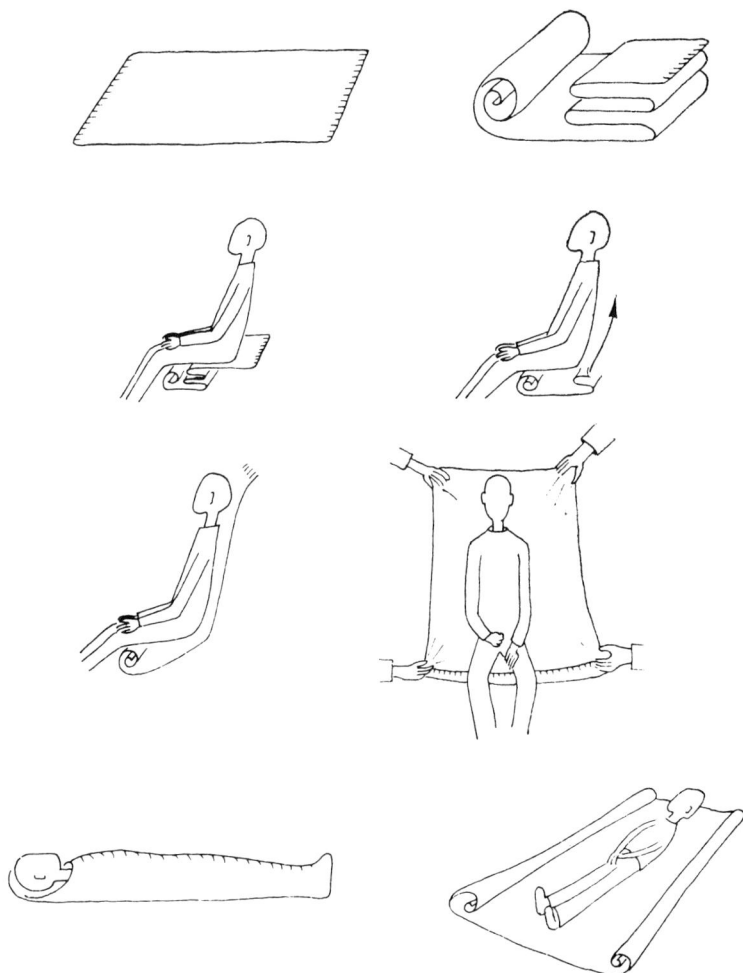

Fig. 6.6. Improvised stretcher, blanket lift.

which can be slipped carefully under the patient's knees. With the
roll behind the knees, the folded portion is brought backwards under
the buttocks (which need to be lifted slightly) and then unfolded upwards between the seat and the patient. The patient is now cradled,
but has not been disturbed, and he can be lifted out sideways supported

and controlled by handholds at a distance. After extrication the patient may be lowered to the ground with the blanket protecting him below and above. By infolding its sides the blanket can now be used as a stretcher.

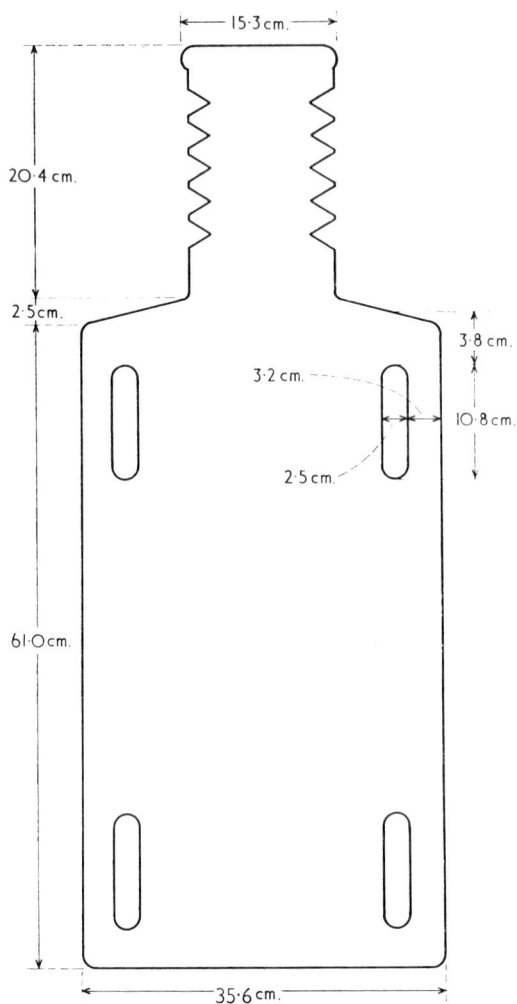

Fig. 6.7. Dimensions of spinal board for road casualties.

Spinal board for road casualties

The short spinal board used during extrication of the injured from wreckage and the journey to hospital was originally described by Dr J D Farrington (1967) and Fig. 6.7 shows an adaption of it (drawn to scale). The board is made from good quality $\frac{1}{2}$ in (1·25 cm) plywood, with all the edges rounded and the board well waxed to facilitate sliding into position. The head-piece has 'saw edges' to prevent head bandages slipping. Two 8 ft (2·6 m) Britax safety straps and buckles are used to position the patient on the board. Overall width of the board is 14 in (35·6 cm).

Before the board is put into use, the patient must first be fitted with a cervical collar. The board is then slid gently behind the patient, making sure that the lower end is well below the level of the sacrum. The two Britax straps are passed through the upper handholds, behind the board, out from the lower handholds, and around the patient's thigh from the outside to the inside, and then under and over the thigh to the chest buckle (Fig. 6.8). The straps must be applied as high as possible in the groin. The forehead can be held in position by triangular bandages or a Velcro type band.

The injured and the board now being one unit, any movements for extricating the patient will not worsen a spinal injury. It sometimes helps to tie the ankles together and to have them supported by a rescuer if fractures have occurred below the knee. The handholds in the board are useful for lifting purposes, but within the Road Accident After Care Scheme the 'blanket lift' is used with the short spinal board (see above). Once the casualty is lying on the ambulance stretcher the buckles are loosened to allow the legs to extend. The board provides a firm base for any type of stretcher.

Blind oral intubation in the deeply unconscious patient (Fig. 6.2)

It is now generally accepted that the lives of many injured persons can be saved if greater attention is paid to maintaining a good airway, and that the chances of effective rehabilitation can be enhanced if positive pressure ventilation is also given. The best way to control respiration is by passing a cuffed endotracheal tube, which also prevents the backflow of blood and vomit into the lungs. Although every doctor should carry a laryngoscope and be proficient in its use, the prospect

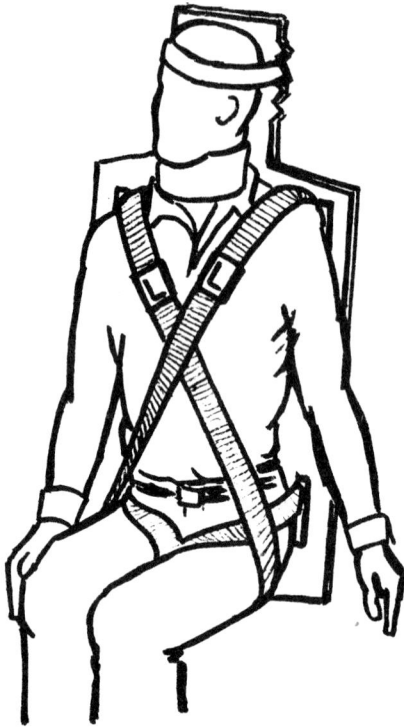

Fig. 6.8. The spinal board in use.

of performing a laryngoscopy at the roadside in poor light and at ground level is a daunting prospect to many.

Knowing that in future more people will need to be intubated by general practitioners or even by trained paramedics, this comparatively simple method of blind intubation has been perfected. The advantages are that it can be used in poor light, at ground level, on any patient, and requires only a rubber tube and a pair of hands. It is indicated in patients who are deeply unconscious or recently 'dead', and in whom the cough reflex is absent or minimal. It should be possible to widen its scope if a relaxant is also used.

With the patient supine, the operator kneels astride or alongside, facing the head. The head is centralised and the forefinger of the left hand is thrust into the mouth to the base of the tongue so that the epiglottis lies over the finger nail. The middle finger is pushed against the posterior pharyngeal wall, acting as a guide for the tube, preventing it from entering the oesophagus. The right hand introduces the tube between the fore and middle fingers, the bevel initially facing backwards and downwards. The bevel impinges upon the pulp of the middle finger and is directed automatically in front of the oesophagus and behind the epiglottis into the larynx. At this stage the right hand rotates the tube through 90°, thus bringing the bevel between the vocal cords. A gentle push passes the tube beyond the cords into the trachea. As soon as an obstruction is felt at the bifurcation the tube is withdrawn $\frac{1}{2}$ in (1 cm) and the cuff inflated. The whole procedure takes only a few seconds. Should some laryngeal spasm occur as the tube touches the cords the tube should be withdrawn slightly and after a moment given another gentle but firm thrust downwards.

Practice at this procedure upon the cadaver will prove its simplicity and give confidence. The intra-oral manipulations are not much more than those required to remove dentures or pieces of food from the posterior pharynx. Depending upon the sizes of individual's fingers the positions of fore and middle fingers may be reversed, or the base of the tongue may be hooked forward to ease the passage of the tube.

The cervical collar (splint)

For use in suspected cervical or thoracic spinal fracture in conjunction with the spinal board.

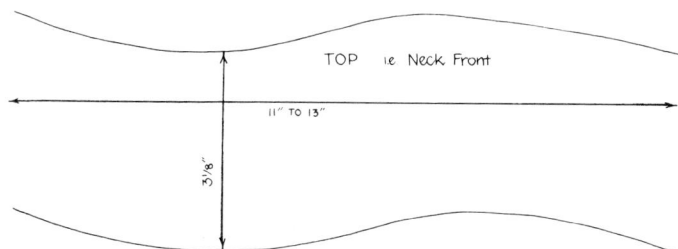

Fig. 6.9. The cervical collar.

Materials

Hard cardboard or, preferably, Vinolay.

Cover with 3 in (7·5 cm) rib unbleached stockinette, 50–60 in (1·25–1·5 m) long, so that this will tie around the back of the neck and can be gently knotted at the front.

Pack the side marked 'Neck Front' with cotton wool in order to make a soft pad of the collar.

Supplier of stockinette 3 in rib, unbleached stockinette 25 yds per roll:
 Seton Products Ltd
 Tibiton House, Medlock Street
 Oldham, Lancashire.

IPPV

Cerebral oedema develops rapidly in brain injuries and is aggravated by any hypoxia, so that the brain damage may become permanent. It is therefore essential to prevent hypoxia in the earliest stages and this is done by ensuring a clear airway and by assisting ventilation with bellows, or mouth-to-mouth respiration. This is a measure in which every rescuer should be practised.

INTERNATIONAL DEVELOPMENTS IN EMERGENCY CARE

When our charitable scheme first started we stipulated that there were to be no financial, administrative or professional barriers. It would seem that there have been no national barriers either. Interest in improving emergency care has brought representatives from many countries to study our methods and to inform our members of their own problems and achievements. Through the kindness of many people it has also been possible for some of our members to study and lecture abroad, extensively so in my own case.

America

Awareness of the needs to improve national standards which we experienced in the 1960s was paralleled in America, and it is fascinating to see how closely the efforts of our two countries have resembled one another.

Dr J 'Deke' Farrington, orthopaedic surgeon of Minocqua and Chairman of the Sub-committee on Transportation of the Committee of Trauma of the American College of Surgeons, developed a volunteer accident rescue team in his own township. It is an adaptation of his short spinal board which we have used.

American physicians and surgeons realised that the profession should give a lead in upgrading care by categorising responsibilities and capabilities of hospital admitting units; and by teaching and equipping ambulance attendants to give much better pre-hospital care. They are to be congratulated upon the dynamism with which they have tackled the problem, and upon their success so far (American Academy of Orthopaedic Surgeons, 1971; American Medical Association, 1971; Farrington, 1970).

In 1971 the American Trauma Society was initiated 'to strive to bring together physicians, ambulance profession, insurance industry, safety engineers, public health officials, communications experts, medical scientists, law enforcement and fire protection professionals, teachers, the press, the Armed Forces and other Governmental agencies, and particularly an informed and interested laity. These concerned groups and individuals, working together, can create programs in all spheres of scientific, clinical and community endeavor and thereby meet the challenge of accidental injury'.

West Germany

The government has tackled the problem of emergency care realistically, accepting Prof Gögler's statistics (1965) of lifesaving by adequate medical care as a norm to be achieved regionally. The 'cost' of a human life being £50 000 or more (in sterling equivalent) the expense was considered justified.

A proportion of all cars have to carry first aid-equipment by law, and display a sign to this effect.

In most areas excellently designed ambulances (Binz) are constantly available from strategically placed depots, and doctors also travel with the ambulances if necessary. However, this places a strain on hospital resources and interest is being shown in the RAAC method of using peripheral general practitioners. The ambulance attendants are trained to a high standard, and defibrillations and intubations en route in the ambulances are routine.

During my latest visit in 1972 I participated with the Heidelberg teams and was very impressed by the care given. Particularly noteable was the detailed analysis of each accident on the following day, the Professor and his helpers studying a series of photographs taken from predetermined angles. A final year medical student is provided with an official Mercedes Benz car, a full photographic kit to cover each accident, and medical equipment should his help be needed.

Anyone wishing to study the organisation in Heidelberg must be prepared to spend several days and nights on the project, and to travel with the teams if invited. I found the conditions on the autobahns more frightening than our worst UK motorways; a warning perhaps of what we might expect now that we are subject to the onslaught of high-speed continental juggernauts.

The use of helicopters to transport doctors from hospital and to evacuate patients from the scene is a daily occurrence, but they are not called at night or in bad weather because of the greater risks to personnel. In Mainz Professor Frey, an anaesthetist, has perfected a complimentary service using doctors and attendants in tandem. The doctors travel from hospital either by ambulance or helicopter to about one in ten road accidents. Professor Frey's medical attendants receive a six-year training course to become proficient, and they intubate and infuse under medical supervision.

Following an international symposium on mobile intensive care units and advanced emergency care delivery systems, at Mainz in September 1973, the scientific committeee comprising Drs Frey and Ahnefeld (Germany), Nagel and Safar (USA), and Poulsen (Denmark), published a series of 'Recommendations' which are all-embracing and applicable to any country.

One recommendation, on the need for training medical students in emergency care and advanced life-support, has been an accepted goal in UK for many years, supported by the British Medical Students Association at Birmingham in 1971. It has been slow in implementation. Professor Hoffman (1973), thoracic surgeon of Middlesbrough, reviewed undergraduate teaching on major trauma and cardio-pulmonary resuscitation at 74 medical schools in 22 countries. This project was staged following his personal survey of 12 hospitals in the North of England in which less than half of the 76 doctors were competent to give advanced cardiopulmonary resuscitation. Hoffman recommends that such teaching should start in the second preclinical year and be a continuing process into postgraduate education. On this, all seem to be agreed. At Catterick we have welcomed many students and postgraduates into our practices, hospitals and ambulance stations. Some are now consultants in their own Accident/Emergency departments, and many from abroad, especially Australia, are actively involved in immediate care of their communities.

Scandinavia

The sense of responsibility in communities for their own injured is particularly strong in Scandinavia, where tuition in life-support begins at primary school and countrywide annual staged exercises ensure continuous progress. The lead given by Dr Poulsen (Arrhus) and his colleagues has received firm Government backing, and Asmund Laerdal of Stavanger has perfected lifesize plastic teaching models of great ingenuity. His 'Resusci-Anne' and resuscitation equipment are in daily use worldwide. The clear thinking and kindly humanity of these men make them much sought-after members of international committees.

In Denmark Dr Poulsen is Director of Hospitals, and he is anxious to involve general practitioners in helping with immediate care. At present this is covered by a private organisation, FALK, which employs nearly 3000 permanent staff.

Russia

In 1974 three British surgeons made a careful study of Accident and Emergency Services in Russia (Hindle, Plewes and Taylor, 1975), and were impressed by what they saw. All densely populated areas have district hospitals and satellites from which ambulances with doctors and feldschers in attendance can be dispatched. A high standard of resuscitation is given and there is no shortage of doctors to undertake such work. In USSR there are 35 doctors to every 10 000 population (UK 10 per 10 000), and emergency care has equal standing with other specialties.

Israel

The Arab/Israeli war has prevented further correspondence with the

Israel Association for Traffic Accident Casualties, a voluntary association formed in 1969. The Israeli Army medical teams have perfected immediate care for casualties with remarkable results. This hinges upon rapid relief of respiratory distress, assisted ventilation to reduce brain hypoxia, and quick restoration of blood volume. Little of this work has been published in the UK and my information has been gleaned from surgeon friends abroad who have volunteered to visit Israel to serve at the front line dressing stations. Eventually our Israeli colleagues should have much to teach us in the application of immediate care (Naggan, 1976).

Lebanon

Again, little contact has been possible because of the war situation. The main load for immediate care is borne by the Red Cross, their medical director Dr Baaklini helping to organise and instruct teams of ambulance men who are placed at strategic points in the cities and in mountainous regions. They have Volkswagen ambulances each with a driver and attendant. Because of the difficult terrain and distances to main hospitals Dr Baaklini has been inviting the help of practitioners in outlying villages, and offers to equip them. In 1972 an ad hoc committee was formed to consider extension of immediate care, its members being high ranking officials. It is likely that their services are now fully extended, and one hopes for favourable reports when peace comes.

India

In 1972 I was invited to study the problems of immediate care in India, and Bombay in particular where in that July alone 49 had been killed and 529 injured. The problems of patient care in the sub-continent are great, but the devotion shown to their countrymen by the doctors struck me forcibly.

A pilot scheme has been launched in Bombay involving 5 medical schools, family practitioners, police, and upgraded ambulance service. The Dean of Seth Medical College visited us in 1974 and reported that the City Authorities had raised the equivalent of £500 000 sterling to aid the project.

Pakistan, Karachi

Dr Omar Jooma, an internationally respected neurosurgeon, has been waging a one-man campaign to help the plight of those with head injuries following accident. He has trained his junior staff to a high degree to assist him in the pioneer work of his specialty. Two Volkswagen ambulances with attendants go to any accident within a six mile radius of his hospital. In order to gain the cooperation of the populace, simple instructions are painted on either side of each ambulance, in two languages, giving the telephone number to use in an emergency.

Dr Jooma started his scheme in 1970 and in the first year showed an 89 per cent reduction in mortality. It was a privilege to meet him and his colleagues of the College of General Practice of Pakistan, who have combined with the police to extend the project.

The exemplary work of the St John Ambulance Association in Karachi must be mentioned. On a voluntary basis they are building, equipping and staffing a 200 bed hospital at an outlying industrial complex towards the Gobi desert. In 1972 the first storey, a dispensary, two part-time doctors, an ambulance and a permanent attendant had been provided. Funds for this project are raised at Karachi St John's Headquarters by organising cheap community entertainment for all age groups every evening. Whole families are able to attend regularly and this effort has also served to reduce juvenile delinquency.

Spain

In April 1970 the International Association of Neurosurgeons held conferences at Edinburgh and Madrid. One of the papers presented covered the pilot scheme for emergency care in Madrid (Head Injuries, 1971). This was set up in 1964 and has since been emulated in Barcelona, Valencia, Seville, Zaragoza, and Bilbao. The Madrid service covers 156 square miles (400 square kilometres) and attends two million people. It is open from 5.0 pm to 9.0 am on working days, and the full 24 hours on holidays. On working days there are two ambulances with attendant doctors from 9.0 am to 5.0 pm to attend to extreme emergency cases.

The city is divided into 8 sectors coordinated from the main centre at which there is a staff of seven doctors, one of whom is medical director. The supporting staff consists of 5 radio operators, 10 telephonists, 60 drivers and 19 orderlies. The total number of doctors in the scheme is 91, and there are 31 ambulances. Should casualties be unable to come to the peripheral centres, ambulances with doctor and nurse in attendance would make home visits.

The main centre is at La Paz Hospital, on top of which is the heliport landing stage, the operating theatres being immediately below. The average time from call out to initial medical care is 25 minutes, reduced in extreme emergencies to 15 minutes. The police are responsible for medical care at the numerous road accidents. They have ambulances with trained attendants, and these combine with the helicopters (Alloutte–11) which can convey the patients to hospital, or doctors to the scene. Personal experience with the air and ground services left the impression that this system should be studied carefully by countries with similar social and geographical problems.

Thailand

Improvements in emergency care are being tackled systematically in Bangkok. The police are in full charge of all rescue, and their responsibilities extend to the fire and developing ambulance services also. The canals (klongs) and the long straight roads running alongside give dual troubles of road accidents and drownings. Government expenditure is limited but voluntary effort and private donations are contributing to paramedical training and to the formation of emergency departments at various hospitals.

Community medicine is the special interest of the physician who is Dean of the Ramathibodi Medical School and his surgeon brother. They have developed a small emergency department and health clinic. Medical students are directly involved in community care through an ongoing process of field work during their undergraduate and postgraduate training. Many eventually become practitioners in the villages which they influenced as students.

Singapore

The island of 224 sq miles (580 sq km) has many government and mission hospitals, each with its own ambulance for non-traumatic cases. Medical care is administered from five areas. Immediate care is given mainly at the Outram Road Hospital which deals with about

100 casualties each week, and specialist care units are being developed. Improvements in immediate care are being conducted by a neuro-surgeon and his casualty specialist colleague. They have the support of the local family practitioners but the latter have problems which could make service along the lines of RAAC impossible to achieve.

Hong Kong

Here one cannot anticipate true family doctor participation because of the social problems. The main effort might be towards improving the ambulance service which is the responsibility of the fire service (two control areas). In major accidents family doctors might be able to help the auxiliary medical service. In 1971, 3000 people were seriously injured, and 50 are injured each day in industrial accidents. Cover for 4 million people is provided by 67 ambulances, 67 per cent of calls being emergencies. Because tenements are high and the lifts are too small to allow a stretcher, there must be three men to a stretcher. Fortunately religious superstition guards against any abuse of the ambulance service.

Australia

In 1972 I was privileged to address the Fifth World Conference on General Practice in Melbourne, a main topic of which was emergency care. All aspects were covered, many countries were actively involved, and an international committee was formed for interchange of information and mutual support. At first this was based at the Royal Australian College of General Practitioners' premises in Melbourne, but it has now been transferred to WONCA (Chairman of the Standing Committee on Emergency Care, 17 Milner Road, Rondebosch 700, South Africa).

The vastness of Australia means that many of its people are steeped in a tradition of hospitality and caring for others, engendered from living in places where distances, terrain and climate create man-size problems. The aeroplane is the obvious means of travel between city and city, inter-state, and where neighbours can be 500 to 1000 miles apart. The work of the Royal Flying Doctor Service in the outback is well known, and the standards of its pioneer John Flynn, who started the service in 1929, are being upheld.

The main population is in the large cities on the seaboard, many people spending their lives travelling intra- rather than inter-state. The motor car accounts for many deaths and injuries on the periphery of cities, and it is in such situations that general practitioners are coordinating to give immediate care. The Royal College of Australian Practitioners at Sydney has offered to help integrate the present schemes set up by members at Fremantle, Sydney, and Melbourne. Later in this book there are accounts of the work of Drs Pacy and Bush who are accepted leaders in their respective fields.

Accident and emergency departments are being staffed by experienced general practitioners, and the advanced care given by the St John Ambulance Brigade is appreciated and relied upon throughout the country. As the medical profession is enlarged through immigration it is possible that doctors might take an even greater part in helping their St John colleagues. In South Australia the St John organisation has neared perfection in its abilities to serve the community and standardise its air/ground services. In the State of Victoria with its greater commitment a State-run ambulance service has developed, which works in conjunction with its St John voluntary counterpart. One can have nothing but admiration for the way in which all these services are meeting their respective problems.

Integration must come but this need not prove difficult if dealt with as decisively as was the compulsory wearing of seatbelts, which halved serious head injuries in the first year.

Rhodesia

There is a close link between the Salisbury and Birmingham medical schools. The students at Salisbury are multiracial, and those now qualifying of high calibre. I saw the excellent work of one young graduate at an outpost hospital near the Zambian border where victims of terrorist activities, friend and foe alike, received treatment.

South Africa

The lead in emergency care has been taken by consultant surgeons and their anaesthetist colleagues based on the hospitals of the main cities. A study on resuscitation of road accident cases was to have begun in September 1973, but this coincided with the introduction of a speed limit on all roads because of the petrol shortage. Multiple injuries from high speed impact suddenly disappeared from emergency departments.

I was impressed with the routine use of innominate/subclavian vein puncture by hospital doctors on shocked patients, and this is a procedure which might well be adopted elsewhere. I remember attending one young man in our own RAAC Scheme who had multiple fractures which made normal roadside infusion impossible. Fortunately the hospital was quite close, otherwise we might have lost him; but subclavian infusion could have been given.

An immediate care scheme run by young doctors under the direction of Dr Alan MacMahon and based on the Tygerberg Hospital, Capetown, is now well established. The director of the Groote Schuur Accident Unit Dr R H Baigrie favours extension of the resuscitatory services to the scenes of accidents. He and surgeon colleagues of Durban and Johannesburg have visited many centres in Europe and have held symposia on emergency care in the Republic.

New Zealand

The most encouraging adaptations of emergency care along the lines of the UK Schemes is apparent in New Zealand, actively supported by Government and Health Departments. The two islands have much the same geographical features as the UK but the population is much less, and the distances between major accident treatment centres is greater.

A pilot project was started by general practitioner Dr Morgan Fahey in 1973 in and around Christchurch (Fahey, 1975). This scheme, with ten practitioners working alongside St John Ambulance staff, has been so successful that Dr Fahey was awarded a Wolfson Travelling Fellowship, augmented by Government funds, in order to come to Europe and America to study individual schemes.

St John Ambulance Officers have made similar journeys, as has the senior surgeon of Southlands Hospital Invercargill, Dr G Davidson, who is organising rescue services over areas similar to those of Scotland. It is envisaged that New Zealand will be the first to show other countries the benefits that can accrue from amalgamation of charitable local emergency care schemes actively supported by government (Fahey, 1975).

THE NEXT FIVE YEARS

Despite the world economic recession there will still be accidents and people in need of care. It has been shown that their needs are being met world-wide by pioneer, farsighted, charitable efforts. Governments generally are not given to pioneer experiment. It will still be the responsibility of individuals to foster the sort of work which has proved successful so far. The public will undoubtedly support such efforts.

In order to have cohesion and mutual support there should now be an international body to whom those actively interested could refer. At present there is the WONCA committee for general practitioners, and the International Trauma Foundation for surgeons (28 Cadogan Lane, London SW1).

In the United Kingdom the Area Health Authorities should foster links between the consultants in accident and emergency departments and the peripheral rescue services, including general practitioners. The strained financial resources of the National Health Service need to be augmented by charitable funds if nationwide emergency services are to be improved and remain viable. The new Community Health Councils might be actively involved in this venture.

REFERENCES

American Academy of Orthopaedic Surgeons, Committee on Injuries (1971), *Emergency Care and Transportation of the Sick and Injured, and Syllabus for Slides on Emergency Medical Care.*

American Medical Association (1971), Categorisation of Hospital Emergency Capabilities.

Documenta Geigy (1969), *Rescue on the Road.* International Symposium Report.

Easton (1969), Medical organisation at road accidents. *Brit. med. J.*, **4**, 150.

Easton (1972), Report to the Royal College of General Practitioners, British Council, Department of Health and Social Security, The Nuffield Foundation.

Easton (1972), The general practitioner and the rural accident services. *Injury*, **3**, 274.

Fahey (1975), Wolfson Travelling Fellowship Report.

Fahey (1975), The Establishment of Decentralised Accident Teams in Christchurch, *New Zealand Medical Journal*, **82**, 191.

Farrington (1967), *Bulletin of the American College of Surgeons*, **52**, 121.

Farrington (1970), The Challenge to the Physicians of Today. *The Journal of Trauma*, Vol. **10**, No. 4.

Frey, Prof Dr med R (personal communication), Institute of Anaesthesiology, Johannes Gutenberg University, D-65, Mainz, Germany.

Gögler (1965), *Road Accidents*. Documenta Geigy, Series Chirurgica.

Grant, Murray and Farrington (1971), Robert Brady and Co.

Head Injuries (1971), Proceedings of an International Symposium held in Edinburgh and Madrid. London: Churchill Livingstone.

Hindle, Plewes, Taylor (1975), *Brit. med. J.*, **1**, 445.

Hoffman, Prof (1973), *Resuscitation*, **2**, 123.

Johnson (1974), Immediate Care Schemes. Upjohn Travelling Fellowship. *Journal of the Royal College of General Practitioners*, **24**, 847.

Naggan (1976), Medical planning for disaster in Israel, *Injury*, **7**, 279.

Platt, Lord (1962), *Ministry of Health, Accident and Emergency Services.* London: HMSO.

Winch, Hines, Booker, Ferrar (1975), Disaster Procedures Report, Moorgate Crash. Personal Communication. (Published in *Injury* May 1976.)

7

The Accident Flying Squad—
Resuscitation and Release

ROGER SNOOK

In spite of safety measures and improved design the road transport system of western civilisation continues to extract its daily toll of casualties. Until such time as preventative measures can considerably reduce or eliminate the problem, it is imperative that prompt and proper management of road accident casualties be regarded as a priority.

Treatment must be considered from the moment of injury and should include the appraisal of such factors as the summoning of help (and) the techniques of first aid, resuscitation, extrication, handling, transportation and arrival at hospital.

Road accidents involve many problems, but one in particular which is common to all areas, is that of extrication of the trapped casualty.

In 1961 the City of Bath Fire Brigade and Ambulance Service brought into operation a special emergency equipment vehicle to deal particularly with the extrication of trapped casualties. This vehicle is a compact. self-contained unit carrying a comprehensive set of cutting, lifting, jacking, winching and lighting equipment together with its own built-in electrical power source. The rescue tools are carried in lockers around the sides of the vehicle for ease of access, and the complete unit forms a compact, mobile workshop that can be taken into the close proximity of the trapped casualty. In use it has proved invaluable at many accidents both on the roads and in other situations. During the course of the first eight years that the vehicle was in service the number of times it was required at road accidents to release trapped and injured casualties increased threefold, giving a clear indication of the need for such rescue facilities.

Accidents at which casualties are trapped are particularly significant for several reasons. Investigations have shown that the force required to distort the passenger carrying compartment of a vehicle and trap the occupant will be sufficient to cause serious injury in 50 per cent of cases. Sixty per cent of casualties trapped in vehicles are held by the legs in the upright position, exaggerating the effect of shock from injury. To this must be added the fact that the patients' hospital treatment will be delayed by the period of the time required to effect their release. On average this is in the region of 35 minutes, but can be as long as 4 to 5 hours in the more difficult situations sometimes encountered. The application of rescue techniques to allow the early release of these casualties is therefore of considerable importance, but does not completely resolve the problem as the patient is still being delayed from reaching medical treatment at hospital. In view of these findings it was decided that medical attendance at the scene of accidents could usefully complement that of the rescue vehicle, giving the benefit of earlier assessment, treatment and pain relief, as well as more rapid release.

Clearly there are several ways in which medical aid may be organised to attend accidents, one of the simplest methods being always to carry a set of medical equipment in a car which could then be driven direct to the scene without waiting for specialised transport.

Two particular advantages of organising medical attendance by this means are immediate availability and freedom of movement when on call. Also with this degree of flexibility such a scheme is equally suited to the hospital or general practice situation. A doctor, together with a set of medical equipment and car could usefully be regarded as one 'unit' and any number of these units could collaborate to cover a large area. For instance one such unit could be based at a District General Hospital accident department and could include some of the more elaborate medical equipment required occasionally. More peripherally individual general practitioner units could provide cover for the rural areas, each unit corresponding to the doctor's practice area. A third type of unit could be based on a health centre where the duty doctor would carry the medical equipment and radio set in his car for his tour of duty and then pass both on to a colleague, this saving duplication of expensive items.

In conjunction with the University of Bristol it was decided therefore to cost and evaluate a single unit 'Accident Flying Squad'. Evaluation was to include the time involved, distance travelled, number of calls answered and equipment required to attend accidents in any situation where medical aid might be of benefit, whether casualties were trapped or not.

During the initial stages of organisation in 1965 it became clear that a few details would require careful attention. In particular the problems relating to transport were considered.

The first of these points concerned the use of a private car for such purposes. No particular problem was encountered with the insurance of the vehicle, this being covered by an existing comprehensive policy. Personal insurance was however considered advisable as some extra risk could result from becoming involved at accident sites. The main problem in driving to an emergency centres around vehicle identification and communication. Provided other road users can quickly recognise a vehicle being used for such a purpose they will invariably offer priority. Regulations do not permit the use of blue flashing light by doctors so a flashing green light was developed by the author for this application. This design was subsequently adopted by the BMA as the 'Mediflash' for use by registered medical practitioners when answering emergency calls. The light unit was designed to be held on the car roof by powerful magnets, thus avoiding a permanent fixture. The unit could be attached quickly when required and powered by a parking light socket or cigar lighter plug. In use this means of identification has proved quite satisfactory although a brighter bulb, if permitted by the regulations, would be advantageous. On the few occasions when the light is not noticed by the inattentive motorist, use of the car horn, though not distinctive, quickly draws attention to the light which is. The light has always been used to help maintain a steady progress through traffic as opposed to achieving maximum top speed. Endorsement of this policy, coupled with rapid mobilisation, is to be found in the average attendance times of the ambulance and accident flying squad. The mean time from receipt of call to arrival at the incident being 8 minutes for the ambulance and $9\frac{1}{2}$ minutes for the Accident Flying Squad.

Speed in mobilisation is heavily dependent on efficient communications. To ensure continuous availability, radiotelephone communication is essential. Various degrees of sophistication are offered with most installations and can considerably influence operational efficiency.

Initially the Accident Flying Squad car was equipped with a simple two way radiotelephone on the ambulance service frequency. The potential of this immediate method of communication was quickly recognised and the system expanded to include those facilities that would influence operational efficiency. The complete system now includes the provision of direct speech between the ambulance control room and all the vehicles; between the vehicles themselves and between the vehicles, control room and hospital accident department. A means of transmitting a 'selective call' tone code from the ambulance control room to actuate a buzzer and call light on the Accident Flying Squad radio, together with the provision of a small portable personal set allows even greater freedom when on call. The main radio is a multi-channel set and includes crystals allowing communication with the County ambulance service, a neighbouring general practitioner scheme for attending accidents and emergencies, and the ambulance service national Emergency Radio Channel designed for use in public disasters.

In addition to this the Accident Flying Squad car is equipped with a radio on the City Fire Service frequency.

Operationally the radio equipment has proved invaluable and on one occasion contributed to saving a patient's life. Direct speech, as opposed to passing messages through a third person, saves both time and misunderstanding. When used to arrange for crossmatched blood to be brought urgently from hospital to a casualty trapped, for instance, under masonry for several hours, the provision of such facilities can be seen to be fully justified. The survey of the radio system showed that 28 per cent of calls received by the Accident Flying Squad were used to mobilise medical aid. This either follows the initial 999 emergency call or the arrival of the first emergency vehicle at the incident. The indications for initial attendance are the same as for the Emergency Equipment Vehicle; the suggestion of a serious accident, or one occurring at a well known black spot or involving a car overturning, leaving the road, catching fire or trapping the occupants.

Applying a degree of selection to calls in this way could be interpreted as taking the risk of missing accidents where medical aid may be required immediately. In practice however this has not been found to be the case. If anything the reverse seems to apply for the part urban part rural area involved. In the first place selection has resulted in attending a higher proportion of accidents where medical aid is required. The more important point however concerns the relationship with the ambulance men. Organising attendance to be available, rather than automatic, encourages the ambulancemen to consider the assessment of the patients even more keenly. Similarly the policy of teaching the ambulancemen to help actively in such procedures as aspiration, intubation and infusion of fluids rather than relying on a team of nurses from hospital for this help, is also felt to be important. Both policies have the advantage of including and advancing the skills of ambulancemen.

This has been taken to its logical conclusion in the Bath area by the Accident Flying Squad officially becoming a part of the Fire and Ambulance Service, with all operational expenses being funded by the local authority. By way of return the medical experience gained from attending accidents can be reinvested as informed training for advancing the ambulancemen. As the standard of training of ambulancemen increases so will the need for informed medical participation in it. Medical participation will also be of value to the emergency services in the field of testing new equipment such as the Laerdal Venturi aspirator 'Jet Sucker' working from a pressurised can (Vickers Medical). Other recent developments include the Hare Splint and the Scoop stretcher (F W Equipment Ltd, York). The Hare Splint is designed on the principle of the Thomas' Splint with adaptations to allow it to be fitted without removal of clothing. The Scoop Stretcher is a light alloy unit that unfastens to form two halves longitudinally. After normal first aid measures including immobilisation of fractures, the two halves are gently eased under the patient and clipped together. The patient can then be lifted with the minimum of disturbance and the device used to place the patient on the more conventional trolley stretcher.

New developments must also include the new ambulances now being evolved, as well as medical aspects of new fire brigade rescue equipment. An example of this is in the use of a new putty like substance known as Heat Ban, which acts as a heat conduction barrier, allowing a wider choice of metal cutting equipment together with a reduction in patient disturbance by avoidance of vibration during cutting operations.

Medical involvement in training and in evaluation of new techniques allows a firmer working relationship to be established with the emergency service personnel which is of considerable value at the accident scene. For instance, on arrival at a serious accident reliance can be placed on the training of ambulancemen to direct medical attention to those patients most in need.

In assessing the casualties at a road accident it has been found helpful to look at both the patients and the vehicles involved to recognise patterns of injury corresponding to vehicle damage. Notice is taken of the relative sizes of vehicle involved, the direction of impact, and the presence of damage or deformity in the proximity of the occupants. Such information can be of value as a diagnostic pointer when working under the adverse conditions of a patient fully clothed, with poor lighting, and restricted access.

Correlation between vehicle damage and occupant injury has been described in medical literature for some years, one of the best known reports being that of Smillie (1954) describing the dashboard fracture of the patella. Many other accounts of patterns of injury have followed involving the various regions of the body.

In a frontal collision the movements of an unrestrained occupant can be seen to follow a predictable sequence. This has been demonstrated by several research groups investigating vehicle performance during collisions. Injuries may include those involving the knee (Smillie, 1954), the hip (Grattan, 1969), the lower limb (de Fonseka, 1969); the cervical spine (Snook, 1973b); the thorax (Goggin, 1970); Deiraniya, 1970); the face and head (Harrison, 1966). In addition investigations by the author have confirmed an increased incidence of head and neck injuries in rollover accidents, an association between side impacts and major intrathoracic or abdominal injury, and between occupant ejection and serious head or multiple injuries. In addition pedestrian casualties are often found to have severe injuries of the lower limbs. An example of the way in which this can be of value is in the quick recognition of injuries requiring careful handling or early fluid replacement.

At the risk of stating the obvious, treatment depends on availability of equipment, so from the onset a careful appraisal was made of the various items of equipment required (see Table I).

Originally the equipment carried consisted of a collection of items in various bags, and inevitably the one left in the boot of the car was just the one required at the scene. Presentation within the bag was also important to avoid having to search through a jumble of items to find the one needed.

To avoid making the mistake of carrying two or three of everything the resuscitation equipment is now presented in one box. This is divided into compartments each of which contains the equipment for a particular procedure. Sufficient items are included for the treatment of one casualty. An additional case carried in the boot of the car with

TABLE I

Accident Flying Squad equipment

Resuscitation box painted white with reflective 'Scotchlite' band and 'Doctor' label, and containing:

Surgical
Sterile cutdown and surgical set in linen pouch, including: 2 linen towels, scalpels, scissors, aneurism needle, artery clips, forceps, needle holders, mosquito forceps and bone saw
Disposable syringe and needle, prepacked swabs, Mersutures, local anaesthetic and adhesive surgical drape

Airway
Intubation set in roll-up linen pouch including: laryngoscope, endotracheal tubes, Magill introducing forceps, syringe, clip, gag, tongue depressor, infant aspirator (disposable) catheter mount and Cobb connector, Knights connectors, Mason gag with Ackland jaws, KY jelly, Argyle Trochar Catheter, Heimlich chest drain valve
Ambu sucker and two Yankauer suction mounts
Laerdal Resusci bag including extra oxygen nipple and endotracheal adaptor, mask and airways
Portogen oxygen cylinder
Brook airway

Intravenous
Pulpet electronic aneroid sphygmomanometer
Portex iv cannulae and suction catheters
Angiocath intravenous cannulae ($\times$ 6)
Baxter pumping drip set ($\times$ 3)
Macrodex plasma volume expander ($\times$ 6)
Hartmann's solution ($\times$ 2)
Sodium bicarbonate 4·2% ($\times$ 2)
MSA elbow immobiliser
Refrigerated box containing O Rh negative blood
(Blood Transfusion Service property)

General
Keeler Practitioner Ophthalmoscope
Everready flat torch
DDA Register
Drugs including:
Adrenaline 1 : 10 000, Aminophylline, Atropine, Calcium Chloride 1%, Cyclimorph, Dextrose 25%, Ergometrine, Fortral, Hydrocortisone, Isoprenaline, Lasix, Lignocaine 1%, Pethedine, Piriton, Valium
Syringes, needles and 'mediswabs'
Blood crossmatch tubes (hospital property)
Lister bandage scissors
Wakeling battery rechargeable cardiac monitor and Multi-point dry electrodes
Philips 85 miniature dictaphone
Kodak Instamatic camera and flashcubes

Additional equipment carried
Entonox (premixed nitrous oxide /oxygen inhalant analgesic gas) cylinders, valve, mask and mouthpiece
Pneumatic splints
Roehampton burns dressings
Spinal boards and straps plus Plastazote cervical collar
Blankets (1 wool and 1 heat retaining foil)

First aid kit including
Aseptor pads, No. 8, 9, 16 standard dressings BPC, 3 in conforming and crepe bandages, triangular bandages, 1 in oxide strapping, safety pins and scissors
Reflective waistcoat type jacket
4 warning triangles
Large torch
Minor rescue equipment including: hacksaw, jemmy bar, tools, rope, asbestos gloves
Fire extinguishers, dry powder and BFC (Bromochlorodifluoromethane)
Fire blanket
14 volt floodlight
Mediflash
Pneumatic horns
Radiotelephone (selective call 10 channel)
Portable radiotelephone
Photographic equipment (personal property)
Information on toxic chemicals and poisons and set of antidotes
Selective vehicle detector remote traffic light switch
Studded snow tyres

the remainder of the equipment, contains a stock of expendable items to allow immediate replenishment of the resuscitation box. In this way all the necessary equipment for resuscitation is available in the close proximity of the patient, and can also be taken in the ambulance without fear of leaving an essential item behind.

The resuscitation box is designed to open up and display all the equipment for immediate use, and to be stable in a moving ambulance. The lid, when open, is held at an angle to prevent it slamming shut in such circumstances.

The main part contains the equipment for infusion of fluids, aspiration and ventilation together with the cardiac monitor and general items. Three compartments in the lid contain an intubation set, a surgical set for 'cut down' or amputation, and a block of foam holding ampoules of emergency drugs.

The intravenous giving set is opened to allow the inclusion of a venous tourniquet, needle and cannula, swab, syringe, specimen bottle and lengths of adhesive tape. All the items required for infusion therefore are ready to hand.

A drip set containing an integral manual 'Squeeze' pump was chosen not only for rapid administration of fluids but also for those situations where the height at which the bottle could be held was restricted. An example of this was encountered at a road accident in which a driver was trapped in a car with its roof partly collapsed and buried under the load of an overturned lorry. An alternative method utilises a plastic pack of fluid. If the giving set is connected and held upside down, and the plastic pack squeezed it will fill completely, displacing any air. Connected to the patient the fluid can then be given rapidly by squeezing and without fear of air embolism. The only disadvantages with this method are the difficulty in estimating the amount of fluid given, and ensuring that the drip is still running properly.

Dextran in saline with a molecular weight of 70 000 or Hartmann's solution is considered the most suitable fluid for emergency use, combining a long shelf life with tolerance of climatic temperature changes. No problems have been encountered with subsequent cross-match as a specimen of blood is always taken before administration. Similarly no difficulty has been encountered in cannulating a vein and obtaining a specimen of blood as the peripheral venous shutdown of hypovolaemic shock is seldom established by the time of arrival. This does not however preclude the carrying of a cut-down set, which could be required if there was any delay in finding the patient or calling for medical aid.

Of particular value in putting up an infusion is the MSA (Medical Supplies Association) elbow immobiliser—a simple device consisting of two plastic covered metal strips that are held in place along the length of the antecubital fossa by a Velcro strap. It holds the elbow straight during and after cannulation, making it possible to use the larger and more easily entered veins of the antecubital fossa.

The equipment for ventilation was chosen for its small size and weight. The 3 lb (1·3 kg) Portogen cylinder contains sufficient oxygen to last for 20 min at a flow rate of 4 litres per min. Used in conjunction with the Laerdal Resusci bag it enables approximately 33 per cent oxygen to be administered by mask or endotracheal tube. The concentration can be raised to approximately 50 per cent by using oxygen 'reservoir' with the Resusci bag. One particular advantage of this Laerdal ventilation equipment is that it can be folded up for storage.

The various items required for intubation are kept in a linen pouch which is divided into sections so that a missing item will be conspicuous by its absence. The aspiration equipment includes an Ambu mechanical suction apparatus with disposable Yankauer suction mount (Eschmann Ltd) and plastic suction catheters. Although not quite as powerful as an electrically operated aspirator this unit has proved quite adequate in practice. At one accident, for instance, it was used for pharyngeal toilet before intubation of a patient in the middle of a field. The patient was found lying on his back, unconscious and inhaling vomit as well as blood from a compound fracture of the mandible. After intubation, tracheal aspiration was also effective and instrumental in ensuring the patient's survival.

The monitoring equipment carried includes a rechargeable battery-operated oscilloscope and dry multipoint electrodes together with a Pulpet electronic anaeroid sphygmomanometer. The former has proved useful at drowning incidents and has also been used during the resuscitation of a patient with carbon monoxide poisoning from a burst gas main. The electronic sphygmomanometer is however, much the more essential of the two devices, being used for repeated monitoring of blood pressure to assess progress, particularly in the case of patients trapped for any length of time. A reading can be taken in 10 seconds and so causes little more than a pause in the extrication procedure. Even in severe shock this instrument has been found to give reliable readings and will, for instance, record a systolic blood pressure as low as 50 mm Hg.

Entonox, (see Chapter 1), premixed nitrous oxide and oxygen in equal and fixed proportions, is carried as part of the medical equipment and in our scheme has displaced the opiates for the majority of conditions requiring analgesia before arrival at hospital.

Principal amongst its advantages are the rapidity of onset, effective relief of pain, relief of anxiety and muscle spasm, freedom from side effects, and ease of discontinuation. A series of seventeen cases was observed personally including monitoring of pulse, blood pressure and rate of bleeding from wounds or into fracture sites. No significant alteration of any of these parameters was noted. Analgesia was sufficient to allow movement at a fracture site to effect earlier extrication in one case and relief of arterial occlusion at a fracture dislocation in another. A small cylinder was found to last between 20 and 40 minutes depending on whether use was continuous or intermittent. The only precautions to be taken in its use relate to external temperature. It must not be used after exposure to sub-zero (°C) temperatures without rewarming and inverting the cylinder. This is necessary as at temperatures below $-7°C$ the mixture begins to separate and may not be given off in 50:50 concentration (Bracken, 1968). A particular advantage of this agent is its use during the extrication of trapped casualties (Fig. 7.1). During the author's $3\frac{1}{2}$ year research period 41 trapped casualties were treated. Thirty-seven of these were due to road accidents and of the 37, 23 of them being trapped by the legs and feet by deformity of the structures in front of them.

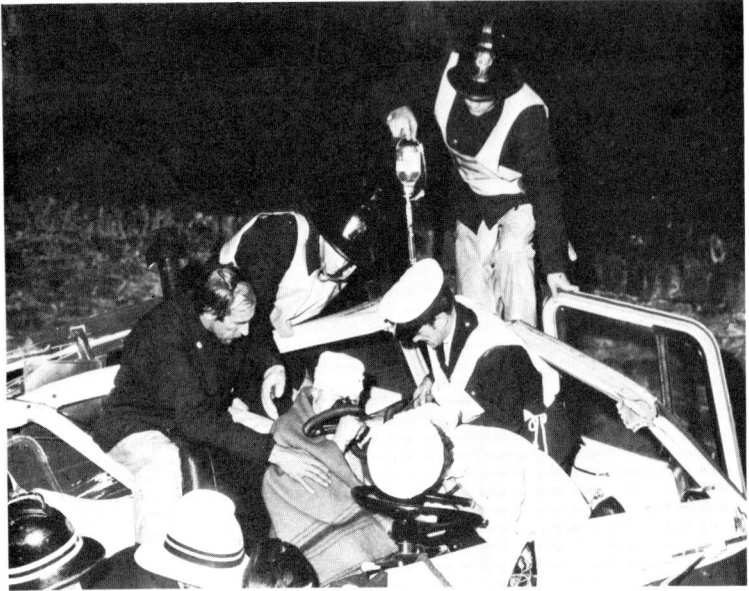

Fig. 7.1. *The driver of this crushed lorry is trapped by the legs and seriously injured. Entonox is being taken for analgesia and a dextran infusion is running. Medical aid included handling the injured lower limb during extrication. (Reproduced by permission of the* Bristol Evening Post.*)*

The techniques used to release the casualties include cutting the pedal stems, gear stick, steering column or other rigid structures. Where feasible the seat mountings are also cut to help to release the lower limbs. See Table II for equipment carried by the Fire Brigade emergency vehicle.

TABLE II

City of Bath Fire Brigade emergency vehicle equipment

The vehicle is based on the 4-wheel drive long wheelbase Land Rover and incorporates a 5 KVA centrally mounted 110 v DC generator and the following specialist equipment:

Electrical equipment
2 Black and Decker 1500 W angle grinders
1 Black and Decker metal shear
1 Black and Decker sabre saw
1 Black and Decker electric drill
3 17 in 1000 W Searchlights complete with tripods
4 cable reels consisting of 1 × 100 ft reel, 1 × 75 ft reel and 2 × 50 ft reels
1 3-way portable junction box for use with cable reels

Hydraulic equipment	*Winching equipment*
1 8 ton Flexiforce hydraulic rescue set	1 standard Land Rover front mounted
1 20 ton Flexiforce hydraulic rescue set	capstan winch
1 Blackhawk hydraulic shear	1 100 ft Terylene line
1 8 ton hydraulic bottle jack	2 × 3 in sheathed pulleys
1 25 ton hydraulic bottle jack	2 'D' shackles
1 7 ton trolly jack	1 double leg chain sling
1 box wooden chocks (30) 6 lashing lines	

Other cutting equipment	
1 complete set oxyacetylene equipment	1 pair HT pliers
1 bow saw	1 sledgehammer
1 hack saw	2 picks and shafts
1 pad saw	2 crowbars
1 multi-blade saw	2 spades
1 pair bolt croppers	1 bass broom
1 sheet metal cutter	1 comprehensive tool kit
2 'Police accident' signs	1 set 'Britool' sockets
2 protective jackets	3 pairs industrial gloves
6 portable flashing lamps	2 plastic buckets
1 first aid kit	1 Nife hand searchlight
2 dry powder fire extinguishers	1 20 ft extending alloy ladder
6 asbestos blankets	1 sheath knife
1 pair asbestos gloves	2 pairs safety goggles
1 pair HT rubber gloves	

A new vehicle has just been commissioned and is based on the forward control Land Rover. It has an increased generator output, and a hydraulic drum winch instead of the capstan winch. In addition to the equipment above a Mitralux P 131 dual purpose, high density flood light, 16 ft telescopic mast, and tripod are also carried and the oxyacetylene cutting set has been replaced by a Gaspak Mk 2 portable oxypropane cutting set.

Hydraulic rams may also be used to push a collapsed dashboard away from the casualty or to expand gaps in the metalwork where appropriate. The hydraulic apparatus carried on the rescue vehicle is especially versatile and can be assembled in a variety of combinations to meet the particular problem. In four cases, after a certain amount of cutting or jacking of the crushed vehicles, it was possible to effect the earlier removal of the patient by the careful manipulation of a broken limb. This combination of extrication and medical procedures can avoid the need for amputation in the vast majority of instances. Only in two instances was the need for such a procedure encountered and in one of these the amputation was performed on a fatally injured casualty trapped in the cab of a petrol tanker with a ruptured tank. The justification for this was in avoiding the risk of fire or explosion, the alternative being to cut the crushed cab.

Other extrication techniques include shearing through the pillars at window height to allow removal of the roof and cutting hinges to remove doors. Creating a large opening in a vehicle is a particularly useful technique in the instance of the patient having a spinal injury. This allows adequate access for a number of rescue personnel to lift the patient carefully, and also allows the use of a spinal board such as the compact fibreglass Tynemouth spinal splint (Vestric Ltd, Runcorn). In use this splint has been found easy to apply and very effective. It consists of a narrow fibreglass board with attached body and head straps. When slipped behind the patient together with contouring foam pads and strapped in place the patient can be moved with much less fear of worsening an unstable injury. For the cervical region an excellent deep moulded collar can be made from a thermal plastic foam—Plastazote. Entonox is usually given to patients with spinal injuries only after the spinal splint has been applied. This is to avoid abolishing the 'safety feedback' of pain which guards against incautious movement. Once splinted care is taken to lift the patient **in** the splint and not **by** the splint to avoid the problem of the board sliding up the patient's back.

Pneumatic splints are carried by the Accident Flying Squad and have been used on many occasions both to splint fractures and to control bleeding from extensive wounds by applying an even pressure over a large dressing. For those wounds which are too big for even the largest standard dressings, one or more sterile 8 in $\times$ 8 in Surgipads (Johnson and Johnson) and an inflatable splint or crepe bandage have always proved effective in practice. Roehampton burns dressings are also carried, being useful as a compact, sterile foam pack that can be cut and fixed to cover large areas if necessary. Fortunately fire at road accidents is rare though the risk can never be ignored. To this same end a fire blanket and extinguishers also form part of the equipment carried.

Particularly useful in the winter are the heat retaining foil space blankets that are also waterproof and reflect a certain amount of light, ensuring visibility. Care should be taken in the summer to avoid overwarming the patient with these though, as this reverses the reflex compensatory action of vasoconstriction in the skin.

Other items included in the equipment are non-medical though equally important. Chief amongst these is the reflective waistcoat jacket. Home made from white 'Ambla' upholstery material this jacket has a distinctive green fluorescent yoke, bearing the legend DOCTOR in reflective letters. For night-time visibility the lower edge of the jacket has a wide band of reflective fabric placed to show up in dipped headlights even when the wearer is bending over. In view of certain unfortunate tragedies in which rescue personnel have been seriously or fatally injured by passing vehicles it is a personal rule that this jacket is put on at the moment of stepping out of the car however serious or trivial the accident. To the same end the car is fitted with 4-way hazard warning lights, and reflective warning triangles, an 'Accident' sign and portable flashing lights are carried to protect the scene for those occasions when arrival precedes that of the emergency services.

A few minor rescue tools, such as a jemmy bar, hacksaw, rope and asbestos gloves are also carried to allow access to be gained to a patient in the event of being first on the scene. Wellington boots and a plastic 'mac' are also carried for adverse weather conditions and a reference book on industrial poisons together with a set of large scale maps are also carried.

The car is also fitted with a miniature transmitter that allows traffic lights to be switched to, or held at, green on an emergency call, this being part of an experimental system installed at a road junction in Bath (Snook, 1972a). Finally a set of studded snow tyres are available for winter use together with headlight wipers for use in snow and rain, and rearguard red lights for use in fog.

The fact that during the $3\frac{1}{2}$ year research period every piece of equipment on the emergency equipment vehicle has been used except the oxyacetylene cutter, and every piece of medical equipment on the Accident Flying Squad has been used, except the cut down set and trochar chest catheters for decompressing a pneumothorax, proves the need for such detailed organisation.

Teamwork is a vital ingredient of the scheme for morale, efficiency and safety. Research has included the development of a technique in conjunction with the Fire Service for opening jammed burst proof doorlocks in under one minute (Snook, 1973a). Organisation evolved a communications system that allowed the Police to bring crossmatched blood to the scene of a serious accident. Discussion between the services reinforced the belief that information should be shared and exchanged. This is evident in the increased fire risk from oxygen when used by a doctor in a crashed vehicle, without the knowledge of the fire officer.

Such points place even more emphasis on the value of interservice training and the active role the medical practitioner can play in this.

The results (Snook, 1972b) of the research project showed that medical aid at the accident scene could be organised, was effective and inexpensive. During the course of $3\frac{1}{2}$ years 132 accidents were attended, 82 per cent when off duty and 18 per cent when on duty in the hospital. The incidence of calls on average was one every 9·5 days and the mean time spent on each call was 31 min. The mean time required per week to answer calls and maintain the equipment was 65 min. These figures show that such a scheme should not cause any significant interference with normal duty.

The mean distance travelled to the incident was 4·7 miles and the mean time taken to arrive at the scene was 9·5 minutes compared with the corresponding ambulance timing of 8 min.

Of the casualties seen 140 were slightly injured, 128 were seriously injured and 34 were fatally injured. 17 per cent of the seriously injured required definitive medical treatment, and medical aid was of direct value to individual patients at 29 per cent of all accidents attended. At many of the remaining accidents the presence of a doctor was of value in confirming the absence of serious injury and in taking photographs and gaining experience for use in training lectures.

The total cost of providing the scheme including the capital cost of all the treatment (except the car) and all running expenses except a medical attendance fee was calculated to be £178 per annum when averaged over a period of 7 years.

Having assessed the cost of providing medical attendance, the Road Research Laboratory's costings of road accidents (Dawson, 1967) were used to assess the 'saving value' of such a scheme to the community. This was calculated to be £22 000 per annum after deduction of all running expenses including a fee based on rates paid to Police Surgeons.

The scheme described has been evolved to operate in conjunction with the emergency services of the area in and around the City of Bath. It would be wrong however to conclude that any one method of organisation is 'best'. Each scheme should be adapted to the needs of the particular area. It is not so much the detail as the fundamental concept that is important. Medical involvement in the operational and training aspects of rescue is of undoubted value and the scheme in the author's area is continued, being justified on both economic and humanitarian grounds.

REFERENCES

Bracken (1968), Safety precautions to be observed with premixed gases, *Brit. med. J.*, **3**, 715.

Dawson (1967), *Cost of Road Accidents in Great Britain*. Road Research Laboratory reports LR 79 and LR 396.

Deiraniya (1970), Traumatic Rupture of the Thoracic Aorta, *Injury*, **2**, 93.

de Fonseka (1969), Fracture of the right lower limb of drivers due to the penetration of the front wheel, *Brit. Jour. of Surg.*, **56**, 320.

Grattan (1969), Injuries to hip joint in car occupants, *Brit. med. J.*, **1**, 71.

Goggin (1970), Deceleration trauma to the heart and great vessels after road traffic accidents, *Brit. med. J.*, **2**, 767.

Harrison (1966), Injury patterns in various classes of road users, *Med. and Biol Ill.*, **16**, 4.

Smillie (1954), Dashboard Fractures of the Patella, *Brit. med. J.*, **2**, 203.

Snook (1972a), Automatic Traffic Light Control, *'Fire'—Journal of the British Fire Services*, **65**, 3.

Snook (1973a), Medical Aid at Road Accidents, *'Update'—Journal of Postgraduate General Practice*, **6**, 239.

Snook (1972b), Accident Flying Squad, *Brit. med. J.*, **3**, 569.

Snook (1973b), Medical Aid at Road Accidents, *'Update'—Journal of Postgraduate General Practice*, **6**, 1141.

8

Hospital Based Schemes — Luton and Dunstable

LAWRENCE PLEWES AND JOHN HINDLE

The Accident Service at Luton was completed at the same time as the first section of the M1, and by some strange coincidence the motorway passed within a few hundred yards of the Luton and Dunstable Hospital. Since then we have had the experience of seeing over a thousand people injured on this highway (Fig. 8.1). In this chapter we will draw some conclusions about mobile operating theatres, the accident surgeon's optimum place in the major accident plan, the organisation of the accident service, equipment and training.

The M1 has provided us with considerable experience, some of which has been unusual. There is no doubt in our minds that a central barrier has cut down dramatically the terrible carnage produced by one car out of control crossing over to the other side of the motorway, crashing head-on into many vehicles travelling at speed. We have had several examples of 'planing' when the combination of heavy rain, severe cross winds and worn tyres on a car travelling fast result in loss of contact with the road surface and inability to negotiate even the very gentle curves of the M1. We are convinced that fatigue is the prime cause of most severe accidents (aside from fog) and it is surprising how many drivers admit that they must have fallen asleep when asked about the cause of their accident. We are accustomed to the invariable 'no' in answer to questions about safety harness wearing by casualties with multiple injuries. We are also getting used to the triviality of injuries sustained by the person who was wearing a harness even in very severe crashes, although we are told about the stretchability of most harness material. As

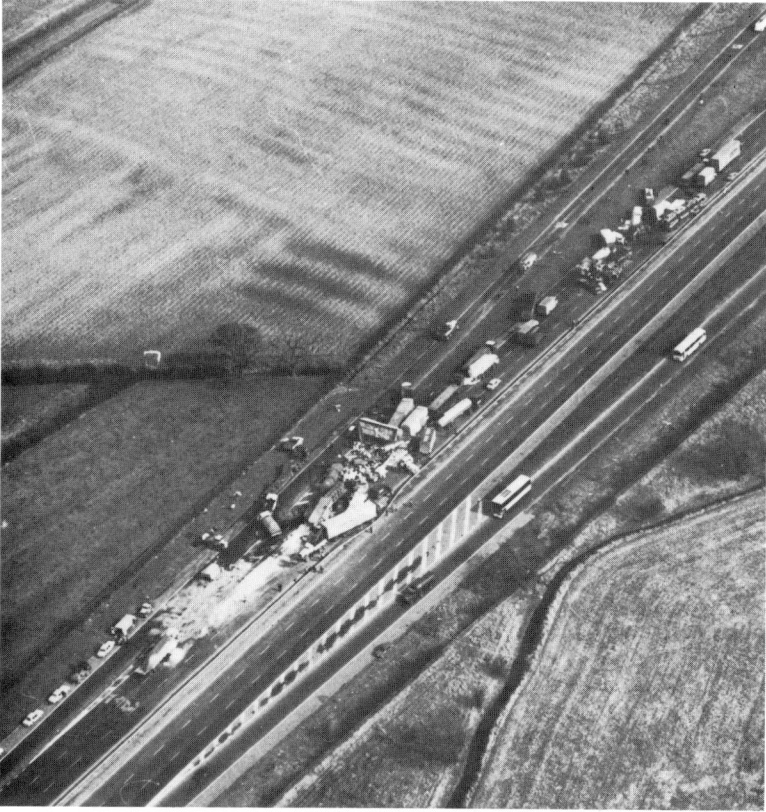

Fig. 8.1. Photograph of pile-up on the M1 as a result of fog — by permission of Aerofilms Ltd.

the motorway gets more crowded and we see more examples of concertina crashes, we know that accidents are going to increase unless something is done to educate the motorist in motorway discipline, with particular attention to distance between vehicles, especially in fog or heavy rain.

THE PLACE FOR SURGERY

William Gissane (personal communication), who was the pioneer of accident services in Great Britain, has said, 'The place for surgery is at the hospital and not at the roadside'. This was after having tried a well-equipped mobile theatre (a converted bus) for a considerable period of time. The main reasons were the delay that resulted in getting the patient to hospital, and the cost in time and money keeping personnel at the ready. For much the same reasons J C Scott (personal communication) gave up the mobile surgical theatre based on the Oxford Accident Service after an eighteen month trial. As more senior doctors became interested enough to go to the scene of an accident, this policy of avoiding surgery at the accident site has become firmly established in urban areas, and attention has shifted from the mobile theatre to the establishment of the doctor's role at the roadside, improvements in the design of the ambulance and adequate ambulance personnel training. Most people agree that ambulancemen feel more confident when they see a senior consultant is with them, particularly when the consultant has helped in their training. The need for amputations of trapped limbs has gone since the introduction of rapid cold cutting equipment has speeded up the release of these victims.

The needs for crowded urban areas involving short distances differ considerably from the requirements for large country areas. In the first place, ambulances in areas of dense population always arrive within a few minutes of the call. Secondly, the doctor's car may fail to get through roads that can be blocked solidly by stationary cars. In 1955 there was a train crash at the Luton railway station. It was announced on the radio and several consultants set out from the hospital only to find that the roads were blocked for a distance of half a mile. Since then the doctors have always travelled by ambulance or police car. Thirdly, in 50 per cent of accidents there is no necessity for a doctor to be present, and it is the practice at Luton to pay attention to the alert and wait for the request for help by radio. Where the M1 passes through Luton, conditions on this road are such that it would be dangerous and foolish for anyone from hospital to try and get to the accident on his own.

For these reasons the Accident Service at the Luton and Dunstable Hospital has been developed with the aim of improving the reception facilities, organising the planned work load with a view of coping with sudden rushes of activity, and designing the physical shape of the department to allow change of purpose according to needs, e.g. multipurpose rooms.

ORGANISATION OF THE ACCIDENT SERVICE

The design of the department

This was based on four basic principles:

(1) There should be enough senior staff in the department with planned out-patient sessions and short operating lists.

(2) Most of the space would be multipurpose.

(3) Facilities in the department should be designed for immediate use in accident work.

(4) General practice should not be one of the functions of the Accident Service.

Workload

The first and most important object was to accommodate a staff with senior loading and with sufficient planned work to keep all sections functioning, so that emergencies could be dealt with promptly. Thus, the surgical team dealing with admissions has two short planned lists each day, leaving time before and after each list for accidents. In the event of multiple casualties, the lists can be cancelled making two consultant surgeons, a senior anaesthetist, two senior house officers and theatre staff available at once. The second principle concerns the physical design of the Accident Service. This was originally published in the Nuffield Provincial Hospital Trust publication Casualty Services and their setting (1960). It was based on a study in depth of an accident service superimposed on a surgical (orthopaedic) department with planned out-patient appointments and operative sessions (Fig. 8.2). Thirdly, the plan included features which had been agreed by all as essential, yet seldom included, in the accident department, such as adequate X-ray facilities in the reception area. In the cleansing theatre there is enough room for the many experts required to help in the resuscitation, assessment and definitive treatment of the patient with multiple injuries. The consulting area, where minor injuries and orthopaedic problems are dealt with, has been fitted with examination cubicles which can be used for the reception of major accidents — another example of a multipurposes design which has proved itself in several M1 pile-ups.

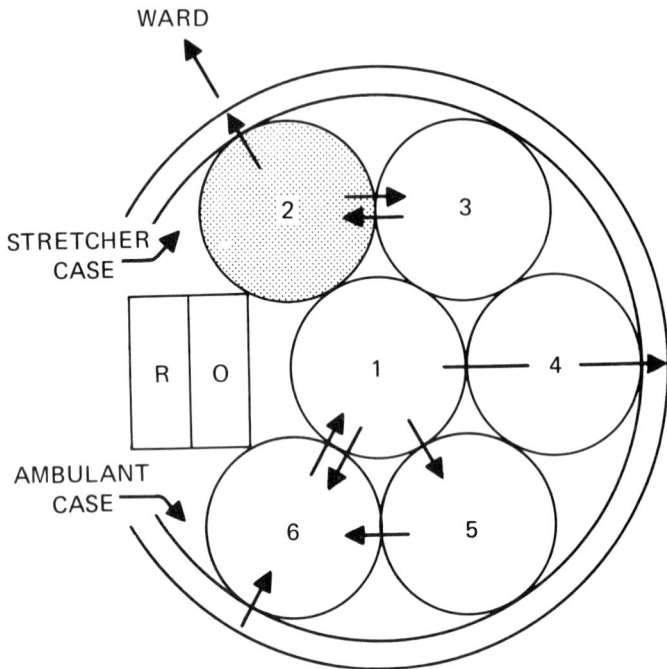

Fig. 8.2. The cluster plan for Accident Service:

R Reception—multipurpose; register stretcher and ambulant cases; keep records; type letters; make return appointments; Ambulance Officer kiosk.

O Office—for surgeon; for sister.

1 Consulting room; twin desk; curtained multipurpose cubicles, one room to be soundproofed; multiple gadgets; no steriliser.

2 Multipurpose for cleansing; resuscitation; anaesthesia; recovery. Semicubicled couches; piped gases; ceiling or wall mounted X-ray; open cupboards; additional exit to ward.

3 Theatre suite without sterilising equipment, recovery and anaesthetic rooms adjacent—prepacked units for soft tissue and bone.

4 Dressings and injection room; prepacked sterilised supplies—curtained cubicles; exit around X-ray to waiting room.

5 X-ray unit with automatic X-ray processing; finishing line opening into 1.

6 Multipurpose waiting room without canteen. Service corridor around periphery.

Function

The function of a modern department requires clear definition. It should not be cluttered with patients with minor complaints and ailments which could be treated much better by the family doctor. Not only is this type of work undemanding on staff who will be expected to work to a quite different pace from time to time, but the whole tempo and morale fails to reach a high level. An active policy of discouraging these casual attenders from coming to the accident service has been successful in keeping the rate of general practice to below 1 per cent. It can only be done by determined consultants who are working full time in the department. A junior casualty officer will not make much impression in solving this problem, and his successors may not be interested enough to try.

Rationalisation

To maintain a high standard there must, of course, be sufficient clinical material to keep a well-trained staff extended (i.e. a population of 250 000 or more). This means rationalisation of services, particularly in dense urban areas. There are many casualty departments struggling to maintain a service in competition with nearby hospitals, whose management committees either cannot understand the need for combining with their neighbours or refuse to consider shutting down a small, inefficient service because of the public outcry against such proposals. The fact that such rationalisation can be done smoothly was demonstrated very adequately in Bradford, to the Accident Services Review Committee (BMA, 1970). A well planned public relations operation prepared the people of Bradford for the closure of three separate small casualty receiving rooms and the establishment of one large, good accident department. When the operation was completed the public knew they were going to get better diagnosis and treatment and willingly put up with the extra travel involved.

Accident work is sporadic and although a certain number of daily return appointments can be planned, the average department catering for a population of a quarter to half a million will not have sufficient work to warrant the appointment of three full time (or maxium part-time) consultants, the minimum necessary for a twenty-four hour service. A basic turnover of surgical work, both consultative and operative, is therefore necessary to provide a steady background of routine planned work, against which a sudden rush of emergencies can be fitted in without difficulty. A major disaster commands the undivided attention of all personnel and the previously prepared schedule is cancelled immediately. The resulting inconvenience to patients with appointments and planned operations are accepted by most people when the reasons are adequately explained. At Luton it has been shown that as many as twenty-seven people with multiple injuries can be dealt with after a pile-up on the motorway.

Planning

All accident services have a plan for dealing with major disasters. This plan will provide for mobilisation of hospital resources and prevent the known bottlenecks, i.e. access to the disaster site, reception at the accident service and excessive pressure on the telephone exchange (see Fig. 8.3). It should also include arrangements for cooperation by nearby general hospitals and special units.

It is improbable that any worthwhile emergency scheme can be planned on paper and then be expected to work without modification. The present plan for motorway accidents at Luton has undergone considerable modification since 1959, when the first eighty miles of the M1 were opened. A call for help would then be answered by an SHO getting into any convenient vehicle with an assorted collection of surgical and anaesthetic equipment, and arriving at the scene of the accident with little idea of his objectives. All too frequently his nerve was shattered by the devastation he saw and the realisation that he was unable to use the skills he had learnt once he was removed from the calm and space of his normal working environment; he was frequently kept at the scene of the accident for several hours with nothing specific to do, whilst his parent unit was left uncovered. The first lesson learnt was that for every trapped casualty there were seven or eight untrapped who would be taken to hospital and would need urgent treatment there; for this reason we have a rule that under no circumstances must anyone go to the accident unless the accident service is left with adequate medical cover.

Objectives

The objectives of the doctor at the scene of the accident must be clearly established at the outset:

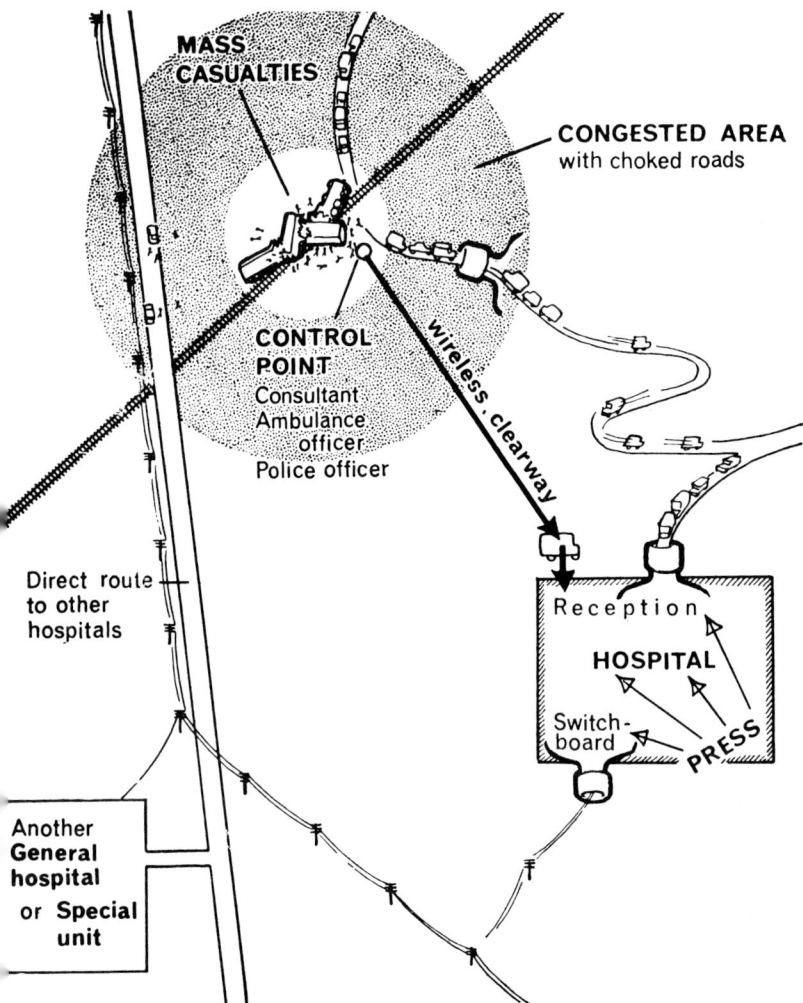

MASS CASUALTIES

CONGESTED AREA
with choked roads

CONTROL POINT
Consultant
Ambulance
officer
Police officer

wireless clearway

Direct route
to other
hospitals

Reception

HOSPITAL

Switch-
board

PRESS

Another
General
hospital
or Special
unit

Accident Service organisation
To show the inevitable traffic congestion around accident, difficulty of telephone communication—usual bottleneck at reception at hospital, special accommodation for Press, direct route from accident site to alternative hospitals, alternative communication by wireless.

Fig. 8.3. *Plan for major disasters, from* Accident Service *(1966) by permission of Pitman Medical Publishing Co Ltd.*

(1) He must not get in the way—the ambulance and fire services are adept at rescue and first aid, and an untrained doctor may often interfere with their work. He must regard himself as complementary to their work and not try to direct it. This problem will be eased if rescue and medical personnel have opportunities for discussion and combined training.

(2) The doctor's main role is the relief of pain which will assist in the removal of the casualty from the vehicle. The introduction of Entonox has made this task much simpler. Intravenous or intra-muscular analgesics may be hazardous or may interfere with the diagnosis of intra-abdominal injury after release.

(3) Management of the obstructed airway is of prime consideration and much of the equipment carried by the doctor is particularly directed to this end.

(4) Resuscitation may be possible before release but on many occasions cannot be started until after removal from the vehicle. The difficulties which are encountered when attempting such a simple procedure as a venepuncture when only part of a limb is accessible, make one appreciate that setting up of a drip in wind, rain or cold may be quite impossible.

(5) Information should be sent to the base hospital about the problems that will be sent in and the numbers of patients that have yet to be released. This enables a plan to be made and allows time for preparation of theatres and beds.

(6) Those brought up on service lines or who worked in the FMAU (Forward Medical Aid Unit) will remember principles of 'triage'. We have found that under motorway conditions setting priorities in this way is quite impossible—the impaction of one vehicle into another means that victims can only be released in turn, regardless of severity of injury. After release it may be necessary to decide on priority of removal to hospital but usually, by this stage, sufficient ambulances are available.

WORK IN THE ACCIDENT DEPARTMENT

Stage I   Fifteen to thirty minutes after accident

Arrival of five to fifteen lightly injured. These may be brought in by ambulances or in private cars. This is usually the first indication that there has been a major accident, and often the first warning of the magnitude of the incident will be given by the ambulance drivers bringing the patients in.

Stage II   Thirty to sixty minutes after accident

After initial confusion some form of order has been established, documentation of patients has been completed and treatment commenced. This usually coincides with the arrival of the first few seriously injured casualties and, at this stage, there is usually a request for medical assistance at the scene of the accident.

Stage III   One to four hours after accident

A steady flow of serious casualties and the first detailed assessment of the situation by police, ambulance and the medical officer at the scene of the accident. By this time the major accident plan has really got under way, the police will have arrived to set up an information centre, enquiries from press and radio will start to come in and the organisation of operating lists, and reorganisation of work in other departments of the hospital will have been established.

PROVISION OF A COMPREHENSIVE ACCIDENT SERVICE

The Accident Service Review Committee, since its inception in 1960, has produced two reports containing proposals for a comprehensive accident service. Since then a working party, set up to review progress in the service, reported their findings in September 1970 (BMA). Their main conclusion was that progress in the provision of accident services from 1962 to 1970 was very disappointing. So far only one of the working party's proposals has been implemented—opportunity has been given for many senior casualty officers to achieve consultant status. Up to August 1973, forty-five senior casualty officers had been appointed consultant in charge of accident and emergency departments. There are probably not many more individuals in the field with adequate experience and of suitable calibre to fill further posts of this kind. The Department of Health is now planning the establishment of training posts of Senior Registrar status in this new specialty, but there are no signs yet of any urgency.

The decision of the Department of Health to appoint consultants in charge of accident and emergency departments was in no small measure due to the enthusiasm and persistence of the Casualty Surgeons Association. The members of this association are determined to upgrade the casualty department to an accident and emergency department, with a standard of work at least equal to that of more established specialties. The Association was formed in 1967 and has regular meetings about organisation and to discuss clinical papers. The attendance rate is exceptionally high. The Association is pressing the Department of Health to get on with the training programme at senior registrar level for young surgeons who wish to make a career in the accident and emergency specialty.

Ambulance personnel training

Although all ambulance attendants receive basic training on joining the service, it is very broad and in the main theoretical. The accident and emergency department must, of necessity, work in close cooperation with ambulance personnel, and the medical staff in that department are probably the ones most fitted to assist in advanced training.

All ambulance personnel should have the opportunity to work in accident and emergency departments to widen their knowledge and to make them appreciate that they are the first link in a long chain leading to patients' eventual recovery. Frequent short discussions on selected subjects can widen the knowledge of the attendants and allow the interchange of information. Admission to the operating theatre will enable them to practise the techniques of pharangeal toilet, insertion of oro-pharangeal airways and the use of an Ambu bag on a paralysed patient. This not only gives them confidence in their own ability, but helps the surgeon to assess the capabilities of the attendants with whom he will work. Consideration has been given to the possibility of teaching endotracheal intubation and intravenous techniques to selected personnel, but no uniform views have so far emerged. Audiovisual teaching aids are invaluable in any training programme and every department should have access to a good slide and film library.

There is little doubt that the opportunities for discussion in these training sessions has already led to improvements in equipment and the methods of documentation throughout the ambulance service. The introduction of suction apparatus, air splints and Entonox as standard equipment is in no small measure due to the enthusiasm of trainers and trainees throughout the country.

Equipment

On some occasions more than one doctor will be needed at an accident. These doctors may well be separated by a quarter or half a mile from each other and it is essential that they each have a basic set of equipment, although supporting equipment may well be available at one central point. The equipment used at the Luton and Dunstable Hospital is carried in an Ambu Zipp bag, as shown in the photograph (Fig. 8.4). Among its contents are a small portable sucker, airways,

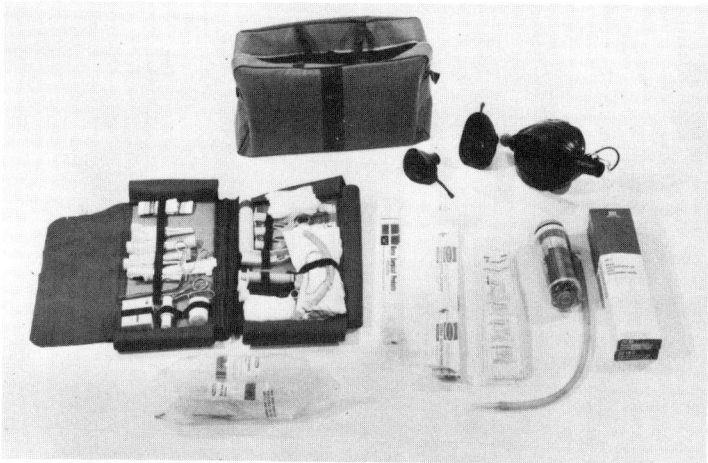

Fig. 8.4. Ambu Zipp bag. Contents include a small portable sucker, airways, endotracheal tubes, a Ferguson mouth gag, supplies of Hartmann's solution with drip sets, and Fortral ampoules.

endotracheal tubes, a Ferguson mouth gag, supplies of Hartmann's solution with drip sets, and Fortral ampoules.

Protective equipment

White boiler suits with identity flashes are provided for all personnel going to the accident. Industrial hard hats are advisable, and the need for protective footwear must be considered in view of accidents involving tankers, as well as damage to ordinary shoes from foam, oil and grit on the road surface.

REFERENCES

Accident Services Review Committee (1970), *Report of a Working Party*, September 1970, p. 24. British Medical Association.

Nuffield Provincial Hospitals Trust (1960), *Casualty Services and their setting.* London: Oxford University Press.

9

Hospital Disaster Planning

PETER SAVAGE

Disaster is an emotive word which describes events ranging from the mundane to the cataclysmic (Garb and Eng, 1969). Earthquakes, tornadoes, floods and other natural phenomena have always taken a large toll of human life, while man's activities contribute to road, rail and air crashes, explosions and structural collapses. There remain the possibilities of atomic, bacterial and chemical warfare.

While the term 'disaster' is in common usage in North America, the more phlegmatic British have favoured the words 'major accident' to describe the events to be considered in this chapter. However, recent bomb incidents in UK cities have been anything but accidental and clarification of terminology is urgently required. In this chapter I shall therefore be using the word 'disaster', and the definition of a disaster I have adopted is the arrival with little or no warning of many more casualties of all types and degrees of severity than a hospital is designed or staffed to handle at any one time (Thorpe, 1965).

The worst disasters in the United Kingdom this century occurred in 1913, when 439 miners were killed in the Caerphilly mine disaster, and in 1915 when 226 people died following a multiple train collision. Since 1951, however, most reported disasters have resulted in between 15 and 49 casualties (Table I) (Rutherford, 1973). The type of disaster a hospital may have to face depends on the hazards in its catchment area, the proximity of motorways, railway lines, airports, and the nature of local industry. In addition, all hospitals should be prepared to meet an internal disaster such as a fire, explosion or bomb threat, and although disasters on a community, regional or national scale have not occurred in the United Kingdom for many years, the eruption of urban guerilla warfare is now taking its toll of human life and limb.

247

TABLE I

The number of victims and casualties admitted to hospital following disasters in the United Kingdom 1951–71 (after Rutherford, 1973).

	Number of incidents	
Size of disaster (number of casualties)	*Total number of victims*	*Number admitted to hospital*
100+	8	1
50–99	9	3
15–49	20	17
15	5	12
Not known		9

Historical review

In 1954 the Ministry of Health issued a memorandum advising Regional Hospital Boards and Boards of Governors of Teaching Hospitals on the arrangements hospitals should make for dealing with major accidents (Ministry of Health, 1954). The main points of this memorandum were that ambulance authorities should be told which hospitals in an area were able to receive casualties; that suitable hospitals should provide mobile medical teams to go to the site of an accident; and that one doctor at a hospital should be in charge of all the medical arrangements.

These suggestions were adopted throughout the United Kingdom (Fairley, 1969; Miller, 1971). One general hospital in an area is designated the main receiving hospital, while others in the same area act in a supporting role. A doctor at the receiving hospital takes charge of the medical arrangements at the hospital, while a colleague goes to the scene of the disaster as site senior medical officer. The receiving hospital is usually responsible for sending a mobile team of doctors and nurses to the disaster scene.

Unfortunately, many hospital major accident procedures have never been adequately tested, and flaws in planning have only been revealed during an actual disaster. Many of the concepts enshrined in the Ministry of Health memorandum are now outdated and a new medical disaster policy document reflecting modern practice in disaster management is urgently required to both guide and stimulate hospitals and health authorities.

The disaster planning committee

Disaster planning is time-consuming and unpopular, and there are always more pressing demands on an individual's time and energy. Although a plan may be devised by one or two enthusiasts, an effective disaster planning committee has the advantage of bringing the corporate experience of many disciplines to bear on the problem and ensures that the committee's decisions are more likely to be accepted by those involved in making the plan work. Membership of the disaster planning committee should include representatives of all those departments which will be directly involved in organizing the hospital should a disaster occur (Table II).

The main objective of the committee is to develop the hospital disaster plan, but it should also ensure that the plan is coordinated with regional, area and district community plans. The committee should liaise with the emergency services (fire, police, ambulance, rescue), local

TABLE II

Membership of a hospital disaster planning committee.

Nursing

        Senior Nursing Officer
        Nursing Officers in charge of
                Accident and Emergency Dept
                Outpatients Dept
                Operating Theatres

Medical

        Chairman, Medical Executive Committee
        Chairman, Division of Surgery
        Disaster Coordinator
        Accident and Emergency Consultant
        Junior Medical Staff Representative

Administrative

        Hospital Administrator
        Hospital Engineer
        Head Porter

Departmental Heads

        Radiology, Laboratory, Physiotherapy, Social Workers, Medical Records, Pharmacy, Chaplain, Security /Fire Prevention Officer government departments (public health and welfare), the emergency departments of the public utilities (telephone, electricity, gas and water), general practitioners, first aid societies, the Salvation Army and organised volunteer units (WRVS, Boy Scouts, Girl Guides, Rotary, etc.), as well as with the other hospitals in the neighbourhood (American Hospital Association, 1966 and 1971; Brickson, 1968; Craig, 1969; Savage, 1971).

The design of a disaster manual

The ideal disaster manual is easily identified by a distinctive cover, and its contents should be arranged so that information may be obtained as rapidly as possible. A brief resumé provides a review of the policies and procedures to be followed should a disaster occur, and is followed by detailed annexes, appendices and action cards. All pages should be dated in the left lower corner, and a loose-leaf binding facilitates revision. Any revision requires the replacement of a whole page (Fellerman, 1969; Housley, 1972; Klinghoffer and Hughes (undated); Savage, 1976).

THE HOSPITAL

(Richardson, 1975; Rutherford, 1975; Sillar, 1974; Spencer, 1973)

The alert

Although it is usually assumed that a hospital will be alerted by one of the emergency services, this does not always happen, and the disaster plan may have to be activated from within the hospital itself by a doctor, nurse or administrator. The installation of a direct telephone line between the alerting authority (usually the ambulance service) and the hospital obviates the necessity of verifying the alerting message, otherwise it is usually wise to confirm its validity. The telephonist should obtain details of the location and nature of the disaster, the time of its occurrence and the estimated number and type of casualties, and this information should be recorded on a standard form (Chesbro, 1961; Kennedy, 1965; Vosburg, 1971).

A hospital disaster plan must be flexible enough to compensate for the completely unforseen mischance and adapt itself to the unscheduled timing and the unstructured nature of a catastrophe (Richwagen, 1967). There are many advantages in having a plan that responds in a phased manner. For example, a phase I (or green) alert mobilises staff to support the accident and emergency (A and E) department when faced with a sudden influx of a small number of casualties of limited duration. A phase II (or amber) alert mobilises personnel and resources to support both the A and E department and other areas of the hospital to deal with a number of casualties requiring inpatient care following a small scale local disaster. A phase III (or red) alert mobilises the whole hospital to meet a large scale local disaster. Completely different plans are not required for each phase, but more stages of the same plan become operational as increasing demands are made on the hospital.

Once the disaster alert has been authorised, the telephonist activates the appropriate plan. During normal working hours (working day), hospital staff may be alerted by using the bleep or public loudspeaker system, internal telephones, or by the sounding of a special siren or alarm. At night and weekends (silent hours), the majority of staff will have to be contacted at their homes. The telephonist needs two separate call out lists, depending on whether a disaster occurs when the hospital is fully or only partly staffed. Many valuable minutes may be lost in making contact with a large number of staff outside the hospital, and a pyramid notification, or fan-out system of alerting personnel has many advantages. The telephone operator alerts only the departmental heads or one of two named deputies, who in turn are responsible for informing other members of that department. Each head and his named deputies keeps an up-to-date list of the home telephone numbers of their staff on their person and in their respective offices and homes. The design of a fan-out system that includes information concerning geographical proximity of individuals and the availability of personal means of transport, allows the greatest number of staff to be alerted and to get to the hospital.

The accident and emergency department

The accident and emergency department of a hospital receiving disaster casualties must have an efficient system of 'triage' (sorting the injured), together with facilities and staff to perform life-saving procedures. The department will normally be prepared to deal with the effects of trauma, burns and acute cardiorespiratory failure, but extra supplies of drugs, dressings and equipment should be readily available to augment those kept in the department as part of the hospital disaster plan, or only when specifically requested (Brictson, 1968; Hirst and Savage, 1974; Nissan and Eldar, 1971).

The reception area

When planning the reception (Owens, 1968) of disaster victims, thoughts often turn to other parts of the hospital building which could be converted to receive patients, particularly if the existing casualty department is structurally inadequate. Generally, however, the advantages of using existing facilities far outweigh any theoretical benefit of a larger reception area. The A and E department is signposted and familiar to hospital staff and ambulancemen, and those who work in the department know where equipment and supplies are kept. The constant risk of overloading the A and E department is reduced by setting up treatment areas in other parts of the hospital, and by rapidly moving patients through existing facilities.

Casualty flow paths (Fig. 9.1) (Hacon, 1964)

In order to avoid confusion, three groups of people entering the hospital must be controlled; casualties, hospital staff and members of the public. The design of the ground floor of the building will determine to what extent these groups can be separated, but unnecessary cross-movements should be avoided. Vehicles entering the hospital grounds will need police control from the outset, and road access to the A and E department's ambulance entrance should be by a one way system.

Triage

In normal clinical practice the casualty with the most critical injury is treated first, no matter how poor the prognosis. Unfortunately this concept may not be practical in a disaster, and priority must be given to the needs of the many at the expense of the few (Debra, 1967; Fogelman, 1958; Hacon, 1964; Hight et al, 1956; Morton, 1970; Mudano, 1970; Savage, 1970; Soltis, 1960).

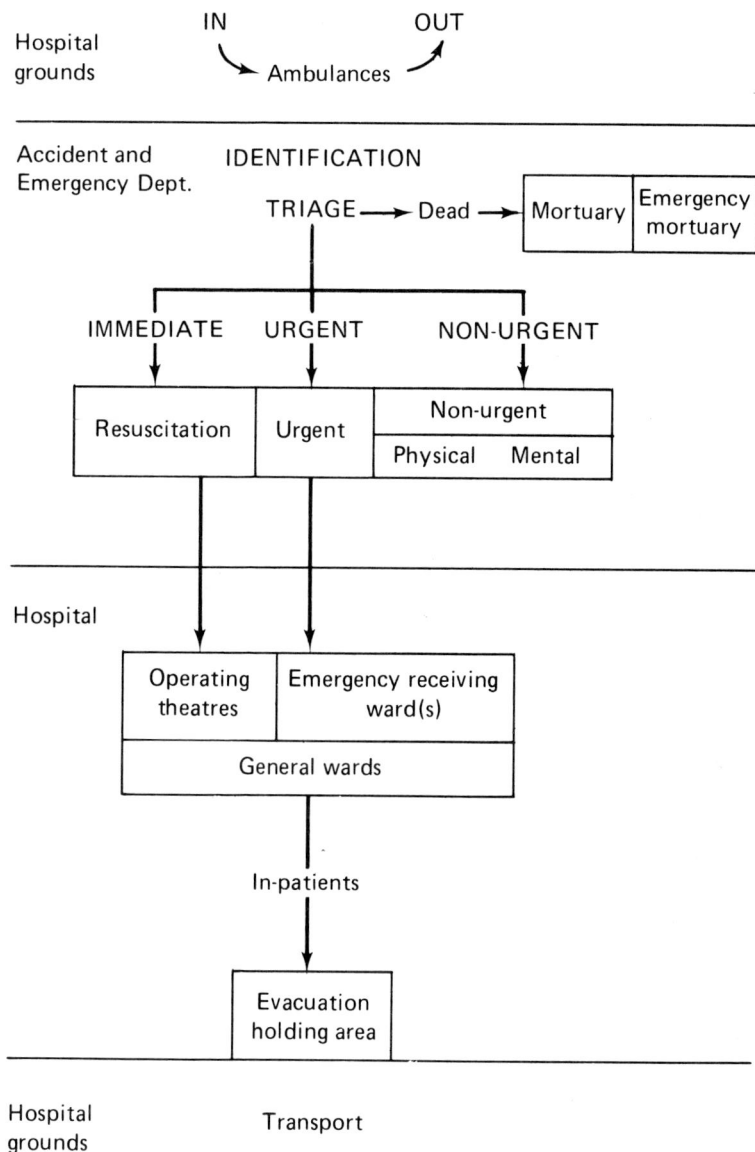

Fig. 9.1. Casualty flow patterns, emphasising the avoidance of cross-movements (after Hacon, 1964).

There are two main methods of triage. In the first method, teams of doctors and nurses examine all casualties thoroughly, carrying out initial treatment, recording diagnosis and instructions, and deciding on the casualty's eventual disposal. The second method depends on a rapid assessment of the extent and severity of the casualty's injuries by an experienced doctor (or in his absence by an experienced nurse), and the assignment of that casualty to an appropriate treatment area. The triage officer (or medical assessor) in this method is stationed at the entrance to the A and E department and does not carry out any treatment. Where the design of the department is suitable, and there are sufficient experienced staff available, triage may be performed at two entrances, one for stretcher cases, the other for walking casualties.

Many different triage classifications have been used in assessing casualties' injuries. The more detailed schemes have the advantage of greater accuracy in patient assignment, but often require an intimate knowledge of the classification by the triage officer. The simplest method of triage is to sort casualties into those that are dead and those needing immediate, urgent (delayed), non-urgent and palliative (expectant) treatment without specifying any particular criteria for their classification. (The words in parenthesis are the North American equivalent terms.)

Identification of casualties (Hospital Council of Southern California, 1972; Morton, 1970)

During a disaster all casualties entering the accident and emergency department must be immediately tagged with a numbered label kept readily available for such an emergency. Once tagged, this number identifies that casualty's property, medical records, X-rays, blood samples and cross-matched blood.

Documentation of casualties (Cashman, 1970; Elson and Eastwood, 1969; Savage, 1975; Sittin, 1964)

Accurate clinical records are particularly important during a disaster. The use of printed casualty cards or notes is common practice in many hospitals and not only allows clinical data to be recorded in a clear and precise way, but prevents duplication of investigations and treatment. A special set of consecutively numbered cards or notes should be available in the accident and emergency department together with similarly numbered pathology and radiology request forms and a plastic bag and stout envelope for the casualty's clothing and valuables.

Primary treatment areas (Jackson, 1959; Owens, 1968; Soltis, 1960)

Following triage, casualties are directed to appropriate treatment areas. Those in need of immediate life-saving measures are taken to a **resuscitation room** where facilities are available for establishing an airway, controlling haemorrhage, supporting fractures and treating shock. It is emphasised that casualties should remain in the resuscitation room for the shortest possible time, further investigations and treatment being carried out in another treatment area.

Urgent cases needing diagnosis, investigation and initial treatment of their injuries receive attention in an **urgent treatment area** which may be in the A and E department itself, in an adjacent department, or in a hospital ward or intensive therapy unit. This treatment area may also receive casualties from the resuscitation rooms and prepare them for surgery.

Non-urgent casualties may be investigated, diagnosed and treated in a **non-urgent treatment area** using any convenient part of the hospital, and they may be separated into the ambulant and non-ambulant. Report centres for patients needing tetanus prophylaxis, and those returning from the X-ray department will be useful (Caro and Irving, 1973). Special arrangements should be made to isolate those patients with minimal physical injuries but who are emotionally disturbed, and those who are so critically injured that they require only palliative treatment.

Staffing requirements in primary treatment areas

A **resuscitation team** of one doctor, two nurses and two aides may deal with 15 patients an hour, but should not be expected to look after more than 5 patients at a time. A minimum of two teams with a third relief team should be available. One **pre-op team** of a doctor, two nurses and one attendant can supervise 30 patients an hour in the urgent treatment area. Very little in the way of treatment should be required apart from the application of additional splints and dressings and the detection of shock or other serious complications. Once the emergency receiving ward is cleared and triage completed, many of these patients are transferred to await surgery. Non-urgent cases are supervised in the non-urgent treatment area by one doctor, two nurses and two aides. Casualties dying in the palliative treatment area will need medical and nursing supervision, and facilities for administering narcotics. A **transportation team** of porters and domestic staff are delegated to move furniture, set up the triage and primary treatment areas and unload special trolleys of supplies and equipment. The team also moves casualties from ambulances to the triage and other treatment areas as required. A **registration team** from the medical records department undertakes the documentation of non-urgent casualties, and collects money and valuables.

These staffing arrangements are only an initial stage in preparing to receive a number of casualties and as the pattern of the disaster unfolds, the triage officer and the disaster coordinator may redistribute medical, nursing and other staff as necessary.

Secondary treatment areas

Patients requiring in-patient care will be taken from primary treatment areas either to the operating theatre or to special **receiving wards** which have been evacuated of as many patients as possible. By designating specific wards for disaster victims, hospital staff, supplies and equipment may be concentrated in a small area of the hospital (Freni and colleagues, 1957).

An experienced surgeon acts as **operating theatre controller**, re-assessing patients as they arrive in the theatre suite, re-treating shock and supervising the pre-operative preparation of patients. He assigns each casualty to an operating team according to their talents and is available to provide advice and relief for these teams. Each **surgical team** is made up of one surgeon, one assistant surgeon, one scrub nurse, one circulating nurse (shared between two theatres if necessary), one attendant, and one anaesthetist. The number of teams naturally depends on the number of operating theatres and surgeons available, but no team should operate for longer than 12 hours, nor on major cases for more than eight hours. An anaesthetist, two nurses and two aides form a **recovery team** to supervise the postoperative recovery of patients after anaesthesia.

Emergency admissions are cared for by **casualty teams** of one doctor, four trained nurses, four student nurses and two aides, each team being in charge of 20 patients, while patients already in the hospital are looked after by **in-patient teams** of one doctor, three trained nurses, two student nurses and two aides, each team being in charge of 25 patients.

Medical management of disaster victims

In a disaster (Berlin, 1974; Trauma Research Group (undated)) there may come a stage when the number of casualties needing medical attention exceeds the facilities available to such an extent that normal standards of care have to be temporarily abandoned. An efficient system of triage ensures that those patients whose medical condition is most critical receive more attention than those whose injuries are not so severe. It is part of the duties of the disaster planning committee to lay down guidelines on medical management. Clear instructions should indicate how a large number of burned patients are to be managed, which intravenous fluid is to be given to treat shock, and the indications for blood transfusions. Radiological and biochemical investigations will need to be limited, and a decision made on whether wounds are to be closed or left for delayed primary suture, and how tetanus prophylaxis is to be carried out.

Personnel

The services of everyone working in a hospital may be called on during a disaster. The majority of individuals, while performing tasks with which they are familiar, will need to know where and to whom they report for instructions. Some members of the staff have special duties and their explicit written instructions can take the form of action cards which have been drawn up in advance. Only a few senior members of the medical, nursing and administrative staff need to have intimate knowledge of the overall disaster plan.

Actions cards

An action card (Hirst and Savage, 1974; Savage, 1972; Thomas, 1969) incorporates written information, advice and instructions. Some cards may be kept on permanent display while others are immediately available to be handed to individuals should a disaster occur. Standard 4 × 6 in (10 × 15 cm) cards are a convenient size, and different coloured cards may help to differentiate between instructions for various grades of staff working in the same department.

The disaster coordinator

One individual has overall control of a hospital during a disaster, and he may be a senior member of either the medical or administrative staff who will usually be the chairman of the disaster planning committee. Senior representatives of the medical, nursing and administrative staff, together with their assistants, should work from a control centre.

The control centre (Fig. 9.2)

The control centre should be a suitable room situated close to the accident and emergency department, the main entrance of the hospital and the wards, without being in the actual front line. It is an advantage to have a number of adjacent rooms available to serve as report and information centres, and all rooms must have adequate communication facilities.

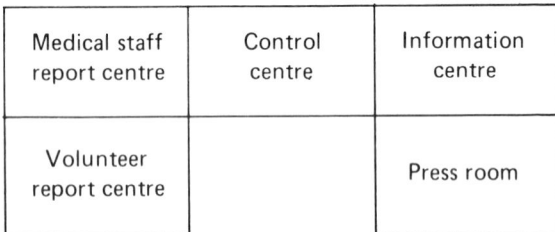

Medical staff report centre	Control centre	Information centre
Volunteer report centre		Press room

Fig. 9.2. Control centre and adjacent offices.

Medical staff (Fig. 9.3)

The initial medical response will depend upon on-duty resident medical staff supported by on-duty consultant staff. Provided an efficient

Disaster coordinator

A and E Director	Duty Consultant Gynaecologist	Duty Consultant Anaesthetist	Duty Consultant Surgeon	Duty Consultant Physician	Off-duty Medical staff
					Medical staff report centre
	Receiving ward	ITU/Theatre	Operating Theatre Controller	Trouble shooter	
Triage Officer					
			Surgical teams		
On-duty Junior Staff					

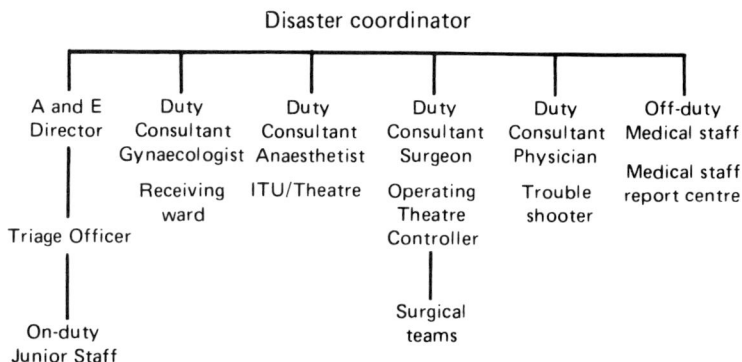

Fig. 9.3. Medical staff organisation.

casualty management plan is in operation, there is a danger of having too many doctors rushing to the A and E department. At the alert, all on-duty junior staff report to the A and E department where they are given action cards deploying them to predetermined treatment areas. The most experienced doctor acts as **triage officer**. On-duty consultant staff also report to the A and E department, but after making sure that the plan is operating smoothly, each consultant has his own area of responsibility. The A and E or orthopaedic consultant acts as the **A and E director** coordinating and directing all activities in the department, advising medical staff on clinical matters and generally trying to bring order out of chaos. The duty consultant gynaecologist takes charge of the receiving ward, while the duty consultant anaesthetist supervises casualties awaiting surgery. The duty consultant surgeon acts as **operating theatre controller** arranging operating lists depending on the degree of urgency of individual cases, and the experience of the surgical teams available. The duty consultant physician could take the role of **'troubleshooter'**, visiting all parts of the hospital identifying and helping to solve any particular problem, while generally giving advice and encouragement.

Nursing staff (Fig. 9.4)

The nursing administration is responsible for allocating nursing staff, initially to the accident and emergency department and primary treatment areas, and subsequently to the receiving wards and the

Senior Nursing
Officer

| Nursing Officer Nursing report centre | Sister Emergency receiving ward(s) | Sister Operating theatres | Sister A and E Dept. |

Off-duty nursing staff

Sisters General wards

Sister OPD

Nursing members of Mobile Medical Team

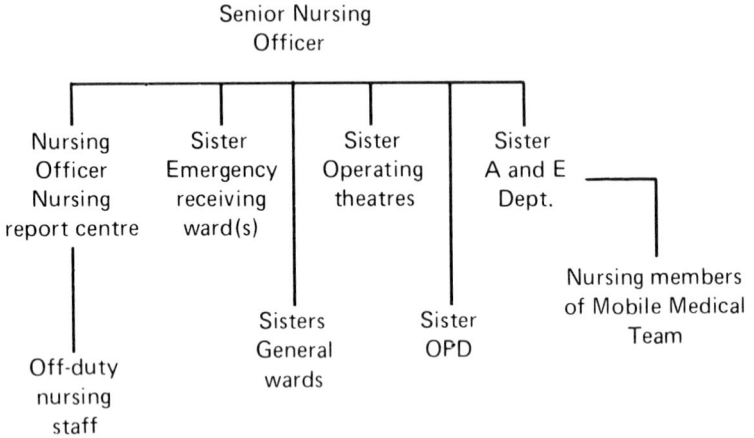

Fig. 9.4. Nursing staff organisation.

operating theatres. General wards will have to remain adequately staffed, and extra nurses may be required to supervise those patients being discharged home or transferred to other hospitals. Nurses on duty should remain at their posts to await instructions, while off-duty nurses report to nursing administration.

Administrative staff (Fig. 9.5) (Thorpe, 1965)

The hospital administrator has many areas of responsibility during a disaster. Extra medical **supplies** of dressings, drugs, anaesthetic agents, oxygen, special kits of equipment, extra beds and trolleys may be required both in the treatment areas and in the wards. Emergency sources of water and electricity should be secured, and space allocated for storing extra supplies. Visitors and hospital personnel will need food and other refreshments.

Alternative means of communication to the hospital switchboard must be readily available including ex-directory lines, public telephones, radio telephones (Hall and Garden, 1967), walkie-talkies (Glaub, 1960; Rowe, 1967), and the use of messengers. Intercoms between the control centre, the triage point and the operating theatre will be useful, and telephone jack plugs should be installed in areas where extra telephones are needed.

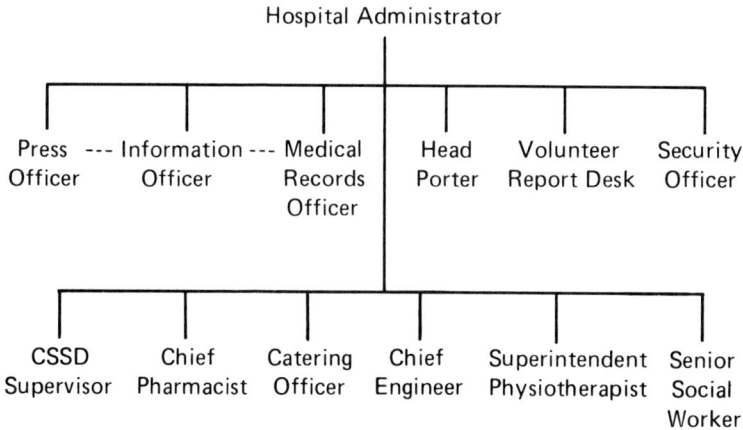

Fig. 9.5. *Departments and individuals responsible to the hospital administrator during a disaster.*

Pedestrian and vehicular **traffic** must be controlled both inside the hospital building and in the hospital grounds, and previously prepared signs will be needed to indicate the route to selected areas of the hospital. The **security** of both personal and hospital property requires supervision, and the assistance of the police may be necessary (Colette, 1968). Auxiliary sources of **transport** should be organised to bring members of the hospital staff from their homes, and to transfer patients to other hospitals.

All hospital **personnel** need to know their duties during a disaster, and the methods of calling in off-duty staff, the means by which they travel to hospital, the post to which they report, and the allocation of their tasks must be recorded in the disaster manual. **Identification** of non-uniformed employees is desirable. The hospital clergy and social workers have a valuable part to play, while volunteers need identification and direction to areas where their assistance will be most useful.

The **documentation** of casualties, both dead and alive, and the preparation of casualty lists requires special attention. The failure of emergency services and hospitals to provide early and accurate casualty lists is often criticised by the general public, and the prompt publishing of an official list of survivors is an important step in allaying concern.

If the hospital has an internal disaster, the **evacuation** of patients must be provided for.

Many of the hospital administrator's duties will be undertaken by his assistants and heads of departments who will individually be responsible for detailing the duties of employees working under them within the general framework of the disaster plan. However, three special administrative posts need to be created. The **hospital information officer** works with the police in the information centre and should be provided with secretarial assistance and an adequate number of telephones. Information about admissions will be channelled through this office to form the basis of casualty lists. The **volunteer report centre officer** organizes those who come to the hospital to volunteer their services, while a **press officer** who understands the problems and is sympathetic to the needs of press reporters, presides over the press room which should also have adequate telephone facilities.

THE DISASTER SCENE
(Fairley, 1969; Kennedy, 1962; Snook, 1975; Spencer, 1962)

All areas of the United Kingdom now have standard community plans whereby the senior police officer becomes the incident officer and co-ordinates all aspects of the rescue work at the site (Fig. 9.6).

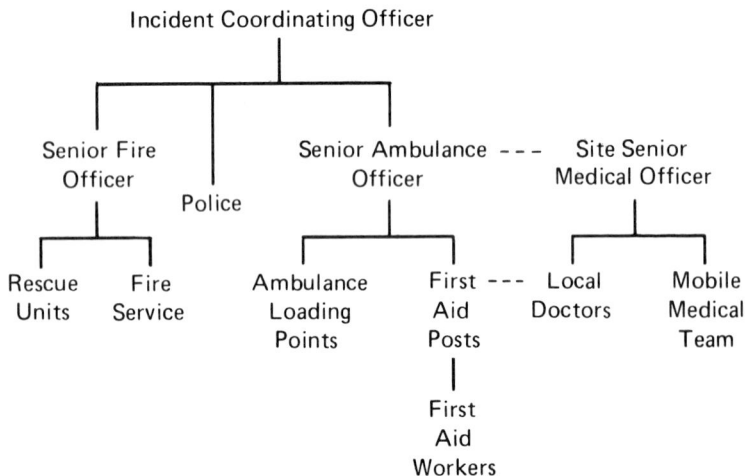

Fig. 9.6. Personnel control at the scene of a disaster.

Usually each of the three emergency services (fire, police and ambulance) will send their own identifiable control vehicle. Each of the emergency services is responsible for a particular part of the rescue operation although these duties often overlap. The fire service is responsible for rescue work and the police for controlling traffic and crowds. The ambulance service provides first aid and transport for the injured, and it is to the ambulance control vehicle that medical, nursing and first aid personnel should report. The responsibility of making the decision that an accident has reached the proportions of a disaster in terms of the number of casualties falls upon the ambulance service. The dispatcher at ambulance headquarters must have clearly defined instructions on which to act, and whether this depends on an estimate of the number of injured, or on the number of ambulances sent to the scene will vary from area to area. Once a disaster has been declared, hospitals and other relevant agencies are alerted, and a special disaster programme is instituted at the site.

Site senior medical officer

The main responsibility of the site senior medical officer (von Guyerz, 1974) is one of liaison between the emergency services and the local hospitals. He should be a senior doctor who is not only familiar with the community and hospital disaster plans, but is known personally to the senior members of the three emergency services. Although there is no place for the site senior medical officer to undertake clinical care of casualties, he should be immediately available to advise on methods of dealing with particular clinical problems, especially the extrication of trapped victims. To this end he must be equipped with a portable radio so that he may be contacted anywhere on the site. This radio together with protective clothing is best supplied from the ambulance control vehicle.

Mobile medical teams

The contribution of hospital doctors and nurses at the scene of a disaster continues to be questioned (Aston, 1969; Holloway and Stolfi, 1972; Rowe, 1967; Savage, 1976; Shaftan, 1962; Snook, 1975; Spencer, 1962). Although their presence is of great help and comfort not only to the injured victims, but also to the rescuers, these members of the medical and nursing professions, inexperienced in mass casualty care, are often more useful back at the hospital working in a familiar environment. Study of many different disaster plans reveals that two different roles are often envisaged for the medical team. The first role continues the tradition of the casualty clearing station with doctors and nurses being transported to the disaster scene accompanied by a variable number of large hampers filled with every conceivable item of equipment. In their second role, the team functions in effect as a resuscitation and amputation squad, carrying only the minimum amount of equipment necessary to assist in the extrication of trapped casualties. Whichever role the mobile team is expected to fill, their efficient operation demands that they be suitably equipped, trained and organised if they are to handle a disaster situation adequately. Medical and nursing staff need waterproof clothing and footwear and protective helmets. All clothing should be clearly marked to identify the wearer, and personal identity cards are often desirable. Disaster equipment should be in readily usable and transportable form, with prepacked sterile dressings, drugs for injection in syringe form with needle attached, and other supplies arranged in functional units.

The ambulance service

To the ambulance service falls perhaps one of the greatest challenges of a disaster. It will usually be obvious to the first ambulance crew whether the accident qualifies as a disaster. Once this fact is recognised, ambulance headquarters are informed by radio, and a special disaster programme is instituted. The major points of this programme are carried out by the first ambulance crew on the scene. The ambulance crew is suitably positioned to indicate to other ambulances the site of the **ambulance loading point;** the ambulance crew carry out a strict **triage** on all casualties brought to them; and as other ambulances arrive, casualties are loaded in order of priority, and are taken to different hospitals in the area, thus **spreading the load.** To carry out this programme ambulance crews will need special training (Sanders, 1956). With the arrival of more senior ambulance officers and the ambulance control vehicle, the first crew and their ambulance is released for general duties.

Spreading the casualty load

The key to disaster management lies in spreading the casualty load both in space and time. All hospitals in an area will be able to indicate how many patients of varying degrees of injury their accident and emergency department can cope with during the first half hour of a disaster, and with prior knowledge of these facts, the ambulance service can distribute casualties in such a way that overloading the facilities of one particular hospital is minimised, if not completely avoided.

Communications

Failure of communication (Allenbaugh, 1972) is a recurring problem in all disasters. With the technology of the 1970s it is possible to connect a radio link with a telephone switchboard enabling someone using a hospital telephone to speak with ambulance control, an ambulance vehicle, or even an individual with a portable radio at the disaster site. Nothing less than this degree of sophistication is acceptable if confusion is to be avoided.

THE PSYCHOLOGICAL EFFECTS OF A DISASTER

The psychological effects of a disaster (Allerton, 1964; Bennet, 1973; Farber, 1967; Glass, 1959; McGonagle, 1964; Shader, 1965) on victims, rescuers and hospital staff are often misunderstood or completely ignored. There are many everyday situations where individuals put their health and life at risk, but anxiety about these events is minimised by denying the possibility of disaster occurring. When the impossible happens, anxiety is replaced by fear, and the degree to which this effects an individual's behaviour will depend on a number of factors. These include the extent of previous preparation and training, the duration of warning before the disaster occurs, the levels of communication before, during and after the event, and the quality of leadership available.

Following a disaster, 10–25 per cent of victims are fairly calm, 50–80 per cent behave in a 'normal' dazed manner, while 10–25 per cent act in a confused, anxious somewhat hysterical fashion often associated with purposeless physical activity. All that is required for the majority of victims demonstrating the physiological response to fear is sympathetic individual support. Some individuals will be severely affected by the impact of their emotional experience and will complain of nausea and vomiting. If feasible they should be given a simple routine job to do, or made comfortable to await specialist medical attention. Occasionally a victim will appear to be emotionally numbed, standing or sitting silently without movement, and failing to show any emotional response. Others may overreact, be argumentative, talk rapidly and make endless suggestions.

It is important for planners to recognise that these psychological disturbances may be found in treating as well as treated individuals, and that under conditions of stress that abound in disaster situations, there are the 'acting' individuals who are best suited to carrying out familiar tasks, and the 'thinking and planning' individuals whose judgement is not compromised. The emotional response of an individual is not related to his intelligence or seniority.

INTERNAL DISASTERS

All hospital disaster plans should include sections for dealing with a disaster befalling the hospital itself.

Fire and explosion

The effects of fire in a hospital (Caunt, 1962) are minimised by the structural design of the building, and the provision of doors to limit the spread of smoke. Fire drills should be a regular feature of hospital life for all grades of staff.

Should evacuation of part or all the building be necessary, a standard procedure is required for both the horizontal movement of patients from an area of danger to one of safety on the same floor, and for the vertical evacuation of patients, usually down to street level. A roll call of all patients involved in an evacuation is mandatory. Emergency lighting must be provided in case of electric power failure to all or part of the building.

Bomb threat

If a hospital receives a bomb threat (Berlow, 1968), special note is made of the caller's emotional state in trying to assess how genuine the threat is, together with any background sounds that may help in identifying the location of the caller. If the exact site of the bomb is not given, a search must be made of the whole building. There is nothing to be gained by trying to keep secret the fact that there has been a bomb threat, and by searching the area in which they work, nursing staff will immediately recognise any unusual or unfamiliar object. Once a possible bomb has been identified, the immediate area must be evacuated, power, gas and fuel lines leading to the danger area turned off, and guards placed outside the danger zone until police experts have dealt with the device.

SPECIAL PROBLEMS OF CIVIL DISORDER

(Crosby, 1967; Frank et al, 1969)

During a riot, the number of people injured and seeking medical attention may reach disaster proportions and a receiving hospital will need to take special precautions to protect hospital staff and property from attack. Casualties reaching the hospital may not only include rival factions but also injured members of the police and security forces to whom the general feeling may be one of antagonism. These groups need to be separated in the treatment areas. When crowd control gases have been used, care must be taken that casualties whose clothes are saturated with the gas are not admitted to an enclosed space until they have been undressed and hosed down with water.

DISASTER EXERCISES

(Brua and Allman, 1962; Campanale, 1963 and 1964; Engelmohr, 1963; Housley, 1972; Kennedy, 1962; Letournean, 1962; Rieman, 1972; Thompson, 1969)

There is only one way of knowing whether a disaster plan works, and that is by testing it in a real or simulated disaster. Although a full scale disaster exercise is an invaluable experience, it is usually an expensive, unpopular and time consuming event. Fortunately other exercises and drills produce almost as much information on the effectiveness of a disaster plan. The main attribute needed by a designer of disaster exercises is imagination, and considerable planning may be necessary to test all aspects of a plan. Reports in the national and local press will provide many examples of accidents that could form the basis of an exercise.

Paper drills are carried out in discussion groups, and take place either 'off-site' in any convenient room, or 'on-site' in their normal geographical setting (e.g. wards, accident and emergency department, control centre, etc.). The number of individuals or specialist groups taking part will vary, as will the degree of complexity of the drill which may last 30 minutes or a complete day. In a paper drill, a disaster situation is outlined and individuals are invited to describe how they and their departments would respond.

A more authentic exercise makes use of simulated casualties, either labelled with their diagnosis, or actively acting the symptoms and signs of their injuries. These exercises can be limited to one part of the hospital, usually the accident and emergency department. The extension of this type of exercise is the full scale hospital or community exercise in which all the emergency services take part. In these larger exercises an element of surprise is important together with as much realism as possible.

The most valuable part of an exercise is the 'critique' at which all actions and responses are examined to see what changes need to be made in the disaster plan. The critique can be carried out immediately after a paper drill or later the same day after a small scale exercise, but for larger hospital or community exercises, or after a real disaster, 7–10 days should elapse to allow the emotional impact to settle before the behaviour and actions of individuals and departments are examined.

REFERENCES

Allenbaugh (1972, Emergency radios restore order to chaos, *Hospitals*, **46**, 60.

Allerton (1964), Mass casualty care and human behaviour, *Med. Ann. Distr. Columbia*, **33**, 206.

American Hospital Association (1971), *Principles of Disaster Preparedness for Hospitals*. American Hospital Association, 840 North Lake Shore Drive, Chicago, Ill. 60611.

American Hospital Association (1966), *Readings in Disaster Planning for Hospitals*. American Hospital Association, 840 North Lake Shore Drive, Chicago, Ill. 60611.

Aston (1969), Road accidents and the family doctor. Equipment for use at roadside accidents, Brit. med. J., **4**, 214.

Bennet (1973), Community Disaster in Britain, in *The Year Book of Social Policy in Britain*, Ed. Jones. London: Routledge and Kegan Paul.

Berlin (1974), The role of the medical services, in *A Guide to Disaster Management*, Ed. Sillar. Glasgow: Action for Disaster.

Berlow (1968), What to do when you get a bomb threat, *Mod. Hosp.*, **111**, 89.

Brictson (1968), The Organization of Medical Services to Cope with Disaster, System Development Corporation, 2500 Colorado Ave., Santa Monica, California, 90406.

Brua and Allman (1962), The value of frequent realistic exercises in disaster control, *Milit. Med.*, **127**, 505.

Campanale (1963), Realism in disaster exercises—a true challenge, *Milit. Med.*, **128**, 418.

Campanale (1964), Surprise realistic mock disasters, *Calif. Med.*, **101**, 435.

Caro and Irving (1973), The Old Bailey bomb explosion, *Lancet*, **i**, 1433.

Cashman (1970), Recording major trauma, *Injury*, **2**, 11.

Caunt (1962), A mental hospital disaster plan, *Ment. Hosps.*, **13**, 414.

Chesbro (1961), Disaster medical care. The basic hospital disaster plan, *Calif. Med.* **95**, 371.

Colette, M. (1968), Direction during disaster, *Am. J. Nurs.*, **68**, 2145.

Craig (1969), Establishing an effective disaster planning committee, *Hosp. Forum*, **12**, 15.

Crosby (1967), AHA memorandum on riot preparedness, *Hospitals*, **41**, 114.

DeBra (1967), Disaster at Cam Ranh Bay in Viet Nam, *Mod. Hosp.*, **108**, 88.

Elson and Eastwood (1969), Documentation for a major incident, *Br. med. J.*, **1**, 38.

Engelmohr (1963), How well are hospitals prepared for mass disaster *Hospitals*, **37**, 35.

Fairley (1969), Mass disaster schemes, *Br. med. J.*, **4**, 551.

Farber (1967), Psychological aspects of mass disaster, *J. natn. med. Ass.*, **59**, 340.

Fellerman (1969), Reorganising hospital disaster plan to facilitate reference and revision, *Hosp. Topics*, **47**, 44.

Fogelman (1958), The Dallas tornado disaster, *Am. J. Surg.*, **95**, 501.

Frank, Roth, Wolfe and Metzger (1969), Medical problems of civil disorders, *New Engl. J. Med.*, **280**, 247.

Freni, Twomey and Killoran (1957), Medical aspects of the Swampscott train-wreck disaster, *New Engl. J. Med.*, **257**, 408.

Garb and Eng (1969), *Disaster Handbook*. 2nd Edition. New York: Springer.

Glass (1959), Psychological aspects of disaster, *J. Am. med. Ass.*, **171**, 222.

Glaub (1960), Walkie-talkies in the disaster kit, *Hospitals*, **34**, 48.

Greyerz von (1974), The doctor at the disaster site, in *A Guide to Disaster Management*, Ed. Sillar. Glasgow: Action for Disaster.

Hacon (1964), It can happen here, *Can. Nurse Hosp. Rev.*, **60**, 972.

Hall and Garden (1967), Radio-communication and the emergency department, *Br. med. J.*, **3**, 170.

Hight, Brodgett, Croce, Horne, McKoan and Whelan (1956), Medical aspects of the Worcester tornado disaster, *New Engl. J. Med.*, **254**, 267.

Hirst and Savage (1974), Disaster planning. A guide for accident and emergency departments, *Nursing Times*, **70**, 186.

Holloway and Stolfi (1972), Mobile vans as disaster scene emergency rooms, *Hospitals*, **46**, 43.

Hospital Council of Southern California (1972), Patient identification tag, *Hospitals*, **46**, 65.

Housley (1972), Assignment specifications facilitate disaster planning, *Hosp. Prog.*, **53**, 78.

Jackson (1959), The story of operation 'Prep. Pitt.', *J. Am. med. Ass.*, **169**, 361.

Kennedy (1962), Disaster in Missoula, *Bull. Am. Coll. Surg.*, **47**, 350.

Kennedy (1965), Considerations in local disasters, *Bull. Am. Coll. Surg.*, **50**, 117.

Klinghoffer, Damiani and Gioielli. *Disaster Manual for Hospitals*. Public Safety Committee. Illinois State Medical Society.

Letourneau (1962), Evaluating of a hospital disaster plan, *Hosp. Mgmt.*, **94**, 44.

McGonagle (1964), Psychological aspects of disaster, *Am. J. Publ. Hlth.*, **54**, 638.

Miller (1971), The management of major accidents, *Injury*, **2**, 168.

Ministry of Health. (1954), *Medical Arrangements for Dealing with Major Accidents*, HM(54)51. London: HMSO.

Morton (1970), Disaster management of burn patients, *N.Y.St. J. Med.*, **70**, 1647.

Mudano (1970), Green alert, *Natn. Saf. News*, **101**, 42.

Nissan and Eldar (1971), Organization of surgical care of mass casualties in a civilian hospital, *J. Trauma*, **11**, 974.

Owens (1968), Expanding the emergency department, *J. Am. med. Ass.*, **203**, 117.

Richardson (1975), *Disaster Planning Symposium*, Haslar 1974. Bristol: Wright.

Richwagen (1967), The 'predictive' approach to disaster planning—how it failed, *Hospitals*, **41**, 48.

Rieman (1972), Disaster test uncovers flaws, *Hosp. Prog.*, **53**, 70.

Rowe (1967), We can't design the next disaster, *Hosp. Admin. Can.*, **9**, 44.

Rutherford (1973), 'Experience in the accident and emergency department of the Royal Victoria Hospital with patients from civil disturbances in Belfast 1969–1972, with a review of disasters in the United Kingdom 1951–1971', *Injury*, **4**, 189.

Rutherford (1975), Disaster Procedures, *Br. med. J.*, **1**, 443.

Sanders (1956), Training for the management of mass casualties, *Milit. Med.*, **118**, 414.

Savage (1970), Disaster planning. A major accident exercise, *Br. med. J.*, **4**, 168.

Savage (1971), Disaster planning. A review, *Injury*, **3**, 49.

Savage (1972), Disaster planning. The use of action cards, *Br. med. J.*, **3**, 42.

Savage (1975), Documentation, in *Disaster Planning Symposium*, Haslar 1974, Ed., Richardson. Bristol: Wright.

Savage (1976), Disaster Planning. Protective clothing for medical team members. *Injury*, **7**, 286.

Savage (1977), Disaster Manual for Hospitals. (In preparation.)

Shader (1965), The emotional reactions to disaster, *The New Physician*, **14**, 270.

Shaftan (1962), Disaster and medical care, *J. Trauma*, **2**, 111.

Siffin (1964), Medical records for a disaster, *Hospitals*, **38**, 78.

Sillar (1974), Ed., *A Guide to Disaster Management.* Glasgow: Action for Disaster.

Snook (1975), *Medical Aid at Accidents.* London: Update Publications.

Soltis (1960), Disaster plan and drills, *Hosp. Mgmt.*, **89**, 44.

Spencer (1962), Disaster in Steelton, *Bull. Am. Coll. Surg.*, **47**, 351.

Spencer (1963), Mass casualties in the civilian hospital, *Bull. Am. Coll. Surg.*, **48**, 342.

Thomas (1969), How to keep the disaster from becoming disastrous, *Hosp. Mgmt.*, **107**, 50.

Thompson (1969), The organization of a major accident exercise, *Hospital, Lond.*, **65**, 94.

Thorpe (1965), Disaster planning, *Hosp. Prog.*, **46**, 115.

Trauma Research Group of Cornell University Medical College. The Treatment of Mass Civilian Casualties in a National Emergency. Medical Education for National Defense. 2300 E Street NW, Washington DC, 20390.

Vosburg (1971), Disaster alert and the community mental health centres, *Community Ment. Health J.*, **7**, 24.

10

The Armed Services

JOHN WATTS

HISTORY

The art of surgery and the care of the injured arose largely from the need to care for the wounded in war. Although Pope Boniface XI introduced the rule of the road in 1300 AD because of the increase in traffic accidents their number was insignificant and it was in war that such famous surgeons as Paracelsus (1493–1541), Paré (1509–1590), Botallo (1530–1600) and Magati (1579–1647) learnt many of their skills and it was about war that they wrote. In the seventeenth century Richard Wiseman, the English naval surgeon, stressed the need for early treatment of wounds especially the need for early amputation of a dismembered limb, but the battles of those days were set pieces, the victor remained in possession of the field and no organised rescue services existed.

The outstanding figure in the Napoleonic wars was undoubtedly Dominique Jean Larrey (1766–1842) who was not only a brilliant surgeon but a superb organiser. Napoleon trusted and admired him, and made him a Marshal of France for his efforts in the care of the wounded. Larrey stressed the need for early care and speedy evacuation to medical facilities; he introduced the systematic use of special vehicles, the 'Ambulances legère'—lightly-sprung horse drawn carriages specially equipped to carry wounded. On the British side too McGrigor (1771–1858) and Guthrie (1782–1857) were outstanding in the organisation of emergency services, McGrigor in the rear and Guthrie on the field, but much of their organisation was improvised and did not survive into the long peace that followed.

It needed the scandals of the Crimean war, and the work of Florence Nightingale (ca. 1855) to force the changes in organisation of the care of the wounded that led to a peacetime organisation for training in the systematic care of the injured, and the formation of the Army Medical School, later the Royal Army Medical College.

Curiously enough, the introduction of antisepis in surgery by Lister introduced a retrograde step in the care of the wounded, as bacterial contamination came to be regarded as both preventable and controllable; the former by not touching the wounds except with sterile dressings and the latter by the copious use of disinfectants in the wounds.

The Boer war saw the introduction (in 1899) of the Field Medical Company, later called the Field Ambulance, a mobile medical unit to care for and evacuate the wounded from the battlefield, but there was little advance in the surgical care of injuries, apart from Stephenson's use of X-rays for the first time in war. The static trench warfare of the 1914—18 war saw the development of the Casualty Clearing Station, a forward surgical unit which carried out the initial surgery of the wounded to enable them to survive the long evacuation to hospital. One of the outstanding developments in this war was the realisation of the importance of adequate splintage, particularly of the lower limb, as in the first year the mortality from compound fractures of the femur was nearly 80 per cent.

Robert Jones, the father of British orthopaedic surgery was appointed Consultant Surgeon to the Army with the task of advising on the treatment of fractures, as he had gained special experience as medical officer to the company constructing the Manchester ship canal. The most outstanding of his many innovations was to reintroduce the Thomas's knee splint designed by his uncle Hugh Owen Thomas, in the nineteenth century for the treatment of tuberculosis of the knee. By modifying this splint and developing a standard technique of application, he was able to reduce the mortality from compound femoral fractures to less than 20 per cent.

Although the motor ambulance and the tank both made their appearance in the 1914—18 war, the army was slow to mechanise and only in 1938 were the Medical Services fully mechanised, and even then their mobility was inadequate for the intensely fluid operation of modern war.

The pattern of care and evacuation of the wounded established in the 1914—18 conflict remained as a basis, the main innovation being the ad hoc creation in 1941 by Stephen and Williams of a highly mobile, fully equipped surgical team to reinforce the advanced dressing station and enable early surgery to be carried out on those who might otherwise be unable to survive evacuation. This unit later became the Field Surgical Unit, now called the Field Surgical Team.

The management of surgical shock, too, underwent a transformation due to the realisation that reduction of the effective circulating blood volume was the cardinal feature, and that early restoration of blood volume was essential. Whitby in Bristol developed the Army Transfusion Services, and Buttle in the Middle East perfected the Forward transfusion teams that provided the early, adequate, transfusion which saved so many lives. In Italy, Buttle expanded his transfusion services to supply the American as well as the British forces, since the Americans had relied on plasma expanders to treat shock until their experiences in North Africa showed the superiority of whole blood.

The Korean war first showed the immense value of the helicopter in casualty evacuation, and this experience was confirmed in Cyprus and Viet Nam.

ORGANISATION

Any organised medical service for the injured must be flexible, since the nature of the casualties, their number and location will vary, climatic and geographical conditions may present additional hazards, and over-provision is a waste of valuable or scarce resources. In the military scene, the advantages of discipline, training and a clear-cut chain of command simplify the problems of organising rescue and emergency care, but a study of the military solution can often be of value in considering the civilian problem.

The care of casualties is a continuous process from wounding to recovery but certain stages can be arbitrarily defined.

Initial management (First aid)

Basic first aid is taught to all ranks, and in addition regimental (i.e. not RAMC) medical orderlies are trained by medical officers. Airborne forces follow the American pattern of having medical corps personnel with units, and in the other services the medical orderlies form part of the medical branch, so the survival of the regimental medical assistant in the army may be regarded as an anachronism. Recent changes have taken place in army first aid, bringing a systems approach to training and designing its objectives around an analysis of the tasks and skills required. It is accepted that all first aid represents a balance of risks but that some skills are critical. A basic course of five hours training is given to all ranks and an advanced course of 70 hours (two weeks) instruction to all medical corpsmen, to unit first aid instructors and to regimental medical assistants.

The basic course is practical and concentrates on:

(1) Airway.
(2) Unconsciousness.
(3) Artificial respiration.
(4) External cardiac massage.
(5) Wounds.
(6) Splinting.
(7) Morphine.
(8) Burns.
(9) Priorities in multiple injuries.

Tests are practical and performed on simulated casualties and failure in any 'critical' skill eliminates from the course. Retesting takes place yearly. The new training is still undergoing evaluation and will undoubtedly be modified and improved but already it is showing effective and worthwhile results.

Evacuation

In forward defended localities, unit stretcher bearers evacuate casualties to the regimental aid post where the unit medical officer provides initial professional treatment; it is the responsibility of the field ambulance to see that this post is cleared of casualties as speedily as possible—by hand carriage, jeep ambulance or helicopter. Evacuation may be direct to hospital, or to the advanced dressing station, a forward medical unit capable of extensive resuscitative treatment and easily reinforced when necessary by one or more field surgical teams, to provide full surgical cover. Because of the limited equipment and high mobility of the field ambulance it is, however, more usual to establish a casualty clearing station (equivalent to the American Mobile Army Surgical Hospital) as the point of initial surgery, where full facilities of X-ray, beds and nursing skills are provided.

In addition, field surgical teams and field transfusion teams, highly mobile units providing surgical and resuscitative skills and equipment, are available to operate—usually at casualty clearing station level, but often at the field ambulance in the isolated role, as in airborne operations, or if the line of evacuation is extended. Forward surgery is what has aptly been called the 'surgery of transportation'; that is to say, the carrying out of those surgical procedures which will enable the patient to withstand the rigours of evacuation until he can reach hospital and undergo elective, definitive and reconstructive surgery.

This outline of the medical organisation is based on evacuation by land vehicles, but the use of air evacuation can simplify and modify the scheme. However, a land route is usually necessary since the number of casualties may exceed the facilities for air evacuation, and bad weather or enemy action may prevent it altogether.

Air evacuation was first used as the main chain of evacuation in the Burma Campaign of 1943–45 but came into its own with the development of the helicopter and its use in Korea in 1950–52. Since then, air evacuation has virtually replaced the ambulance car for serious casualties. The helicopter possesses three insuperable advantages for casualty evacuation: speed, comfort and point-to-point carriage. It has revolutionised war surgery almost as much as the three major advances of World War II, namely anaesthesia, blood transfusion and antibotics. In the author's opinion, failure to develop a satisfactory civilian helicopter ambulance service is inexcusable.

TRIAGE

This word, now often applied to casualty sorting in general, was first used to describe the three point system evolved in the Spanish Civil War 1936–39. This first developed the idea of separating the casualty clearing station functions into:

(1) A casualty classification post.
(2) A forward surgical unit, the **No 1 Hospital**, for urgent cases.
(3) The **No 2 Hospital** for less urgent surgical cases.

The Triage team, consisting of two medical officers with nurses, orderlies, clerks and stretcher bearers allotted cases into one of three groups:

THE ARMED SERVICES 277

(a) For operation.
(b) For observation.
(c) For evacuation.

Later the word was extended and applied to any sorting of medical priorities and bids fair to become as misused and misunderstood as the term 'debridement'.

Nevertheless in the care of the injured some assessment of priorities is usually required. The principles of care for the injured are easily stated as being: to save life, to restore function and to relieve suffering. And, of these, clearly the first is most urgent and important. Casualties who survive the immediate injury are at risk from its complications, the most important of which are: **haemorrhage, impeded respiration, wound shock, infection** and **metabolic disturbance**. The first two can kill in minutes, the next in hours and the last two in days. Hence training of forward medical personnel must concentrate on the control of haemorrhage and the maintenance of normal respiration, then on adequate splintage and resuscitation; control of infection and prevention of metabolic disturbance taking third place.

In the First Aid Training Centre at the Depot and Training Establishment of the Royal Army Medical Corps, advanced first-aid procedures are taught, so that the medical orderly can play a more useful role. Advanced knowledge of anatomy, physiology and pathology is not an absolute prerequisite of such practical procedures as tracheal intubation, intravenous infusion and tracheostomy—any more than an engineering degree is necessary before changing a wheel or a sparking plug. Indeed, the recent successful tracheostomy by an RAMC sergeant in Ulster compares favourably with the case of the doctor censured by a coroner for not being able to do the operation in a child with a dummy impacted in the pharynx. That such technical procedures are easily and successfully taught to ambulance personnel has been shown by some coronary care teams, in which the ambulance orderlies are trained in the detection and management of cardiac arrest, both threatened and actual.

Once a casualty's respiratory and circulatory distress has been alleviated by control of haemorrhage, establishment of a clear airway and physiological respiration, and in grave blood loss by replacement therapy, further assessment of the patient's diagnosis and a plan for continuing management can be made. For adequate and effective initial surgery in wounds the 'Friedrich period' of six hours is still a useful guide, although experience in World War II showed that under penicillin cover this could be extended to 12 hours. During the Korean war casualties with major head wounds were evacuated to Japan for primary surgery.

However, in the civilian situation, such delays and lengthy evacuation should never be necessary. It is unfortunately true that the deleterious effects of delay and the rigours and hardships of evacuation are often not fully appreciated so that death, disability and suffering may follow.

In major disasters the military analogy can be pressed too far— much service planning is for a continuing flood of casualties, whereas the solitary disaster involving a number of casualties is an episode which must be dealt with within a few hours. In war the casualty is brought to the doctor, but in a single episode an experienced doctor on the site can not only support and control the efforts of first-aiders, but will often be able to return with the casualties to hospital, and play his full role in the treatment scheme.

The armed services have the advantages of a unified medical chain of command, and an organised, equipped and trained medical service whose primary responsibility is for the first-aid, evacuation and care of the wounded and sick. In addition they are equipped to establish and maintain hospitals and other medical establishments without reliance on local services such as water supply, hygiene and sanitation, light, heating and power. This would be an advantage in dealing with many large-scale civilian disasters, in which breakdown of sanitation and lack of hygiene often present graver continuing risks to health than do injuries. Indeed, after the first few hours, the main need in most catastrophes is for food, water, shelter and sanitation; not for doctors.

The establishment of nuclear power stations makes it advisable that the services' experience and training in radiation hazards should be more widely disseminated. Here the main requirement is for cleansing and monitoring stations to decontaminate persons exposed to radioactive contamination before a hazardous dose is received, and to identify those who have received a dosage of radiation which needs treatment. Fortunately, the time factor here is on a different scale, and radiation symptoms in anyone saveable are unlikely to appear before 24–48 hours. Moreover, the evacuation of casualties, and of the apparently unaffected, from contaminated zones is of vital importance, and again the speed of helicopter evacuation presents a major advantage since the radiation dosage varies with the **duration** of exposure as well as the square of the distance away from the contaminated ground. In default of helicopters, it is worth remembering that the upper floor of a double-decker bus will only be subject to about one-thirtieth of the radiation at ground level; it may therefore be used for command posts and for other personnel who have to stay in the contaminated zone. Evacuation should wherever possible be upwind of the disaster area. The major problem in such a disaster will undoubtedly be panic, and the gravest hazard may be created by persons moving aimlessly in the open with maximum exposure to radioactive dust. Concrete buildings protect to some degree and whenever possible persons should take shelter until orderly evacuation can be achieved. In this, as in the other spheres outlined, service experience has much to contribute to the development of civil casualty care.

11

Flying Doctor Services

JAMES LAWLESS

Medical care of all kinds involves communication and movement. In Britain and similar countries many of the problems have been solved by non-medical means. The telephone is an effective communications system. Tarmacadam roads and the internal combustion engine have between them helped solve some of the transport requirements of the sick. Doctors can drive to the houses of their patients and a woman with, say, a ruptured ectopic pregnancy can be carried speedily to hospital.

Difficulties arise in any arrangements, and the effects of geography and climate often serve to reduce the medical facilities available to a community. Even in the United kingdom some small centres of population are over 100 miles from the nearest hospital, and the problems of transporting a patient over this distance, especially in winter, must be frequently in the mind of any doctor practising under such conditions. In other parts of the world, where distances are much greater, it is not only the evacuation of the acutely ill patient that is difficult but also the movement of the doctor himself. Scattered communities, each one too small to require a full-time resident medical attendant, need access to regular medical facilities. This can be arranged only by the doctor achieving sufficient mobility to cater for the needs of these scattered centres of population. Elsewhere communities may be large enough to provide a sufficient workload for several doctors, and in some cases, even small general hospitals. In spite of this, it may not be possible to recruit the medical personnel required, or cultural and other stresses may make it impossible for them to stay long in the area.

Aircraft and radio transmitters have a part to play in the solution of all these problems, and in some instances they represent the only solution available.

280

As aircraft are of many types to suit varying circumstances, so there are many kinds of flying doctor service. At the one extreme is the occasional, irregular evacuation of an injured man from an isolated mining survey camp perhaps situated in mountainous country. At the other, the provision of a full time medical service with regular general practitioner clinics, a reliable 24-hour, seven-day-week emergency service, and full access to any specialised units required.

Many intermediate arrangements exist. The acutely ill patient has a demand on society beyond all others, and once the need has been made clear by the doctor lay assistance is readily forthcoming. The limitations of such assistance must be appreciated, and a doctor's request must be tempered by a previous awareness of the technical problems.

The doctor may have his own small aircraft for visiting, but one too small for carrying a prone patient with fractured leg or spine. He may then be able to call upon the larger machines flown by police or military.

A local flying club with an instructor pilot, or the owners of a private plane with a professional pilot, might be called upon in some emergencies or to fly a doctor to isolated areas on a regular schedule.

Aircraft and crews can be chartered, and where both an efficient charter company and sufficient funds are available this can be a satisfactory way of providing a service. The crews will be professional, there will be a larger choice of aircraft, the standards of maintenance will be high and risks in flight low.

Even in a large flying doctor service with its standby and reserve aircraft there will be occasions when it will be necessary to call upon the help of a neighbouring charter company or Air Force unit. Such essential contacts must be built up by administrators. Out of a fleet of six aircraft only three or perhaps four would be serviceable on any one day.

Aircraft are attractive because of their speed, and direct line of flight, the distance by air being generally one third less than the same journey by road. Helicopters are the slowest aircraft, twin-engined fixed wing the fastest available, with the many types of single engined machine intermediate. A small helicopter flies at no more than 70 mph and is limited to a range of 200 miles without refuelling. Larger single- or twin-engined gas turbine helicopters cruise at 110 mph over a maximum range of 400 miles. Their maximum endurance in the air is 4 hours but to achieve this the speed has to be kept down to about 50 mph. These are air speeds. A head-wind against any aircraft will reduce its ground speed and its effective range. The slower the aircraft the more critical the effect of a head-wind which reduces ground speed commensurately. Twin-engined light aircraft carrying a pilot plus five passengers (or one stretcher case plus two or three sitting passengers) cruise at 200 mph and have a range of about 1000 miles. Single-engined machines usually carry a pilot plus three sitting passengers but some can carry a pilot plus five. These latter machines will generally take a stretcher. The speed of a single-engined aircraft is not always related to its size. One of the biggest, the De Haviland Beaver, although a very fine aircraft, is also one of the slowest (115 mph). Others achieve 165 mph. The average speed of single-engined aircraft is 140–150 mph.

Timetables rely upon factors other than absolute air speed. Aircraft, even on standby, are rarely airborne in less than twenty minutes. Under irregular or ad hoc conditions, it could take two hours. A pilot and engineer have to be found, the aircraft checked and fuelled, routes worked out, a meteorological report obtained, flight plans filed with the air traffic control authority, and any necessary medical items stowed on board. It is not possible to use small airfields after dusk, and this creates an urgency when calls are received after midday. An aircraft airborne at 4.15 pm may have ten minutes to get down and be airborne again at the other end. A 4.30 pm take off would be too late, and the patient would then have to wait all night for a pick up at dawn, a delay in evacuation of 13 hours. A large flying doctor service has a standby pilot and doctor present in the crew room from 2.0 pm onwards and the standby machine will be outside the hangar field and ready to go as soon as an emergency call is received over the radio network. The maximum fuel load of 120 gallons will be used in flight at the rate of about 24 gallons an hour. Petrol weighs 7 lb a gallon so the fuel load at take off will be 840 lb, equivalent in weight to five average-sized adults. Drums hold 44 gallons, so two or three will be used every time a twin-engined aircraft is refuelled in the bush. The logistics of getting drums of fuel to remote airfields can pose great problems. Drums which have been specially inspected and sealed by the fuel supply companies **can** be flown on board the aircraft, but this is not generally acceptable.

Aircraft need airfields. The bigger and better the airfield the safer and the more expensive the operation becomes. Somewhere a compromise has to be made between safety and cost. This compromise is crucial and no flying doctor service can be evaluated without its most careful consideration. We may all be prepared to risk our lives for one of our fellows, and this is often and rightly done; but it is amoral and inefficient to organise a service dependent on bravery or bravado. At sea level, in a cool temperate climate, with a stiff breeze and a concrete runway, light twin-engined aircraft weighing two and a half tons will leave the ground in as little as 250 yd. However, these are ideal conditions and flying doctor service aircraft, like lifeboats, do not operate under ideal conditions. The airfield may be 5000 ft above sea level, the temperature may be well over 100°F and the airfield surface grass, gravel, loose dust, or mud. Under these conditions the same aircraft will take over 800 yd to become airborne and even a short-field technique, using every skill and taking very considerable risks, will require 600 yd. Depending on the type of machine a further distance, varying from half to the full length of the actual ground run, will be taken by the aircraft before it has reached a height of 50 ft. The airfield will need to be 100 yd wide and, together with the cleared approach areas of perhaps 200 yd at each end, can easily amount to 20 acres in area. This must often be fenced against wild or domestic animals.

Efficient communications are essential in any flying doctor service. A clear radio message carefully evaluated and discussed could save an unnecessary thousand mile flight. **The service's own doctors must talk directly to the originators of the call.** Messages passed via a police or military radio network must of course be acted upon, but they are frequently received third or even fourth hand and this often results in changes and omissions, as well as preventing any discussion of the alternatives with the people on the spot. Modern radio transmitters are good, reliable, and any remote centre of population should have one. Their value is immense not only in emergencies but in the general reassurance that they provide. A person may be 500 miles away but with a radio still feel part of the community. If the transmitter fails the feeling of isolation experienced by the individual is overpowering.

Depending on the terrain and the height of the mast, a VHF transmitter of 20 watts output is effective for twenty to thirty miles. Beyond that distance the best equipment is a SSB FM transmitter (single side band, frequency modulated) of 100 watts output operated from a 12 volt supply. This has a reliable range, depending on frequency, of approximately 700 miles. These sets with four channels are small, about 20 in square and 8 in deep, and weigh only 16 lb. They cost approximately £600. Each aircraft will need to be equipped with a whole battery of radios. At least one long-range transmitter, and duplicated VHF sets are essential. There will be at least two navigational radio aids called a VOR and an ADF, and if the base airfield is reasonably sophisticated there will also be a glide slope receiver. For any night flying in thunderstorm areas a storm radar set is essential. The radio equipment in a light twin-engined machine will cost £3000 to £8000 and the price of a complete aircraft will vary between £50 000 and £100 000.

Aircraft operating costs are always divided into a fixed element calculated on an annual basis and a variable element related to the hours flown. Both added together and divided by the number of hours flown in a year give the total hourly operating costs of the machine, which are generally lower the greater number of hours flown. Aircraft on the ground are like empty, fully-staffed hospitals, very expensive and not much use. A utilisation of between forty and sixty hours a month is reasonable. In the Zambian Service the most ever obtained in a month· was one hundred and twenty hours from a Piper Aztec, but this was under exceptional circumstances and involved some night maintenance. The total hourly cost, inclusive of pilot's salary, varies between £50 and £120 an hour. A machine flown 800 hours a year will be about 50 per cent cheaper per hour than the same machine flown for 300 hours a year.

Examples of flying doctor arrangements start with the ad hoc, occasional, irregular evacuation of a seriously ill patient over a moderate distance of say 50 to 200 miles. An Air Force or Army helicopter is the answer here and those doctors who may have need of this type of service, however rarely, should know how to make the necessary arrangements. It is most important to define the medical requirement and the degree of urgency in unambiguous terms. The needs of a woman going into normal labour with her third child, after having excellent antenatal care and now being attended by a police constable's wife who has delivered a few babies before, are different from those of a mother with a history of a previous Caesarian section who collapses shortly after going into labour and is reported to have a pulse rate of 180/min.

Ambulance services usually define an 'emergency' as a patient requiring evacuation within one hour. The London Ambulance Service achieves an average time from receipt of message to patient pick up of about nine minutes. Depending on the distances involved, an organised flying doctor service will achieve an average pick-up time of one to three hours. The Zambian Service has three classifications of call:

Emergency—A patient requiring evacuation within 5 hours.
Urgent—Evacuation within 24 hours.
Ambulance—which requires evacuation within five days.

In an organised, full-time service the priorities, conflicts and risks are the subject of constant discussion, and the pilots, nurses, engineers, and doctors concerned come to a balanced appreciation of the problems. The responsibility for defining the degree of urgency must always rest with the doctor. The evaluation of risk to the crew, and this includes the patient once he or she is on board, must always lie with the pilot. A nurse should always be on board the plane for any type of evacuation flight. In emergencies, especially acute ones, a doctor should also go along. Ideally, though this is not always possible, it should be the doctor who declared the emergency. To battle along in a tropical storm with severe turbulance, loss of radio contact, and engine air intake icing problems is a formidable experience—on a par perhaps with a slipping arterial clamp in inaccessible depths during an abdominal operation.

In addition to the degree of urgency, it needs to be made clear whether the patient is a sitting or stretcher case. If the patient is a child, the need for him to be accompanied by his mother will have to borne in mind. It will also be necessary to detail any special flying requirements should these be relevant. Aircraft used in most flying doctor service applications are not pressurised. A child with severe bronchopneumonia should be flown at as low an altitude as is safely possible. Children in this condition will often lose consciousness following a gain in altitude of as little as 2000 or 3000 feet above the pick-up point. The density of the atmosphere, which affects both our physiology and the power output of an unsupercharged aircraft engine, is dependent not only on height above sea level but also temperature. This can have a marked effect in hot climates, where the density may be equivalent to a height as much as 2000 feet greater than the actual height above sea level. Cases of severe malaria, anaemia, or haemorrhage will also need to be flown low and, where the disease is endemic, the possibility of inducing a sickle cell crisis must be kept in mind. Head injuries travel well. The pilot has to keep to his flight plan altitude and may only vary it by permission of the air traffic control authority.

The exact destinations for both outward and return flights need to be made clear. For a helicopter, sheets will be used to mark out the landing area nearest the patient. Helicopters **can** land in tiny spaces surrounded by trees and buildings, but it is dangerous for them to do so and increases the risk. Far better to carry the patient 400 yards down the road to the nearest meadow, football pitch, or beach. Because aircraft go in a straight line the best centre for the reception of the patient may not be the one usually considered by road users. A few extra minutes flying time may put a large general hospital or teaching unit within reach, and this may be better for the patient than a small local hospital. The pilot is always in touch by radio with an air traffic control centre. In genuine cases of emergency the controllers are always helpful and will relay, by telephone to the hospital concerned, any information concerning the patient's reception that may be required.

It is extremely difficult to assess variations in the condition of a patient on board a helicopter or light aircraft in flight. Auscultation is quite impossible and taking a pulse rate is surprisingly difficult as noise and vibration seem to interfere with the tactile senses. If it is bumpy, drip bottles swing around with amazing violence and need careful attention. Helicopters, although very noisy, give a much smoother ride than fixed wing aircraft. Ordinary light aircraft do not carry oxygen but the better equipped twin-engined machines often do. This is usually a piped supply to each seat location with a simple form of face mask. Small, portable, positive pressure respirators with their own oxygen supply and a built-in suction device are invaluable and can be carried around in different aircraft as required. Built-in suction from a 'venturi' tube can be fitted to an aircraft but has the disadvantage of not operating when the aircraft is on the ground.

The next stage in complexity, after the occasional use of an aircraft for evacuation purposes, is the regular provision of a medical service by air. A doctor may fly himself, or someone may fly him, to isolated communities on a regular basis. It may be that he goes when alerted or, in addition, he may hold outpatient consultations at fixed regular intervals. Thus a consultant surgeon may go on tour to isolated hospitals operating in each as required. The East African Service flying from Nairobi works mainly in this way, and in Russia consultants from the teaching units do similar tours. Fixed wing machines are more suitable than helicopters for regular long flights over a known land route, and this kind of service will involve the provision of landing grounds close to the visited community. For a single doctor service the people being visited will provide these airfields. The doctor or his pilot will insist on the airfields being kept in good condition, which is not always easy. Civil aviation authorities issue licences for airfields and classify them in a variety of ways. Flights into and out of an unlicensed airfield can usually be made only with prior permission of the authorities. The insurances carried by the doctor on himself and the aircraft will specify the conditions under which they remain valid. All these matters can be circumvented in an emergency but for any kind of regular arrangement the pressures to conform are very strong. Transgressions are dealt with by the removal of the pilot's licence, and professional pilots cannot of course take the risk lightly.

Once the need for a regular service becomes apparent the arguments for organising a suitable professional scheme are very strong. The organisation will generate its own momentum. Its own peculiar problems and the pattern to deal with these, is difficult to change once established. Its aims and features must be established at the outset. Their implications must be understood, the requirements to meet them in men, women and machinery listed, and the funds required evaluated. For example, it may be easy to purchase and install a radio transmitter in an isolated area, and once this is done the acutely ill patient can contact a doctor. Immediately, something has then to be done for that patient. Unless proper arrangements have been made beforehand, the only way to save that patient's life might be to use an unsuitable aircraft, flown perhaps by an inexperienced pilot into a dangerously small, unprepared field or clearing.

Provision of a communications system will always involve the organisation of a patient transport system. For example, if an airfield is under construction and the builders have a radio, then arrangements need to be made to carry any seriously ill patients to the nearest useable airfield until such time as their own is finished. Two or three hundred men might be involved in the construction work, using potentially dangerous hand tools. The surrounding population, within a day's journey on foot (30 miles), could be anything between two and ten thousand people. Thus the amount of serious illness in the locality may be great and the temptation to use the partially constructed airfield at the earliest possible moment very strong. This aspect requires careful judgement both from the doctors, in assessing a patient's condition, and from the pilots in assessing the degree of flying risk involved. For this reason it is helpful if a doctor is on site during the period of construction. This reduces the necessity of evacuation to the minimum and provides the most accurate assessment of any seriously ill patient carried into the camp. On a personal note, I once flew with two colleagues, at some risk, into an airfield to evacuate a patient correctly reported on the radio to have been gored by a buffalo. He had two huge penetrating holes in his left chest and an unpleasant cavity in his neck which, miraculously, had avoided his carotids, jugulars, and most other vital structures. He had been carried by two friends for ten days and was on the way to a spontaneous, if heavily scarred, recovery. Paradoxically the take-off, under very adverse and difficult conditions, was a much greater danger to the patient than his injuries.

The quality of medical care at the peripheral airfield clinic influences the evacuation rate. The greater the degree of diagnostic and therapeutic skill available on the spot the fewer patients will need air evacuation. Doctors are usually in short supply and it can be argued that it is more efficient to keep them mobile and therefore free to concentrate on those patients most in need. This involves the selection by a nurse or auxiliary of those patients who are most in need. While this is easy enough in cases of catastrophic illness the selection of patients who are about to become seriously ill requires judgements and skills more frequently found in a doctor than in a nurse or auxiliary. Questions of this sort need discussion at an early stage and the decisions taken will help decide the format and costs of the service.

When a flying doctor service is first provided the evacuation rate will be high due to the large number of cases that have been receiving no treatment. Later the rate drops but this is sometimes obscured by an increase in total patient visits. In Zambia a new airfield at which patients were seen by a doctor would produce an evacuation rate of 1·5 per cent dropping later to between 0·5 per cent and 1·0 per cent of patients seen. Good care by a medical auxiliary should produce a rate about three or four times higher than this. Thus the percentage of cases needing referral from an outstation staffed by the latter would be about 5 per cent. Poor quality medical care, whether at the doctor or auxiliary level produces lower not higher evacuation rates because many serious cases are missed, particularly among children. Exceptionally able peripheral medical care can of course also produce a low evacuation rate, but as ability is less common than mediocrity this is not the usual reason for a low rate.

The design of a service will determine the ideal type of aircraft required, and economics will decide whether the ideal can be achieved. Perfection in an aircraft can be a very expensive quality. Aircraft have a maximum weight and an empty weight, the difference being called the 'useful load' and this is made up of the pilot, the fuel, passengers, baggage, and any moveable items of equipment that are not normally kept on board the aircraft. The weight of fuel for a 1000 mile range will take up over a third of the useful load, i.e. between 800 and 1100 lb. The pilot, doctor, nurse, patient, and one relative will weigh between 800 and 900 lb. However, the patient and relative will not get on board until the airfield is reached by which time some of the fuel will have been used, perhaps 250 or 300 lb after flying for an hour and a half. A simple medical kit of one black bag plus a portable positive pressure respirator will weigh together about 60 lb. The weight of the stretcher, blankets and any other medical items must also be considered, as must the patients' and relatives' baggage, plus any survival items carried in case of a forced landing.

Weight is always a battle and it is very easy to overequip aircraft to an extent that actually reduces their usefulness. The 'useful load' of the suitable types of twin-engine machines varies between 1800 and 2800 lb according to type and equipment. A full fuel load will often reduce the passenger-carrying capacity to a number very much less than the actual seating available.

Twin-engined aircraft are always desirable. For flights over remote land areas, over the sea or large lakes, and after sunset, they are essential. Aviation maps of many countries will show large areas prohibited to single-engined flying. Even so, single-engined machines may cope better with some conditions, such as small rough airfields, perhaps in the mountains, requiring a short take-off performance, and supply work to partially constructed airfields and survey camps involving air drops of provisions or drugs. Provided they are wrapped in sufficient layers of sacking even glass pint bottles of whole blood can be dropped from a slow flying aircraft. For work of this kind a single-engined machine with a 'conventional', i.e. tail wheel, undercarriage is used. The tricycle (nose wheel) arrangement, particularly in the designs with much weight on the nose wheel, has disadvantages in rough conditions. The nose wheel tends to sink in, often during the early part of the take-off run, the spinning propeller hits the ground necessitating a complete strip and overhaul of both propeller and engine at a cost to the insurance company of anything up to £3000. The aircraft will be unserviceable until a spare engine and propeller can be flown in. Meanwhile, as patients continue to be taken ill and die, a replacement aircraft will have to be hired. To facilitate engine changes in the bush, a frequent occurrence, it is useful if some of the aircraft of a fleet are able to carry a spare power plant and propeller inside the cabin.

Conditions vary, but stretcher cases are less common than sitting cases and the interior fittings of the aircraft are designed accordingly. Even with powerful, expensive twin-engined machines, weight is always a primary consideration and unnecessary equipment only serves to reduce the versatility of the aircraft. Most aircraft manufacturers will provide various stretcher installations. Usually two or three seats are removed and the stretcher clamped on to the seat bearers. The ease of loading varies greatly and when contemplating the purchase of an aircraft this aspect must be subject to actual test and not accepted simply on the word of the manufacturers. Low wing twin-engined machines with over-wing access are difficult. An aft door, level with the trailing edge of the wing, improves the stretcher access and many machines now have doors in this position. High winged twin-engined craft are easier to load but usually have fixed undercarriages making them slower than low wing machines. Reduction in cruising speed is important in itself but also reduces the aircraft's range, a very critical factor in a large country. As a rough rule of thumb, a prospective purchaser should aim for a minimum range of 1000 miles. With allowances for bad weather and at least one diversion to another airfield, and assuming that no fuel is available en route, this gives a possible overall journey of from 350 to 400 miles.

Twin-engined machines can still fly on only one engine and thus afford a considerable safety factor. Manufacturers tend to be optimistic about the single-engined ceiling of their machines and it is important to have a demonstration in the fully loaded condition, remembering that in many areas ground level might be 4500 feet above sea level. Turbocharged engines for higher altitudes are much more expensive, heavier and less reliable. They are at a disadvantage at low altitudes because their extra weight reduces the useful load by as much as 200 lb (one large patient), and there is no increase in power at sea level. However, the sea level power is maintained at height resulting in a very much higher single-engined ceiling, well over double that of the same aircraft with unsupercharged engines.

If the service involves a fairly complex schedule, as the Zambian service does, with many short five or ten minute stops, the engines must restart easily when hot. Some units either will not start at all under these conditions or will only do so with the utmost difficulty.

It is a great help for the service to have its own ambulance with interchangeable stretchers and for the nurse accompanying the patient in the aircraft to go in the ambulance to the hospital. This ensures a proper continuity of responsibility with no confusion and also ensures a good relationship with the hospital. Transfers from one stretcher to another are at best uncomfortable and at worst dangerous and they also increase a patient's feeling of insecurity. The Volkswagen ambulance is excellent, the stretchers fold if required and when extended they will fit into most twin-engined machines without too much difficulty.

Complete and fixed ambulance conversions of the interior of the aircraft itself are available, the Australian service being undoubtedly the experts in this field. A seriously ill prone patient can be cared for in flight and the aircraft can also be used for consultations and examinations on the airfield. There is a wash basin and hot water supply, and the whole conversion, made in Australia, is most practical. Machines of this kind are universally acceptable for the long distance transport of seriously ill patients to specialised centres, and should be available. Journeys by road ambulance over similar distances would be extremely uncomfortable.

Many flying doctor services operate in situations where they provide the only form of regular communication, and their aircraft are often filled with live chickens, picks and shovels, consultant surgeons, maize seeds, patients, paraffin for the clinic Tilley lamps, fowl pest vaccine, spare bow saw blades, bicycle inner tubes, the mail, boxes of drugs, and of course the dusty and usually exhausted doctors and nurses. It will be appreciated why the basic ordinary seating arrangement, with a simple stretcher conversion when needed, is the best form of layout.

Professional pilots are essential for any form of organised flying doctor service and the doctors, even if capable of flying the aircraft, should not be allowed to do so. In the Zambian service the twin-engined aircraft fly 1000 miles a day each averaging a dozen landings and take-offs at a series of airfield clinics on a timed schedule in all weather conditions. In addition to the regular clinic work, emergency calls are dealt with as they occur and aircraft diverted accordingly. Sixteen thousand patients a month are treated and one hundred and forty a month flown to a central hospital. Following discharge, these patients plus one relative are returned by air to their homes. Approximately two hundred in-patients are under treatment at any one time at the airfield clinics. Indeed one of the advantages of a Flying Doctor Service is that it helps to ensure the treatment of many patients at clinics near their homes. Rapidly available help on demand reassures the doctor or medical attendant so that a potentially serious condition can be treated locally. In the minority of cases in which the patient's response is unsatisfactory, help or evacuation is immediately available. Without that certainty many more patients would need to be sent to hospital on a precautionary basis.

Time is often an ally of disease. To save time is always to save lives and to provide help rapidly to those in need has always been the objective of medical practice. Aircraft are often the best means, and sometimes the only means of achieving that objective. Their increasing use would greatly benefit our patients.

12

Remote Highway Crashes: First Aid by Drivers; the Isolated Doctor and His Team

HANNS PACY

Much of the world's population lives in large cities, where medical and emergency services can be highly specialised. In large and sparsely populated countries like Australia the large cities are connected by a few long, narrow country roads running over a thousand kilometres through lonely country areas, state forests, National Parks, fishing, holiday and retirement hamlets, consisting largely of 'second homes', which are occupied in the holiday season only.

Within an area of 2000 sq km may live a population of one thousand, sometimes without a local hospital, and with the only personnel available to handle the frequent accidents on a busy intercity route (in my area, National Route No 1) a single doctor, an ambulance officer/driver, a policeman-cum-coastguard and the local tow-truck operator. The severity of injuries from high speed country crashes compares badly with those in city accidents (see Table I), as also shown in the larger ambulance survey of the Australian Medical Association (Stuckey, 1972). This appears to be consistent with the situation in the Rocky Mountain States of the USA (Morgan, 1972).

It is difficult for a single ambulance officer driving a hearse-like, stationwagon ambulance to supply an adequate service 80 km (50 miles) from the nearest casualty department. Similarly, a single doctor, police officer or tow-truck man could not do much in a serious multiple vehicle collision. However, combined and trained as a team they could achieve a great deal, and it is vital that available talent in such an area should be utilised.

TABLE I

Five times more fatal

	Melbourne City Survey by Ryan and Clark (1972), Med. J. Aust., 1, 1173	Tea Gardens Police District	
		National Route 1 and Main Road 506	Urban and Local Roads
Consecutive crashes	100	111	74
Persons Injured	202	238	84
Serious and Critical	20	92	15
Died	4	23	0
Mortality of Serious Injury	1 : 5	1 : 4	Nil
Approximate average distances: Casualty Dept and full-time			
Fire Brigade	7 km (4 miles)	80 km (50 miles)	80 km (50 miles)
Ambulance	8 km (5 miles)	18 km (11 miles)	4 km (2 miles)
Doctor	2 km (1 mile)	18 km (11 miles)	4 km (2 miles)
Approximate number in area: Ambulance Officers	10	1	1
Doctors	100	1	1

FIRST AID BY DRIVERS

Alerting facilities

Having such a rescue team in a settlement like ours, nine km from
the highway, is not enough. Alerting facilities are of vital importance.
There are no emergency roadside telephones on Australian country
highways and no Government or other institution wishes to create
a precedent by financing them locally. We therefore maintain one
by private donations for our small community. This phone is sited
at the 'Tea Gardens' junction from Highway 1 where the highway
between the hamlets of Karuah and Bulahdelah runs through 24 miles
(39 km) of forest and has neither dwellings nor telephones. This phone
saves our rescue team 15 min in reaching the scene of an accident
from Tea Gardens.

The time factor is vital in modern resuscitation (Figs. 12.1(a)
and (b)), yet the importance of ascertaining how long a victim has
stopped breathing or moving is regularly omitted or understated in
current first aid manuals.

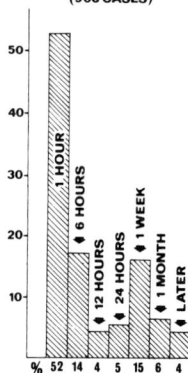

(a)

(b)

Fig. 12.1. (a) Those first fifteen minutes.
(b) The time factor is crucial.

The phone itself consists of a bulletproof steel box containing a loudspeaker—microphone assembly. A push button rings a bell at the local garage in Tea Gardens (the only place occupied 24 hours a day). On lifting the receiver the bell stops and the garage men can hear voices within a 10 m radius from the emergency phone box. A reply through the loudspeaker inside the emergency box can be understood across the highway. From the garage the message is relayed by phone or two-way radio to ambulances travelling in the area, to the doctor's car and to the local tow/rescue truck.

Difficulties occur when messages are relayed by people who have no medical training. It would be far better to have a roadside radiophone which would allow direct two-way conversation between the motorists giving the alerting message and all the members of the rescue team, who could then determine priorities. No doctor is needed for mere cuts and bruises, and no ambulance is needed if only a vehicle is damaged.

The vital first message

The efficient and economic response of emergency teams is determined by the quality of the primary message. The success of medical aid to those severely injured depends upon immediacy of application. A delay of 20 min waiting for the ambulance officer to arrive at the scene would be doubled if he had then to alert the doctor. Therefore it is essential that all drivers be trained to give a standardised, concise, and reasonably complete message. They must know what are the priorities and the immediate action required. A reminder could then be appended to each renewed licence including three message forms.

The following could be a prototype instruction:

READ THIS AND KEEP IN YOUR CAR AT ALL TIMES

HOW TO SAVE VICTIMS OF A ROAD ACCIDENT

1 Park safely

Do not become the next casualty. Leave room between you and the accident for ambulances and doctor's car. Make sure your car can be seen from at least 500 yd away (crests, curves). Leave trafficators flashing. Do not obscure the lights of the car in front of you. At night, light up the scene without blinding oncoming traffic (Fig. 12.2).

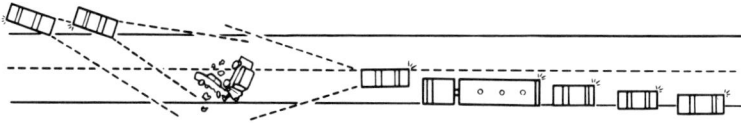

Fig. 12.2. *Protective parking on a straight road.*

2 Assess the essential information

Use the message form appended to your licence (Fig. 12.3).

```
              HELP! ROAD ACCIDENT!

EXACTLY WHERE.......................................
...................................................
CASUALTIES:    UNCONSCIOUS.........................
(State number)                              yes........
                          bluish pale     no ........

               TRAPPED.............................
               POSSIBLY BROKEN BONES..............
               BURNS......... ABDOMINAL............
               LOOK SERIOUS........................
               LIGHT INJURIES.....................
NEEDED:        AMBULANCE, DOCTOR, RESCUE VAN,
(Encircle)     FIRE BRIGADE (trapped), POLICE,
               TOW-TRUCK.

Time of accident...........Time of Message.......
```

Fig. 12.3. *Emergency message form.*

3 Get help, using message form

Send someone to the nearest phone and have another stop all oncoming cars asking whether they have two-way radio and can transmit the message; also whether they have a doctor, nurse or trained first aider in the car.

4   Attend unconscious and bleeding victims first

But first:

REMOVE DANGER

Do not touch a car with a live powerline on it. Switch off the engine of a crashed car. No smoking. Station flagmen 500 yd up and down the road as soon as possible. They must be clearly visible in the dark, showing white shirts, or a newspaper. Place small branches on roadway, or triangles and flares if available. If time, remove debris from path of traffic.

REMOVE DANGER

Where casualties are in danger of being run over, they must be moved a few yards to safety. Lift them by their clothing, one man making sure that there is no movement in the neck during the procedure (Fig. 12.4). If a casualty is moved face downwards one person must ensure support of the head.

5   The unconscious victim

Does not respond to voice.
Does not move when pinched.
Has a fixed stare and a limp, flaccid jaw (deeply unconscious).

IF OUTSIDE THE CAR

Roll casualty onto his side (Figs. 12.5 and 6).
Remove any dentures and clear debris or sticky fluid from his mouth in this position (this alone may start him breathing).
Loosen tight clothing (neck, chest, waist).

IS HE BREATHING?

Look for chest movement, listen for breathing, feel his chest move,

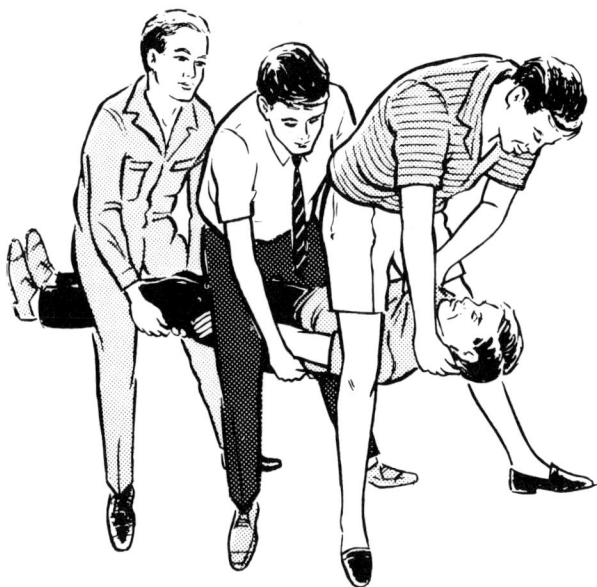

Fig. 12.4. Rautek's carry.

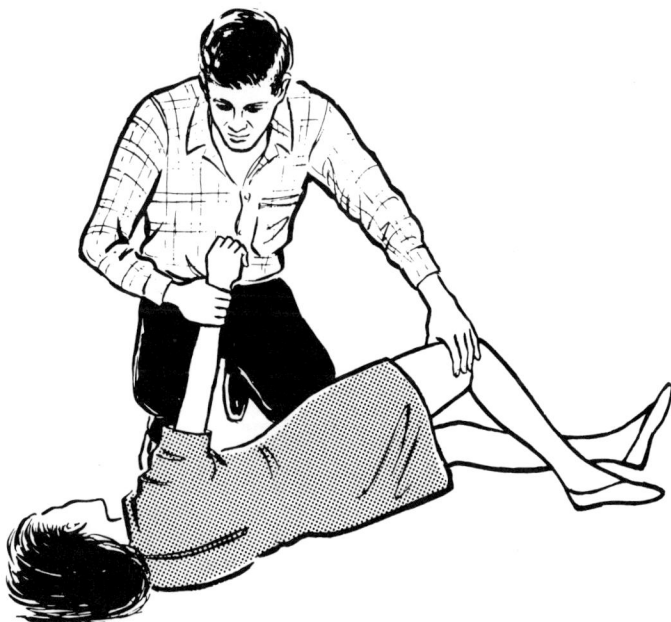

Fig. 12.5. Roll on side.

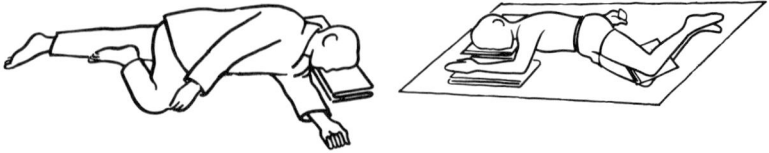

Fig. 12.6. Positioning of the casualty either (a) with both arms forward (avoid kink in the neck) or (b) in the classic 'coma', 'semiprone' or 'modified Sim's' position; no pillow should be placed under the head in this position, but a folded towel may be to prevent lateral flexion.

make sure airway is clear. If he is not breathing apply mouth-to-mouth resuscitation till an ambulance arrives.

IF SITTING IN THE CAR WITH HEAD SLUMPED FORWARD

Remove dentures and clean out his mouth.

Support the back of the head with one hand and his chin with the other, lift his head into the 'head back' position (Fig. 12.7) and maintain this position till the ambulance arrives. The victim's head can be stabilised in this position (which keeps his airway open) by supporting his chin and back of head with an improvised 'cervical collar' made from several sheets of newspaper folded about 4–5 in (10–15 cm) wide, cut to a length which will just go around the victim's neck, and secured with a triangular bandage (rectangular corner outside).

However, if there is bleeding from nose, mouth or throat and if the breathing is very rattly, an attempt must be made to put the

Fig. 12.7. Holding the airway free in a sitting victim.

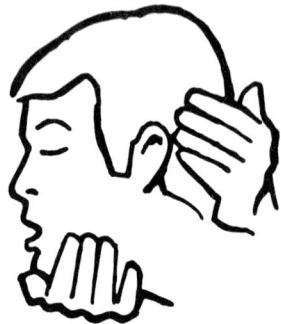

casualty onto his side, inside or outside the car, otherwise he may rapidly choke to death.

Loosen tight clothing (neck, chest, waist).

If not breathing commence mouth-to-mouth resuscitation.

6 Stop bleeding by applying a pressure dressing

(Pad or handkerchief pressed onto the bleeding spot by a bandage.) If this does not stop the bleeding tie a flat stone, matchbox etc over the pad to exert more pressure. Press around, but not onto, large objects sticking out of a wound.

7 Only in a dire emergency (fire) should a casualty be removed from a car

This is a difficult procedure without special equipment such as spinal boards and even with the best of skill (see point 9 (below)) can cause lasting damage to an already injured spinal cord.

8 Look out for broken bones, burns and internal injuries

Having secured breathing and position of all unconscious victims and controlled bleeding, now look for **victims with broken bones or burns and victims with perhaps hidden injuries who are feeling cold and clammy and start to look bluish pale (shock). Suspect internal abdominal injuries where an impact has involved great force and a lap belt or lap-sash belt has been worn** (Fig. 12.8 shows positioning of victims with suspected abdominal injuries).

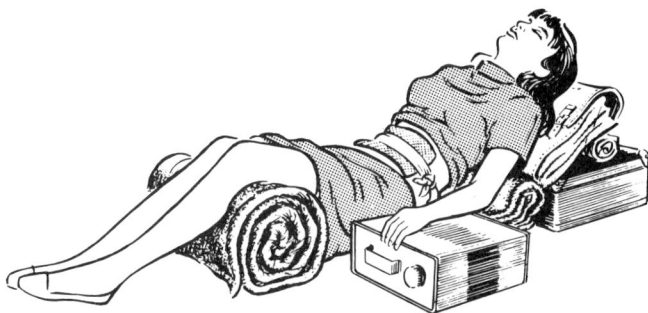

Fig. 12.8. Positioning for abdominal injuries.

Support and stabilise broken bones in the position of least pain and rest victims with suspected abdominal injuries with their knees up in a half-sitting position with the head back and supported. Shocked victims should lie flat with their legs straight and elevated where possible. Reassure all casualties. Get someone to take aside and talk to people with acute nervous reaction. Never give any alcohol.

9   Removal of an injured person sitting in a car, where no spinal board is available (Figs. 12.9 and 10).

(i)   Slide car seat into most backward position possible.

(ii)   Spread a blanket on the ground immediately alongside the door of the car.

(iii)   The first helper stabilises the victim's head in the 'head back' position (Fig. 12.7) making sure there is no neck movement during transfer of the casualty. If no extra helper is available for this task, stabilise the head with an improvised cervical collar (Fig. 12.10).

(iv)   The second helper slides his arms from behind around the victim's chest and grabs one or both of his forearms, bent at the elbow.

(v)   The third helper now takes up the weight of the legs, making sure that in the process of easing the victim out of the car neither the legs are pulled nor the pelvis turned in relation to the chest.

(vi)   The second helper now eases the victim's weight off the seat and moves him sideways onto his straightly held body, which acts like a spinal board. He himself must at the same time turn slightly towards the car, so that the legs can be eased out of the car by helper three without any turning of the legs sideways in relation to the body. If no third helper is available, the procedure may have to be carried out without him trying to minimise traction on the legs (and resulting flexion of the spine) as they are slid out of the car.

(vii)   Avoiding any pulling or sideways turning of the legs, the victim is now lowered supine between the second helper's legs and onto the blanket the ankles being held with slight traction by helper three, to prevent spinal flexion during extrication.

(viii) The edges of the blanket are now rolled up and used as handles

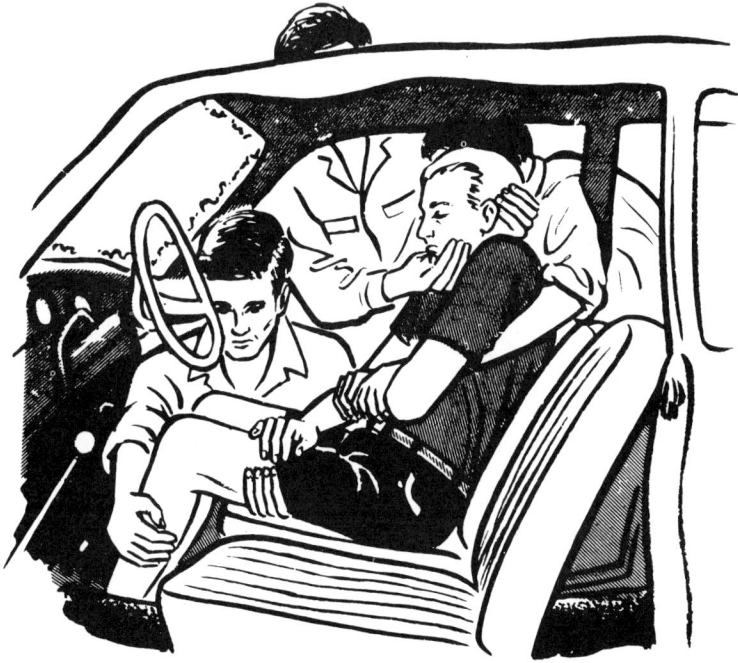

Fig. 12.9. Removal from car by three persons.

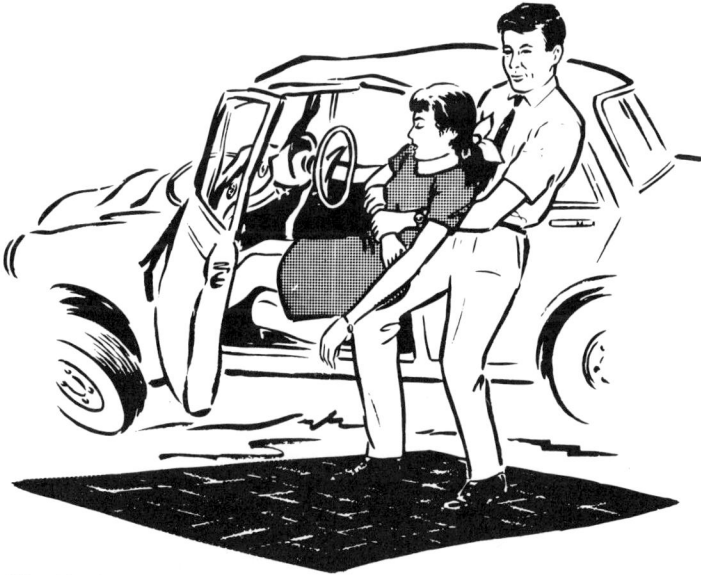

Fig. 12.10. Removal from car by one person. Note the improvised collar.

by about eight helpers (four on each side), with an additional helper holding the head so that it cannot move on the neck. In this 'blanket lift' the casualty can be carried a short distance (body absolutely straight and no sagging) to a safe spot nearby.

An alternative method is Easton's Blanket Lift (see Fig. 6.6) whereby a blanket, folded in concertina fashion is pushed under the victim's seat as soon as helper number two has grabbed and lifted him (Rautek's Grip) and is unfolded behind the victim's back. It is then unfolded on both sides of the victim, the edges rolled up towards him to serve as handles and he is lifted out with the blanket. The big problem with all these methods is of course to avoid bending the spine of the victim forward.

First aid kit for the family car

The contents of a first aid kit for the family car include:

A plastic airway ('Resuscitube') so that the victim's lips need not be touched in mouth-to-mouth respiration.

A clothes peg or strong wooden spatula the thickness of a finger, to be introduced with the finger when cleaning out the mouth (to avoid being bitten). A spoon is handy to remove vomitus.

Four triangular bandages and safety pins.

A block of soft wood $2 \times 4 \times 4$ cm with rounded edges, which can be bandaged over a pressure pad, should this alone not have stopped the bleeding.

Sheets of newspaper, readily folded and cut to make a cervical collar or a 'Pneumopack'.

A pair of strong notched scissors to cut away clothing to expose fractures or bleeding wounds.

A well packed dispenser of sterilised large dressing pads.

A roll of sticky tape (e.g. 'Micropore', or 'Blenderm').

A torch.

A sheet of reflecting aluminium foil to cover casualties ('space' blanket).

Two pencils (one always breaks off).

A supply of message forms (where not appended by law to the driving licence).

Standardised spaces for such a small first aid box (say inside the backrest of a driver's seat) could be a registration requirement for motor cars.

Instruction in first aid

Hossack's (1972) post mortem survey of 500 consecutive drivers and passengers killed in road crashes in Victoria highlighted the need for basic first aid instruction. Seven per cent of those killed were found to have died from inhalation of blood or vomitus before reaching hospital while concussed unconscious. No other serious injury was present. The Commissioner for Motor Transport in New South Wales the year before had already approved the inclusion of basic first aid in the new edition of the Motor Traffic Handbook, the official syllabus for driver licensing.

The importance of driver training in first aid rises with the distance from skilled help. Messages correctly given mean that ambulances are not misdirected and that ambulances and doctors are called less frequently to accidents in which no one is injured.

It is insufficient for every driver to be trained in elementary first aid if this is forgotten over the years. First aid, explained and practised in the course of driver training, must be reinforced by having its essentials printed on the back of the driving licence (mostly annually renewed) which should also have message forms as a tear-off portion.

While extrication of casualties by the untrained is undesirable, it is nevertheless unavoidable in some emergencies and an indication of technique must therefore be part of driver training.

THE ISOLATED DOCTOR

Is it important to have the country doctor at the scene?

In an area like mine, it is vital to have a doctor present at a serious accident. Even if the ambulance officer knew how to intubate, had frequent and continuing practice (how?) in finding bad veins, was skilled in diagnosing a tension pneumothorax, assessing shock and interpreting an electrocardiographic monitor, he would still have to drive the ambulance. To employ two officers per vehicle in a sparsely populated area, considering the number of accidents and the frequency of ambulance usage, has previously not been acceptable in New South Wales on economic grounds. Ambulance officers are naturally reluctant to allow volunteers to drive the ambulance vehicle for which they are responsible. Such volunteers—if available at crucial times—are usually not conversant with emergency driving techniques. Hence the involvement of country general practitioners in sparsely populated areas near national routes is not only a question of skill, but better use of available manpower.

The number of emergency calls I receive is small enough not to interfere significantly with the practice, yet is large enough to maintain and develop interest and experience (Table II).

The following cases indicate where **immediate medical intervention may have been lifesaving:**

16th February 1965: Mr P P, aged 47 years. Deep petrol burns involving about one third of body surface. Extensive intravenous shock treatment before about 50 miles transport to hospital.

14th January 1966: Mrs L W, aged 47 years. Knocked down by car, fractured pelvis, fractured nose, concussion, lacerations, unconscious. Inhaled vomitus, blue. Immediate laryngoscopic removal of laryngeal and tracheal obstruction by suction attached to intratracheal tubes (withdrawing lumps of meat) restoring respiration at scene by doctor 50 miles from casualty department.

17th January 1967: Mrs R T, aged 21 years. Bleeding heavily from vaginal lacerations at 34 weeks pregnancy. Immediate suturing at scene inside vagina was only means of arresting profuse haemorrhage. Delivered healthy female infant at 39 weeks in hospital, about 50 miles away.

2nd June 1968: Mrs N P, 37 years. Bruises and lacerations, alcohol and barbiturate overdosage. Limp coma, fixed, wide, unresponsive pupils, uncertain occasional heartbeat. Blood pressure 80/60 mm Hg. Time cycled positive pressure oxygenation and intravenous shock treatment with saline and Red Cross stable plasma protein solution as well as cortrophin before and during transport to casualty department about 50 miles away.

TABLE II

Not enough to interfere with the practice, yet sufficient to maintain and develop experience.

Accidents in the Tea Gardens Police District

Year	All accidents where medical aid was sought	Traffic accidents reported to police			Traffic accidents where the doctor was called to the scene			
		accidents	injured	killed	accidents	involved	injured	killed
1965	288	82	25	3	8	23	13	3
1966	331	92	51	2	23	50	40	2
1967	320	67	42	0	7	20	15	0
1968	310	50	18	3	10	43	27	2
1969	313	35	22	4	12	36	26	4
1970	325	66	56	9	13	73	47	9
1971	318	76	36	2	14	53	36	2
1972	325	88	53	4	10	36	24	3
TOTAL	2520	556	303	27	97	334	228	25

16th September 1971: head-on collision at midnight. Ten injured, five serious. Mother died at scene with fractured skull, but no brain injury noted at post mortem. Clot found, totally obstructing coronary artery. Father jammed in the wreckage, dislocated hip, multiple chest fractures, haemopneumothorax. Rescuers arrived 20 min after the accident. Freeing trapped victim another 20 min (recovered). Sixteen-year-old-son had a cerebral contusion, no fractured skull, but fractured left mandible with a large haematoma; deep, long laceration of the tongue; surgical emphysema extending to the neck, and fractured left radius and ulna. Deeply unconscious with clonic spasms right and left leg. Intratracheal intubation followed by time cycled positive pressure pure oxygen breathing through cuffed intratracheal tube on the scene and during one hour's transport to nearest intensive care hospital. Slowly regained consciousness after two weeks, then slow recovery. Eleven-year-old brother also had a cerebral contusion without a fractured skull, and a scalp laceration. He had to be transported without intubation and on admission had Cheyne–Stokes respiration and midbrain spasms. His heat regulation failed progressively and, in spite of steroids and intensive care, he died in two days.

13th November 1973: Mr P K aged 19 years. Motor cyclist whose right thigh caught between his cycle and a truck in a head-on collision. Suffered a high three-quarter amputation of his thigh, with 10 cm of his midfemur scattered in fragments over the road. Three doctors, an ambulance officer and police immediately infused 1000 ml of Red Cross Plasma Protein Solution (severe blood loss mainly from the femoral artery) and 1 litre of Hartmann's Solution during transport. On arrival at the base hospital about 2 hours later his blood pressure was 70 mm systolic with a haemoglobin of 7·6 per cent, but he was alive and treatable. His limb, which had been packed in crushed ice on the scene and put into a Thomas Splint however became rapidly gangrenous 14 days after admission and had to be amputated.

Where no doctor was called to the scene

21st November 1968: Two car collision near Swanbay turnoff. Two girls, fractured femurs, their 28-year-old mother, fractured pelvis, some rib fractures, some internal bruising. She suffocated slowly in transit to hospital from a small haemorrhage in her upper trachea. At the time of the message the nearest ambulance was 20 miles south, the nearest doctor (myself) 18 miles north (but not called).

The Government Medical Officer in Newcastle, NSW, who did the postmortem, thought that intratracheal intubation with a cuffed intratracheal tube on the scene by a medical practitioner might have been life saving. By the time the ambulance reached the scene it would have been too late to call a doctor (doctor's two-way radio was then not yet available—fund raising not far enough advanced).

24th January 1965: Mr N P, aged 22 years. Schoolteacher involved in a head-on collision north of the Tea Gardens turnoff on the Pacific Highway about 14 miles from my office, which could not be contacted. He was lying on the road for over an hour (nearest ambulance was then 50 miles away, no roadside phone) slowly lost consciousness and became unresponsive during another hour of ambulance transport. Post mortem showed some minor lacerations and multiple bruising including lungs and brain.

Whilst it may be difficult to say exactly why a person survived and how great the salvage rate in lives from immediate specially trained and experienced graduate medical aid may be, nobody doubts that there is in fact such a salvage rate. Also, while it may be still more difficult to measure how many complications and how much disability can be prevented by immediate medical aid, nobody doubts that it must be a considerably greater amount than the lives saved.

Cost benefit

The cost benefit of a young male saved in terms of compensation payments vis-à-vis the cost of a few medical calls is so astronomical that the provision can no longer be delayed of certain, immediate remuneration of doctors, who are prepared to train and equip themselves, and respond immediately to an emergency call.

The Government Insurance Office in New South Wales, the greatest underwriter of third party insurance in that state, has agreed with the New South Wales Branch of the Australian Medical Association to pay for any treatment given by doctors to their policyholders at the scene of a road accident. This is valid for three months irrespective of whether a claim has been received from the insured at the time.

THE RURAL RESCUE TEAM

In an isolated area this must of necessity be limited by the manpower and resources available. In my area (300 sq miles of land and water, 50 miles from the nearest casualty department, with a partly scattered resident population of 1500) there are—one ambulance officer, a police constable and a tow-truck operator, plus the occasional ad hoc volunteer. None of them is available or in the district 24 hours a day, but most of them are usually on call in case of an accident.

Police

Police secure the scene from 'run up' accidents, control bystanders, clear parked cars to allow ambulances and doctors to get to the casualties, control traffic and investigate the cause of the crash.

In spite of these many commitments police officers have always been most helpful in assisting with the treatment of the injured. Their help has included lifting and carrying, holding up infusion bottles, procuring ice to cool a partially severed limb, using an inflatable splint, stopping all oncoming cars to recruit doctors, nurses and trained first aiders and locating tablets, medical record cards and 'medi-alert' amulets.

Sometimes a police officer drives the ambulance to hospital thus freeing the ambulance officer to look after the patient in the stretcher compartment.

The police also have a radio communication system, which is helpful when the rest of the group attending an accident are otherwise engaged. Reciprocally, the ambulance radio is frequently used to notify police. While police cannot allow private doctors to listen in on their frequency, the ambulance service has allowed private doctors to use theirs to communicate vital medical information to the receiving hospitals, to call ambulances or to be called for by them.

Tow-truck drivers

In the absence of professional fire brigades or special volunteer rescue teams, as are available in larger centres of population, tow-truck drivers show a keen interest in assisting ambulance men and police not only in freeing trapped victims (not part of their normal job), and partici-pating in joint demonstrations, but also in carrying (and servicing) rescue equipment such as heavy hydraulic lifting gear, and sparkless pneumatic cutting tools. Many are expert car dismantlers and wreckers. Such services could be funded and controlled by central government, which could allow only trained truck drivers to operate on specified sections of highway.

Ambulance officers

It is too much to expect a singlehanded officer to both drive an ambulance **and** prevent deterioration in a patient's condition en route to hospital. (Although the expertise and knowledge of ambulance officers are increasing.)

New techniques to facilitate moving, splinting dressing and respirating casualties are being advertised almost daily. There is also the rapid emergence of electronic monitoring and telemetry devices, and car operated communication equipment. In order to save medical manpower there are demands that ambulance officers be taught to intubate and give intravenous infusions.

While most of these innovations are at present economically Utopian in a thinly populated area, nevertheless an ambulance officer has a formidable task to perform.

In New South Wales, as from 2nd April, 1973 the ambulance service has come under the control of an overriding Health Commission coordinating all services concerned with health. Ambulance Officers have now to show certain pass levels at the intermediate high school examinations. They must pass the three levels of first aid courses available to volunteers; and take a three-year diploma course as a male nurse at approved hospitals. Only then can they start training at the New South Wales Ambulance School. To my mind a training course of three years in a hospital is unnecessarily long, but will certainly help relieve the shortage of trainee nurses.

Role of the doctor in the team

The doctor must:

(1) Select those who can be resuscitated.
(2) Ensure immediate and effective medical treatment of breathing problems and shock.

(3) Prevent casualties likely to die or significantly deteriorate, unless treated at once, from being rushed untreated to the nearest hospital.

(4) Direct transport to a properly staffed and equipped hospital, not necessarily the nearest one.

(5) Ensure proper supervision and treatment during transport to prevent complications in transit.

What sort of medical skill is needed?

The quality of immediate treatment given to an accident victim is influenced by the quality of immediate assessment. The advantage of roadside radio phones directly linked to the two-way radio sets of the members of the team in their cars and offices has already been stressed. Such phones convert the fragmented pieces of information relayed by non-medical people into an immediate medical group interview. Isolated general practitioners, used to taking messages directly, have a particular skill in spot phone-diagnosis. During the epidemic tourist season I am able to dispense routinely the expected prescriptions before visiting patients and can give the treatment at consultation.

General practitioners are also at an advantage, in that experience has taught them to deal immediately with group situations involving more than one patient and in a highly relevant environment. They are highly experienced in the art of making cautious quick decisions based on their own observations, in improvising and giving immediate treatment, which is often all that is required in the vast majority of cases.

A road smash scene is such a group situation and it is often impossible to concentrate on one victim at a time. A quick assessment has to be made and priorities decided upon simultaneously.

In unconscious victims with absent or obstructed breathing, **every minute counts**—and allowance has also to be made for the time it takes to set up resuscitators, intravenous drips and monitoring equipment. The injured must be examined from top to toe (without the 'organ system' diagnostic approach of student days) (Fig. 12.11).

Training for this work must therefore be rationalised.

Assessment

Occasional combined exercises with ambulance officers, police and

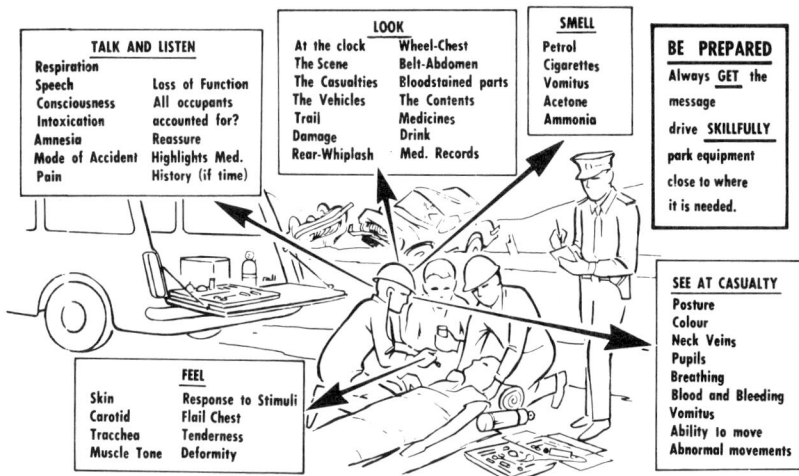

TALK AND LISTEN

Respiration	
Speech	Loss of Function
Consciousness	All occupants
Intoxication	accounted for?
Amnesia	Reassure
Mode of Accident	Highlights Med.
Pain	History (if time)

LOOK

At the clock	Wheel-Chest
The Scene	Belt-Abdomen
The Casualties	Bloodstained parts
The Vehicles	The Contents
Trail	Medicines
Damage	Drink
Rear-Whiplash	Med. Records

SMELL

Petrol
Cigarettes
Vomitus
Acetone
Ammonia

BE PREPARED

Always GET the
message
drive SKILLFULLY
park equipment
close to where
it is needed.

FEEL

Skin	Response to Stimuli
Carotid	Flail Chest
Trachea	Tenderness
Muscle Tone	Deformity

SEE AT CASUALTY

Posture
Colour
Neck Veins
Pupils
Breathing
Blood and Bleeding
Vomitus
Ability to move
Abnormal movements

"THOSE FIRST MOMENTS"....

Fig. 12.11. Those first moments.

rescuers (fire brigades, 'tow-truckies' or volunteers) are essential. Everybody must know what equipment the others have, and its mode of application. If rescue is the first priority the rescue specialist will take charge. Everyone, including the doctor may then need to act as his 'unskilled' labour. Where immediate intubation and infusion is first priority, ambulance and police officers can prepare the doctor's equipment, while he assesses other casualties.

The utmost information must be elicited from the first message without delay. This is the moment to ascertain the exact time of the accident. Later statements vary greatly. Exactly where is the accident? Should the messenger return to the scene with first-aid instructions? (e.g. turn unconscious persons into the coma position). Should any equipment be picked up which is not already in the doctor's car? (most should be).

It is important to arrive at the scene relaxed and in a state of high concentration. Do not arrive in a state of nervous tension from a risky drive at high speed. If the alleged 'emergency' should in fact have been trivial, breach of laws are difficult to justify later. If aroused from a deep sleep at night make sure you remember to put on your glasses (if worn). (Ed—and your trousers matey!)

Slow up and appraise the accident from a distance. It is sometimes possible to surmise the mechanism of the crash, and to select the best parking spot, particularly where one has to back the car to the casualties in order to have equipment handy from the 'instrument table' of a flip-down rear door of a station sedan. Room might be left for the ambulance to reverse in from the other side, its trolley— stretcher serving as an operating table outside the confined space of its stretcher compartment. Equipment may also have to be carried some distance from the road to a victim.

Treatment

Having first concentrated on the unconscious and attended to any breathing and vomiting problems, attention can be given to those with suspected fractures, burns and large wounds, most of whom will be conscious and complaining (which is a diagnostic help). Should the ambulance officer have arrived before he would already be busy splinting, bandaging and reassuring. If possible, have a word also with the lightly injured, because on occasion there will be one among them whose condition might suddenly worsen.

Quickly check whether first-aid as mentioned above has been done, whether the site of treatment is secure from oncoming traffic and whether a search and inquiry has been made for tablets, medical records, amulets, necklace tokens and alcohol. Are all accounted for?

Mouth-to-mouth resuscitation must immediately be delegated, other- wise the skilled rescuer can do no other important thing. Exhaled air respiration must be continued till the ambulance officer can continue with oxygen and a Guedel airway, followed where necessary by intubation.

Where there is a shortage of manpower, artificial respiration may have to be stopped on persons dead and grossly injured. Gross skull deformity is compatible with life.

Cardiac compression

This is always indicated in cases of heart attack, drowning or electrocution, but if it does not produce a readable blood pressure and return of pupil reflexes after 10 min, the situation should be reviewed. In traumatic shock, intravenous volume replacement may be of immediate importance and must not be delayed where artificial respiration and cardiac compression can be delegated. The value of cardiac compression in cardiac arrest due to massive haemorrhage from multiple fractures remains to be documented.

The chances of survival among casualties with multiple injuries, who are deeply unconscious and have non-reacting pupils, yet reach hospital alive, is poor.

Practical details are dealt with in my glove compartment manual (Pacy, 1971), which has been recommended for training medical graduates and senior ambulance officers. The essentials include assessment and prognosis, techniques of intubation, infusion venepuncture (including central veins), and shock treatment without equipment.

Indications for emergency measures

Intubation
Ideally all deeply unconscious patients, but certainly those with head injuries, injuries of their air passages and those who show signs of respiratory inadequacy; dyspnoea, air hunger, rapid respiration, use of accessory muscles, rising pulse or respiration rates, rising blood pressure indicating anoxia and carbon dioxide retention. Apathy and cyanosis are late signs. Adequate clearance of the airway (spooning out material if necessary) must precede intubation. A powerful sucker attached to an intratracheal tube may be needed to affect this clearance (see case '14th January 1966' quoted above).

Intravenous volume replacement

This can be decided on the following points:
The time since the accident.
The visible amount of blood lost.
The length of the journey to hospital and the type of transport.
The vascularity of the bleeding part (scalp, bowel, vagina).
The age and general condition of the patient.

More than one closed fracture of a limb needs 500 ml infusion for each and additional amounts if femur or pelvis are involved.
Rescue of chest and/or abdominal injuries.

Guidelines

The following rules are helpful:

The rule of hands

Deep soft tissue wounds the size of the patient's hand, need a transfusion of 500 ml.

The rule of hundred

A victim with a systolic blood pressure under and a pulse rate over a hundred should not be transported until an infusion has been given.

The rule of nine for burns

Blood volume lost and requiring replacement may be calculated as follows:

One whole arm, 9 per cent.
Whole of head and neck, 9 per cent.
One whole leg, 18 per cent.
Front of trunk, 18 per cent.
Back of trunk, 18 per cent.
Genitalia, 1 per cent.

The risk of overhydration if a head injury is present must be constantly kept in mind.

Paracentesis thoracis

Respiratory inadequacy with signs of tension pneumothorax; blue face; suffusion of conjunctivae; congested neck veins; flail chest; surgical emphysema; deviation of trachea to opposite side; and slow (paradoxical) pulse on inspiration. Listening to breath sounds through a stethoscope is usually difficult and unhelpful. Failure to improve colour on positive pressure oxygen breathing through a cuffed intratracheal tube must always arouse suspicion of a tension pneumothorax, (if it is certain that the tube is in the trachea). Disposable equipment for paracentesis can be carried, in a plastic bag included in the accident bag.

Special problems arising with some injuries

Chest injuries

(Look for deformed steering wheel)

(i) Ensure carefully controlled ventilation and treat for shock.
(ii) Fix parts of the chest wall moving abnormally then close penetrating chest wounds.

Head injuries

Anyone who claims to have amnesia or has lost consciousness transiently in a traumatic accident must have:

(i) Follow-up examination.
(ii) Regular recording of blood pressure, pulse rate and level of consciousness, together with the time they were taken.

Anyone with disturbed consciousness or headaches must have the above recorded half hourly, and must be taken to a suitable hospital.

Abdominal injuries

Any patient with a history of an abdominal blow must have a follow-up examination when symptoms appear, or if none appear, after 6 hours. If there are any symptoms or signs of internal injury, he must be sent to a suitable hospital for clearance.

Think of ruptured spleens and livers when the impact was great and a lap-sash belt was worn, or where the steering wheel was deformed by a driver's body.

Anticipate shock and infuse liberally at an early stage.

Fractures

Do not transport without adequate immobilisation (the best analgesic) and adequate intravenous shock treatment where indicated. Give transport priority to fractures impairing blood supply.

Spinal injuries

Think of whiplash injury to neck, where car is damaged in the rear and there is no head restraint at the back of the seat. Any victim, who complains of significant pain in the neck or is suspected of a vertebral fracture (tenderness of mal-aligned spinal process, or localised spinal pain) must be treated as for spinal injury. Any paralysis or loss of sensation indicative of a spinal injury must be treated as for vertebral fracture.

Two principles govern management:

(i) Ensure immobility.
(ii) Prevent decubitus lateral flexion—(which in paralysed areas can appear within 2 hours). Cushion heels, sacrum, lumbar and cervical lordoses (padded cardboard stretcher).

What sort of equipment?

Apart from the items listed for a first aid box that every motorist might carry, the essential contents of a doctor's equipment is a shock-box and an intubation set. Both can be carried under the front seats of a doctor's car. Where these are carried in a special bag it is wise to have the bag in a bright reflecting colour for visibility on the road and to carry a strong bright vinyl sheet buttoned around the bag, which can be spread out on the ground and upon which small items of equipment are clearly distinguishable even in the light of a torch.

The shock box

This should at least contain one or more litres of plasma expander or substitute, of a kind that can be stored indefinitely at the temperatures in a doctor's car, that does not interfere with subsequent blood grouping and cross-matching, and can leak paravenously in quantity during unsupervised transport without any ill effect.

It must carry injectable Adrenaline (1 ml, 1:1000), an antihistaminic (promethazine 50 mg in 2 ml) and sufficient corticosteroid (1 g methyl-prednisolone or equivalent) to deal with the rare, sudden, but potentially fatal, sensitivity reaction to an infusion. The signs of such a reaction are: backache, nausea (stop infusion); generalised rubor and hot flushes (give antihistaminic); tachycardia, collapse of systolic blood pressure below 90 mm Hg (give 100 mg methylprednisolone); dyspnoea (give massive corticosteroid); cardiac arrest (reanimate).

Other essential contents of the shock box are:

Two or more giving sets.

Plastic wide bore cannulas with trocars in them to fit the giving sets.

Venous tourniquets.

Scalp vein needles for entering small veins, which can then be distended with saline to make them puncturable by a large cannula.

Large bore central venous giving sets for those experienced with the technique (of innominate puncture).

Transparent adhesive strapping which adheres to perspiring (or wet) skin.

'Sporefree' foil-wrapped alcohol swabs.

Sterile disposable syringes 2 ml and 10 ml with lateral cannula insertion, and a range of cannulae.

Ampoules of: 30 mg Pentazocine; 5 mg Dexamethasone (prevention of cerebral oedema); a hypoallergic, antibiotic injection stable at the high temperatures in a doctor's car (such as 600 mg Lincomycin) for the prevention of infection and—where temperatures allow: Heparin (helpful in snakebites and septic shock).

The intubation set

At least two sizes of laryngoscope with working batteries.

Strong wooden spatula or finger armour.

Spoon.

Range of cuffed intratracheal tubes with syringe for inflation and clamp.

Sticky tape, which can adhere to perspiring skin.

Sucker

In my experience a really satisfactory sucker for the doctor's car has not yet been found. Both the foot and hand operated ones are generally weak, particularly when fitted with thin suction tubes. Oxygen powered apparatus is wasteful of oxygen, needed for positive pressure respiration. Suckers should be connectable to intratracheal tubes.

Artificial breathing apparatus

For manual operation the 'Ambu' bag is excellent. It weighs little, packs into a small space, is instantly operational and reinflates spontaneously after being compressed.

There is, however, a case for giving pure oxygen when positive pressure ventilation through a cuffed intratracheal tube is being used. Tissue damage involves damaged circulation and among the tissues most vulnerable to oxygen starvation are brain, heart, liver and kidneys. Loss of blood volume must be replaced but plasma substitutes provide no red blood cells to carry oxygen. Abnormally high partial oxygen pressure in the lungs can improve the exchange in the remaining oxygen carriers and, subsequently into the damaged tissues. Infusable fluorocarbon emulsions as oxygen carriers are not yet commercially available. (Clark, Becattini and Kaplan).

Ambulances in New South Wales are equipped with manually time cycled respirators (the 'oxy-viva') and I prefer these, because with push button control the operator can apply positive pressure in short inspiratory bursts, thus preventing the building up of unduly elevated positive pressure inside the chest, with inhibition of venous return and enhancement of cerebral oedema. He can also detect the enhancement of a latent, previously unnoticed, tension pneumothorax and aspirate the chest. When pressed, I have on occasion delegated this push button control to an instructed volunteer in order to attend to other things. This has worked quite well.

Apart from a whole range of cardiac monitors there is now available (Teknis) a simple respiratory monitor, which is cheap, can be strapped to the victim's chest and confirms that air is actually entering the lungs at a certain (appropriate) rate. In this case the monitor sits on the chest. As a general rule monitoring equipment should be mountable in a fixed position in the ambulance. Trying to control infusion bottles, respirators and loose monitoring equipment in the confined space of a moving ambulance is an impossible task.

Another problem on a long trip is the short life of conventional oxygen bottles when used for positive pressure breathing through a cuffed intratracheal tube as well as for suction. This may partly be overcome by fitting ambulances with larger oxygen containers and providing piped oxygen to the stretcher compartment. However, as far as doctors' cars in remote areas are concerned, Dr Komesaroff of the Royal Hobart Hospital has now invented an ingenious re-breathing ventilator which from one small, light portable oxygen bottle provides positive pressure oxygen breathing for up to six hours. It is certainly an interesting innovation. It includes an intubation set and a mini shock box, but it does need a carrying handle to make it more portable alongside an elevated stretcher.

A helpful innovation is Sarnoff's inflatable cuff, which contains a pressure pack to control bleeding arteries and can also be used as an adjustable neck collar.

A chest drainage set can be easily made up from the disposable catheters, flutter valves and bags commercially available. This, with a local anaesthetic set and a scalpel are packed in the same sterilised cloth and wrapped in plastic. Before performing a thoracotomy, the wise roadside surgeon will verify his suspicions using a simple pneumothorax-type, winged cannula ('Strauss' cannula) to which is attached a surgeons finger cot. I keep this in a sterilised screw cap jar which goes with the set. Such a cannula can be sufficient for a short journey, but because of the small lumen it blocks up easily. It can of course be readily accommodated in a shock box, where no thoracotomy set is carried.

In addition, an isolated doctor attending remote accidents will need to wear protective, light-reflecting clothing and carry a warning triangle, a red flashing light, a helmet with a headlamp, inflatable splints, spare infusion fluid, spare adaptors—for tracheal tubes and respirators —fitting those carried by the ambulances. Plastic transparent sheets are useful for putting over messy parts of the patient, allowing observation for bleeding. A variety of large sterilised dressings completes the choice of equipment which is based on statistical records of needs over a number of years. While I started with a lot of my own equipment in the absence of a local ambulance, I now am relying more and more on the ambulance to carry equipment.

The 'non-traumatic' emergency bag

In this age of proliferating welfare legislation I find it increasingly difficult to carry a doctor's bag to the usual welfare domiciliary visit.

The very weight of government stationery is so great that medical items had to gradually disappear from the bag, which has now been stripped to a stethoscope, a sphygmomanometer, a few ballpens, a small supply of disposable syringes—but is still getting weightier as new application forms multiply.

However, there is still the genuine medical emergency call and for this I have in my car a 'non-traumatic' emergency bag, containing first of all a range of injections and appropriate disposable syringes and cannulas and premoist swabs.

Digoxin (0·5 mg in 1 ml), which can be mixed in the syringe with 10 per cent calcium gluconate (10 ml), deslanoside (0·4 mg in 2 ml) —if veins are small, can be given undiluted; lignocaine (100 mg, 5 ml), heparin (12 500 i.u. in 1 ml), aminophylline (250 mg, 10 ml), adrenalin (2 × 1 mg in 1 ml), metaraminol (10 mg, 1 ml), hydrocortisone sodium succinate (100 mg inject. set), promethazine (50 mg, 2 ml), promazine 50 mg, pethilorfan 50/0·625 mg, hyoscine butylbromide (20 mg, 2 ml), tiemonium iodide (5 mg, 2 ml), pentazocine (60 mg in 2 ml), diazepam 10 mg, chlorpromazine (50 mg, 2 ml), prochlorperazine (12, 5 mg, 1 ml), phenytoin sodium—inject 250 mg with 5 ml solvent, dextrose— inject 50%, 10 ml, diazoxide (300 mg in 20 ml) and clauden (10 ml). I still carry morphine–atropine (15/0·4 mg, 1 ml) morphine–hyoscine (15/0·6 mg) and pethidine (100 mg in 2 ml), but these will probably be discontinued when my stocks are exhausted. A liberal amount of local anaesthetic is packed with the thoracic paracentesis set in the road accident bag.

There is a tracheotomy set which I have not used in 18 years and two 'Koller' vacuum venules for the collection of blood specimens. More frequent, however, is the use of the gastric lavage tube and Syrup of Ipecac. Glauber's salt, liquid paraffin and charcoal complete this side of the picture. A sterilised bladder catherisation set is in the bottom compartment of the bag. This bag is not usually carried out of the car to a road accident.

With all these bags an isolated doctor's car becomes a powerful tool in the handling of emergencies.

Economic versus desirable ambulance vehicles

Ambulances

A modern ambulance is allegedly not a clinic bus or free taxi for the irresponsible contributor demanding medical authorisation for transport, but should be suitable for treatment during transport, have a centrally mountable stretcher, standing room for the attendants and room beyond the head end of the stretcher.

Until recently our small remote community in a thinly populated area through which the busiest national intercity routes run could afford only a cheap converted station sedan to serve both as life support unit for accidents or serious illness and taxi for elderly infirm, to the nearest base hospital town 50 miles (80 km) away.

Now the State government of New South Wales with its Health Commission controlling the ambulance service has already supplied two larger ambulances, two full time ambulance officers, helicopter landing sites at hospitals, and improved communications (October 1976). Approval has been given for another ambulance station 22 miles North on the highway. The Government and Commission is also sending officials to study Immediate Care Schemes abroad.

Advanced life support course for ambulance officers

This three segment, 14 weeks course, which has been modified to meet the needs of New South Wales, is based on the Los Angeles paramedics training course:
1. A primer segment of two weeks at the Ambulance Board Training School.
2. A didactic segment of 6 weeks at St Vincent Hospital in Sydney using the teaching staff of the Medical Schools of the Universities of Sydney and New South Wales.
3. A clinical segment of six weeks duration, during which officers gain experience in a major hospital.

The ambulance constructed by the body builders Binz and Co in West Germany has been selected as the most suitable vehicle.

Helicopters

With the distances and roads involved, the introduction of ambulance helicopters in Australia looks promising, even if one has to realise that 20 existing ambulance vehicles can be obtained for the price of one helicopter. A successful helicopter service operates from the isolated Mornington peninsula in Victoria, where there is a large population to be served.

In my area a helicopter is available at the Williamtown Air Force base, which is on the aerial route from here to the nearest base hospital. But this has so far never been used in a road accident, because of the time consuming authorisation procedure for civilian use of military aircraft and inability to land safely on the narrow National Route No 1 under civilian air safety regulations. There are now some prepared landing spots for a helicopter along the highway and better use of existing helicopter facilities might be possible. However the smaller helicopters have the space disadvantages of small ambulances and when normally on other work are seldom equipped as life support units.

The rescue angle

Only once in a few years is there any need for heavy rescue vehicles on a remote stretch of highway and these have to travel far. The situation is however, not quite as hopeless as it may seem. A minimum of civil defence training for local tow-truck operators, a few blocks and beams, a civil defence steel rope pulling and lifting device, some heavy hydraulic lifting and spreading tools (the 'Porto Power' range) as well as a sparkless pneumatic cutter and saw, powered by the pressure of a nitrogen bottle, together with crowbars and similar tools, will in fact solve most extrication problems. The problem is of course to obtain this equipment, make the tow-truck operators conversant with its use, and have it regularly inspected and maintained. I have not yet been able to find any tow-truck operator prepared to undergo formal civil defence training in a remote place (though one, fortunately, was an ex-army rescue instructor), and funds for the provision of necessary equipment have largely to be begged from the local people. These are the weakest links in a rural rescue team on an interstate national route passing through such an area. There is considerable resistance by residents to be called upon to donate money for equipment which does not benefit them locally. In most areas no equipment at all is available at the necessary close range. The problem could only be solved by limiting the towing of wrecks from national routes and main roads to operators who have undertaken the necessary rescue training and are given not only training, but also equipment and its maintenance at public expense.

ORGANISED SCHEMES BRINGING DOCTORS TO THE SCENE OF ROAD ACCIDENTS

The performance of passing doctors stopped by police at the scene of accidents has been rather variable. Most doctors seem to set up intravenous drips when necessary, but there is certainly ample room for improvement of our undergraduate and graduate training in the proper management of major trauma—our modern epidemic.

Following the tremendous stimulus given by Easton in Britain, several attempts are being made in this country to involve surburban and country general practitioners at the scene of road accidents on a permanent basis. For this purpose certain general practitioners have been appointed Directors of Emergency Services. One is Dr Peter Bush in Melbourne, who holds this position at the Royal Melbourne Hospital and has a scheme involving about 20 general practitioners in the area of the Box Hill District Hospital on the fringe of Melbourne. They converge onto road accidents together with police, ambulance and where needed other rescuers. Another is Dr K J Murphy at the Freemantle Hospital, who runs a similar organisation called 'Emergency Care Western Australia'. The results of these schemes are awaited with interest. The success of them will of course largely depend on rapid transmission of the primary message and whether doctors can respond to it as fast as ambulance and police.

PREVENTION OR MITIGATION OF ROAD ACCIDENTS IN AUSTRALIA

There is a conflict between natural human behaviour and the cars and roads that are available. With 13 million taxpayers having to provide roads for a continent almost the size of Europe, expressway construction between all capital cities is unlikely to have been accomplished by the end of this century. Yet most cars locally manufactured and sold follow designs from denser populated countries with expressway networks. Alcohol in Australia has been shown to be involved in at least half of fatal road accidents (Henderson). Consumption of intoxicants per capita has been going up every year for at least seventeen years. This year the excise on wine has been removed— to stimulate the wine industry. As the consumption of alcohol before eating on the way home from work (and it gets hot in Australia in summer) is a cherished national custom, the question of controlling drunken driving is politically explosive, and an almost impractical avenue to controlling road accidents. This atmosphere also makes effective preventive use of breathalysers by police very difficult. In a rare burst of political courage the State Government of Victoria recently legislated for the compulsory wearing of seatbelts to prevent injuries and deaths. This measure, which was well accepted and soon followed by all other states, has been followed by a 20 per cent fall in road deaths in the first 12 months. This fall has been sustained. While accidents themselves are also difficult to prevent by improvements in roads, injuries and deaths can be prevented by vehicle improvements. Here Australian legal specifications usually follow slowly behind the USA, where most cars sold in Australia are designed. This is likely to yield results. The effect of constant appeals to drivers to slow up, not to drink, to have a rest after driving long hours, to give way, and so on have of course been tried over many years. No really convincing proof of their effectiveness has yet been produced, but it is impressive to notice altered driving behaviour around well known roadside radar speed traps. In spite of all this there is a steady fall of injuries and deaths in terms of vehicle miles. New South Wales has now introduced basic first aid as part of its driver training syllabus. There is no doubt that the death and injury rate could be further reduced by better organised and legislated first aid and medical treatment at accident sites.

REFERENCES

Clark, Becattini, and Kaplan (1972), Can Fluorocarbon Emulsions be used as artificial bloods, *Triangle*, **2**, 115–122.
Easton (1968), Improvised Stretcher, *Brit. med. J.* **3**, 123.
Henderson (1973), The Cup That Cheers, *Autosafe*, **1**, 29. (Sydney NSW: Dept of Motor Transport.)
Hossack (1972), The Pattern Of Injuries Received by 500 Drivers and Passengers Killed In Road Accidents, *Med. J. Aust.*, **2**, 193.
Komesaroff (1972), A New Concept In Emergency Resuscitation–The Oxy-Resuscitator, *Proceedings of the Fifth World Conference on general practice, Papers and Abstracts*, **1**, 21–24.
Morgan (1972) Accident Services in America, *Injury* **4**, 95–101.
Pacy (1972), Rescue and First Aid for our Highways, *Med. J. Aust.* **1**, 704–707.

Pacy (1972), Road Accidents—The Immediate Response when, where, by whom, and how, *Injury*, **4**, 11–17.

Pacy (1972), Problems of Roadside Aid in New South Wales *Australian Family Physician* **1**, 70–75.

Pacy (1973), First Aid for Drivers, *JAMA*, **223**, 1151–1153.

Rautek's Grip (1965), Erste Arztliche Hilfe am Unfallort *Bundesarztekammer Manual*. Koln-Berlin: Deutscher Arzteverlag.

Ryan and Clark (1972), The Emergency Care of Traffic Injury Before Hospital, *Med. J. Aust.*, **1**, 1173.

Stuckey (1972), The Australian Medical Associations Ambulance Survey, *Proceedings of the National Road Safety Symposium 14–16 March*, 1972 Canberra, Concurrent Session 2C, Department of Shipping and Transport, Canberra, A.C.T., Australia.

Teknis Pty. Ltd., Box 45, Kingswood, South Australia, makers of the Respiration Monitor mentioned.

FURTHER READING

Advanced Training Program for Emergency Medical Technician-Ambulance. National Academy of Sciences /National Research Council, Washington, USA.

Ambulance Design Criteria, US Department of Transportation. US Govt. Printing Office.

American Academy of Orthopaedic Surgeons (1972), Emergency Care and Transportation of the Sick and Injured, Americ. Acad. of Orthop. Sgns. Chicago.

American College of Surgeons (1970), Essential Equipment for Ambulances *Bulletin, May 1970.*

American College of Surgeons (1972), *Early care of the injured patient*, p. 425. Philadelphia: WB Saunders Company:

Cole and Puestow (1972), *Emergency Care.* New York: Appleton Century Crofts, Meredith Corporation.

Easton (1970), Road Accidents and the Family Doctor, British Medical Association, Tavistock Square, London.

Gardner and Roylance (1969), *New Advanced First Aid.* London: Butterworths.

Gogler (1960), Unfallopfer im Strassenverkehr *Documenta Geigy, Series chirurgica, Nr. 5*, p. 144.

Huntley (1972), How is emergency care in *your* community?, *Emergency Medicine*, April issue p. 51. (New York).

Hooper (1969), *Patterns of acute head injury*, p. 162. London: Edward Arnold.

Irving (1972), *Traumatic shock*, Folia Traumatologica Geigy. Basle: Ciba-Geigy Ltd.

Jamieson and Tait (1966), *Traffic Injury in Brisbane*, p. 384. National Health and Medical Research Council Special Report Series N. 13, Canberra, Australia.

Jamieson, Duggan, Tweddell, Pope and Zvirbulis (1971), *Traffic Injury in Brisbane*, p. 359. Australian Road Research Board, Special Report Nr. 2.

Ledingham and Mcallister (1972), *Conference on shock*, p. 193. London: Kimpton.

National Road Safety Symposium (1972), Report of discussions at the, Expert Group on Road Safety, Dept. of Shipping and Transport, Canberra, Australia.

Pacy (1971), *Road accidents—medical aid*, a guide for medical practitioners and senior ambulance officers involved at the scene of motor traffic accidents, p. 120. E. & S. Livingstone Ltd. (now Churchill Livingstone), Edinburgh and London.

Proctor and London, (1962), *Principles of First Aid for the Injured*. London: Butterworths.

Rescue, Civil Defence Handbook, Nr. 7. London: Her Majesty's Stationery Office (ask for latest edition).

Royal Australasian College of Surgeons (1970), The management of Road Traffic Casualties, Proceedings of the First Seminar May, Melbourne, 1969.

Skinner, Henderson and Herbert, Compulsory wearing of seatbelts, a feasibility study. Traffic Accident Research Unit, Dept. of Motor Transport, NSW, 1st December, 1970.

Snook (1974), *Medical aid at Accidents*, London: Update Publications.

St Vincent Hospitals Staff, Sydney (1969), *The medical and surgical management of road injuries*, p. 178. Sydney: E. J. Dwyer.

World Health Organization (1968), The organization of resuscitation and casualty services, Document EURO 0256, Regional Office for Europe, Copenhagen.

World Medical Journal. The whole of the Jan–Feb. 1970 issue, which is on Emergency Services and Care.

35 mm SLIDES WITH TAPED COMMENTARY

Easton (1968), Roadsmash Rescue is Your Concern, set of 65 slides and commentary produced by the Royal College of General Practitioners Medical Recording Service (updated 1976).

Easton (1969), Roadside First Aid (set of 31 slides and commentary) produced by the Royal College of General Practitioners Medical Recording Service.

Easton (1972), Every Doctor's Roadside Drill, The Medical Recording Service Foundation, Kitts Croft, Writtle, Chelmsford Essex. CM1 3EH (26 min).

Pacy (1970), Roadside Aid: Are we prepared?, set of 82 slides and commentary. The Medical Recording Service, Royal Australian College of General Practitioners, 43 Lower Fort str. Sydney.
Pacy (1971), First Aid by the Roadside, ibidem.

13

Safety On, In or Under Water

STANLEY MILES

Man is essentially a land animal conditioned to existence in a two-dimensional environment. Natural curiosity and economic necessity have, over the ages, resulted in a considerable exploitation of the seas and inland waters for transport, productivity, warfare and recreation.

In the course of this development many lives have been lost and much hardship endured largely due to lack of concern for or understanding of the hazards. A three-dimensional environment is quite different from man's natural habitat. Storms, tempests and turbulence contrast in the extreme with the serene gentleness of a placid sea. Tides, currents and submerged obstacles are traps for the unwary. Vast distances, silence and loneliness may disturb the reason of the single-handed adventurer or castaway.

The inland waters have special dangers. Their very nearness to centres of population presents risks to playing children and intoxicated pedestrians. They are a handy means for the potential suicide. Natural falls and rapids, man-made weirs, hidden objects and embracing weeds add further hazard.

For swimmers in, and divers under water there are special factors which must be appreciated for success and safety. Tides and currents frequently move swifter than the fastest swimmer. Buoyancy just fails to give man support and his efforts to stay afloat or swim must sooner or later be expended and he will drown. In some parts of the world dangerous marine animals, from subtle death-stinging coelenterata to ferocious sharks or killer whales, are man's natural enemies.

The diver, for adaptation to an environment which will not support life, has special problems with respiration, with the supply of air or other breathing mixtures at pressures appropriate to his depth. He must be protected from the poisonous effects of excess nitrogen, or oxygen or carbon dioxide and return to the surface free from the crippling disabilities of decompression sickness. He must accommodate his senses to changes in the speed of sound, the refraction of light, of diminished vision and a state of relative weightlessness.

It is wise to consider this long list of potential hazards at the outset, to stimulate thought. At the same time it must be made quite clear that, formidable as the list may seem, there is no room whatever for despondency. The opportunities and pleasures which the seas and inland waters offer can be acheived with comfort and safety provided the environment is fully understood and the need to come to terms with it accepted. Much has been learnt from experience and much achieved by study and research. Most activities on, in or under water have organisations which accept mandatory or voluntary responsibility for those participating. They organise training programmes and have established codes of practice. These are the blueprints for survival. It is the 'freelance' individual who frequently comes to grief, or the casual unthinking holidaymaker.

SAFETY ON THE WATER

In the big ships

By and large the big ships, say those of 200 ft (60 m) in length or over, offer the safest means of transport or recreation. For the crew and passengers there are, of course, the ever present risks of injury similar to those of the factory and home increased from time to time by bad weather which if additional care is not taken may result in persons falling against or being struck by heavy objects. Care is needed on the part of the crew to secure all free articles and furniture and for passengers to exercise caution and keep firm hold on guard rails which are readily available. For some, vigilance may be reduced by seasickness for which specific remedies are available and effective.

In big ships, the major disasters result from navigational error and fire, either of which may necessitate abandoning ship and taking to boats or rafts. This is usually a well planned, though rarely well rehearsed, procedure.

The major killers in the water are drowning and hypothermia though injury may well occur if care is not taken when leaving the ship. Usually the first thought on such occasions is to grab the life jacket and rush to the lifeboat station. Equally important is the need to keep warm. Ordinary clothing, even when wet, offers some protection. Thus equally important as the lifejacket is the need to put on as much warm clothing as possible. It was cold, not drowning which killed 1200 victims when the Titanic sank.

If a lifeboat or liferaft can be reached with safety, survival thereafter depends on the search and rescue organisations having been alerted. For this reason it is better to remain in the area of the shipwreck in an inflatable raft with its protective canopy than sail or row off in an open lifeboat to attempt to reach land which may be many miles away.

Water now becomes the prime necessity—each person requiring a minimum of half a litre per day. This is the main component of the liferaft rations and usually supplied in cans. It may be supplemented by the collection of rain or the use of solar stills or desalting tablets. If water is available life can be maintained for six weeks or so without food. If food is to form part of the emergency supply, though most would wish all available space to be taken up by water, carbohydrates appear to give the best calorie value for bulk. Exhaustion, exposure, seasickness, sunburn or frostbite and loss of hope may adversely affect the chances of survival. The presence of highly skilled and mature professional sailors will do much to reduce these hazards.

When help does arrive or shore is reached rehabilitation must be gentle with frequent administrations of nourishing fluids in small quantities, and good nursing.

In small ships

The bulk of vessels falling into this category are the trawlers, the professional fishermen, who face the most perilous adversities of the sea and an industry demanding skilful practice with complicated machinery on a slippery heaving deck.

In recent years much official action has been taken to improve the safety of trawler fishermen by modifying technique, encouraging training and above all supplying adequate survival clothing and liferafts. Fleets in northern waters are now accompanied by support ships with medical officers which give a considerable degree of added security and reassurance.

Also in this category must be placed the ferry steamers and pleasure boats active in coastal waters. Disasters are not common though collisions do occur in fog from time to time. Such misadventures are usually within reach of shore-based rescue facilities and casualties are light. No special recommendations need be made to passengers and government safety regulations are adequate.

In small boats

In the coastal waters round the maturer countries of the world countless amateur sailors of all degrees of skill and experience constantly enjoy the freedom and adventure available to them. The majority remain within easy reach of land but quite a few venture from one country to another, and here and there the dedicated and experienced enthusiast may set out single-handed to cross a major ocean or circumnavigate the world.

These small boats from time to time capsize through lack of skill, exceptional risk taking or violent weather conditions. Prevention of such mishaps is undoubtably the most important investment in safety. This calls for prudence in avoiding adverse conditions by using local knowledge and accepting informed advice, particularly by the weather forecasters. Skill in handling the craft should be gained by practice and instruction from experts. Its seaworthiness and buoyancy should be assured. Crew and passengers should wear approved lifejackets and, in all but the warmest climates, clothing which will protect from hypothermia. The degree of cold which an individual can tolerate varies very much indeed from one person to another, but even round the coasts of Britain survival in the winter months may be measured in minutes for the unprotected. Wet suits or specially designed survival suits are the best investment but warm woollens and oilskins are also a help.

Further measures in larger boats include the 'body line' for security on deck in bad weather. For those going out of sight, or easy reach of land, good communications (radio, flares, smoke candles and emergency signals) are essential. A good inflatable liferaft, large enough to take all on board completes the safety equipment. None of this however can ever be a substitute for **good seamanship** which is, without any doubt, the secret not only of safety but of true enjoyment of small boat sailing.

Speed boats and motor cruisers must not be overlooked. They have the same potential for disaster and need much the same precautions. They are particularly dangerous to swimmers, when close inshore their propeller blades inflicting grave injuries. The helmsman must accept the responsibility for others' safety and be at all times vigilant and alert.

The requirements of the ocean going single-handed sailor are beyond the scope of this book. He is dependent on years of experience, training and maturity and must plan his voyage to the smallest detail and with every possible danger in mind. What can be achieved has been shown by success in recent years. The example of these experts should be an encouragement to all, and the contribution they make to safety of small boat sailing throughout the world is immeasurable.

Other activities on the water

These include canoeing, water skiing and surfboard riding; all exciting sports demanding the highest degrees of skill. Each has its own well-established association which produces codes of safety and offers training for beginners and competitive activities for the experts. But each activity may leave its participants alone in the water faced with the risks of drowning or hypothermia. They should therefore be good swimmers and wear clothing which would keep them afloat and warm. They must also be fully aware of their responsibility to others. The motor boat towing the skier must keep clear of bathers, as must the surfboard rider. The board is heavy and has a sharp keel. When parted from its rider it may be thrown in the air and strike unsuspecting persons nearby in the water.

SAFETY IN THE WATER

A great deal of relaxed pleasure and competitive enjoyment results from man's ability to swim and his affinity for bathing, be it in the sea, some inland waterway or an artificial swimming pool. Unfortunately large numbers of persons drown each year in such activities, very often children, and mostly when on holiday or a recreational outing. All too often the victim loses his life in an attempt to save another.

Invariably these drownings are unnecessary and due to lack of elementary precautions or gross ignorance. In this country about 1500 persons drown each year—three-quarters of them in inland waters.

On holiday beaches most tragedies occur when conditions for bathing are unsuitable. Undertows, tides and currents carry the inexperienced swimmer into danger. Children are not adequately supervised by parents and may easily be lost in a crowd in relatively shallow water and drown unnoticed. Others may be relaxing on inflated toys or mattresses and drift or be blown into deep or dangerous water. Lone swimmers in isolated coves may attempt to swim beyond their capability.

Much can be done to lessen the toll of drowning by education and propaganda. 'Learn to swim' campaigns for children will be successful if lessons are accompanied by instruction in water safety and lifesaving. A respect for, and confidence in the water should be the final aim.

On the beaches in recent years the establishment of lifeguards, patrols, look-outs and rescue boats has done much to save life. Lifesaving clubs offer in themselves an exciting and rewarding activity with ample scope for challenging competitive sport. An efficient lifeguard unit will be alert and competent to rescue anyone in danger and will maintain an indicating system of signal flags to denote where and when conditions are safe for bathing or where there is danger.

The loss of life on beaches is seasonal but inland waters extort a steady toll throughout the year. It is impossible to establish any effective system of patrolling and the only satisfactory safety measure, apart from educating the public and especially children to an awareness of the danger, is effective fencing.

Even small garden pools claim many victims. It is therefore imperative that parents should be aware of this and ensure that in their own gardens their own small children and those of their friends are not exposed to this risk.

Drowning

Nearly all deaths from major mishaps in water are by drowning. It should therefore be considered as a specific process and accepted as a medical condition capable of investigation, diagnosis, treatment and prevention. Drowning itself is a progressive condition which if not reversed will result in death when the victim is said to be 'drowned'.

Even the strongest swimmer will ultimately become exhausted and no longer able to remain afloat. The majority of people at rest in water will sink and those who do not will only have a little of the scalp out of water and be unable to breathe.

It is difficult to advise a person when threatened by drowning whether to try and reach some object, or the shore, or whether he should maintain the minimum effort and keep afloat as long as possible in the hope that help may come. When the drowning threat is accompanied by the risk of hypothermia the correct advice is most certainly to exert the minimum effort and remain in the same place. Increased activity under these circumstances brings more blood to the peripheral circulation and thus markedly increases heat loss with a shortening of survival time. The action to be taken in each case is different, however, and can only be dictated by the immediate conditions.

When the ability to keep one's head above water is lost the process of drowning begins; water enters the mouth and breathing is no longer possible. Copious amounts of water are swallowed which, particularly if salt, may be regurgitated during recovery or unnecessarily expelled by well-meaning rescuers attempting to drain the lungs.

The expansion of the stomach under these circumstances tends to lessen the desire to breathe but in the healthy individual a powerful laryngeal reflex spasm prevents the inhalation of water. Available evidence suggests that in 20–40 per cent of all cases of drowning, the lungs are kept dry by this reaction. In the remainder, and this may well be where the individual has struggled and is exhausted, water is inhaled into the lungs.

Thus two distinct types of drowning may be present: one where no water enters the lung—**dry drowning**; and one in which water is inhaled—**wet drowning**.

In dry drowning there is simple asphyxia, and where resuscitative measures are applied promptly recovery may be complete and uncomplicated. It is these patients who may recall events in their past life or similar phenomena and suffer no real distress throughout the episode.

In wet drowning occasionally the patient may remember a searing pain in the chest before losing consciousness. The resulting asphyxia is complicated by the presence of water in the lungs. This may be salt or fresh.

Work with animals and the physical difference between salt and fresh water suggests that the presence of the former in the alveoli would, because of its higher salt content, draw fluid from the blood which would become concentrated, increase the resistance of blood flow and result within three or minutes in a failed dilated heart.

Fresh water, on the other hand, would act quite differently. Being hypotonic it would be quickly absorbed into the blood stream which would be diluted. This would cause rupture of the red blood cells with liberation of potassium and resulting ventricular fibrillation.

In practice a close study of drowning in man gives little to support these ideas. This difference is most likely due to the presence of a lipid surfactant which lines the alveoli. Its function is to neutralise surface tension in the alveoli so enabling them to remain equally patent. Without it some would collapse and others expand. It is suggested that any water in the alveoli would neutralise this action, allowing surface tension to develop. Thus some alveoli would collapse and others expand. The collapsed alveoli would contain little or none of the inhaled fluid but have an ample blood flow. The expanded ones would be full of inhaled fluid with their circulatory capillaries squeezed empty. Thus any transfer of water due to osmotic differences one way or the other would be minimal.

Provided part of the patient's lungs remained free from inhaled water and resuscitation was prompt, a return of consciousness could be achieved. In the case of wet drowning, however, the water still remains in the lungs where it acts as an irritant, particularly if it contains oil, sand, mud or other debris.

If no action is taken other than resuscitative measures a typical clinical picture will develop within hours. The patient exhibits respiratory distress with pain in the chest, cough and growing cyanosis, followed by ultimate haemoptysis collapse and death. Clinically there is evidence of pulmonary oedema and consolidation. This is **secondary drowning**.

Even when a drowning patient has been resuscitated and regained consciousness it is impossible to be sure whether water has been inhaled. Thus it is essential in every case of successful recovery from drowning, however well the patient, that he or she should be admitted to hospital, as an acute medical emergency, and remain under observation for at least 24 hours.

The treatment of drowning

If drowning has progressed so far that respiratory failure is present, resuscitative measures must be commenced as soon as possible. If this can be done while still in the water, without delaying return to shore or a boat, so much the better. Exhaled air resuscitation is the method of choice, supplemented by oxygen as soon as available. If there is no apparent improvement within six or so inflations it is necessary to check whether the heart is beating. If not, closed chest cardiac massage should be performed in addition and maintained until the heart restarts or until admission to hospital.

On admission to hospital a chest X-ray and clinical examination should establish whether or not water has been inhaled. If this is known or suspected further emergency treatment should include positive pressure oxygen ventilation and intravenous plasma to replace fluid loss to the alveoli, i.e. to compensate for the pulmonary oedema. Antibiotics and possibly steroids should supplement treatment, as well as careful nursing.

Uncomplicated cases should be kept under observation in hospital for 24 hours. If during this period there is no evidence of secondary drowning they may return home.

The immersion syndrome

From time to time sudden death may occur for no apparent reason soon after an individual has plunged into water. Usually this occurs in a young adult jumping into cold fresh water, frequently after taking a fair amount of alcohol. The cause of this event is uncertain but it may well be some form of vasovagal reaction.

Seasickness

The majority of individuals when subjected to the movements of a boat or ship in a rough sea suffer nausea, and many vomit. A few are immune, and these seem to include many people who are deaf.

Man is a two-dimensional animal who maintains his posture by visual fixation on static objects, the sense of position of his limbs and the balance mechanism in his ears.

In the inexperienced this mechanism has profound difficulty in adapting to abnormal motions of the sea, and the flood of incoming sensory stimuli from the balance-controlling nerve endings (visual, auditory and proprioceptive) overflows and impinges on the vomiting centre in the brain—with the well-known reaction.

At sea the susceptible suffer with the onset of motion but settle down in a day or two. Most recover in 48 hours even if bad weather continues. In times of stress, particularly in small boats or after shipwreck, the seasickness may interfere with the need to carry out critical tasks and control is necessary. There is a large psychological element in seasickness and many physical factors may contribute to its onset. Fear, seeing others suffer, the smell of cooking or fuel oil are all contributory. Overindulgence in food and wine before embarking may be disastrous.

For the sailor with responsibility during the bad weather or other crisis repeated small doses of hyoscine hydrobromide (every six hours) is usually effective. The uncommitted passenger may prefer to take to his bunk in a darkened cabin and there, with the help of cyclizine, remain until the storm has passed.

SAFETY UNDER THE WATER

Diving is not a new activity though today more and more men and women are taking it up for commercial and recreational rewards. It began over 2000 years ago with women in the seas around the Pacific Islands diving for sponges, sea food, shells and pearls. They had no apparatus but relied on their breath-holding ability which experience would extend to about five minutes. The depth to which they dived was limited by pressure on the chest to about 100 ft.

Such free diving is still practised particularly by spear fishermen. Over the years it has been supplemented by the commercial diver with metal helmet and heavy boots and the more recent aqualung which enables a diver to take his own air supply under water and so dispense with the need for surface pumps and a supporting team.

Recent advances are taking the diver to greater depths and enabling him to establish underwater bases which will support life for many months at a time. Research foreshadows an extension of these techniques coupled with methods of fluid breathing to reach even greater depths. This however is something for the future and the vast majority of present day underwater swimmers use either a schnorkel tube or an aqualung or similar self-contained underwater breathing apparatus. These techniques offer a great deal of valuable underwater experience and enjoyment but are not without their dangers.

Schnorkel swimming

Most men and women can float effortlessly with just a little scalp above water. This does not allow breathing, but a short schnorkel tube easily gives this facility. The tube should be as short as possible, as its volume inevitably adds to the diver's own 'dead-space air'. This with a pair of goggles and fins (or flippers) on the feet is the ideal equipment for the exciting sport of spear fishing. The diver cruises on the surface with the goggles under water until a fish is spotted, then dives down to chase it until within range of his spear gun.

This sport has one major hazard which has claimed many victims and still does so. Only on the surface is it possible to breathe through the schnorkel tube—underwater the breath must be held. It is well known that breath-holding time can be significantly prolonged by a brisk period of hyperventilation before doing so. This lowers the immediate carbon dioxide content of the lungs and so delays its return to a level at which breath-holding is terminated by carbon dioxide build-up. Normally when breath-holding is so terminated there is sufficient oxygen in the lungs to maintain consciousness until breathing resumes. Where, however, a schnorkel diver has hyperventilated and dived to chase a fish he may be emotionally motivated by his chase to maintain his breath-holding until the carbon dioxide breaking point has been stretched to the limit.

During this time the oxygen content of the lungs may have fallen to a critical level. If the diver then turns to the surface his ascent will cause a drop in the pressure of the air in the lungs with expansion of the chest. As absorption of oxygen from the alveoli is dependent on the partial pressure of the oxygen present this further fall may result in the level being insufficient to support consciousness. If the diver is unconscious when he reaches or nears the surface he will lose his grip on the schnorkel tube and drown.

It is therefore imperative that, however great the temptation, spear fishermen must be convinced that the practice of hyperventilation before the dive is extremely dangerous. It must never be done.

Diving with self-contained breathing apparatus

The diver who goes under the water must adapt himself to a three-dimensional environment in which the pressure on his body is increased by one atmosphere (760 mm Hg) for every 33 ft (10 m) he descends in the sea. Thus when he is 99 ft (30 m) down the pressure is four times as great as that at the surface (i.e. 4 atmospheres). Although man's tissues, like those of a fish, behave as a fluid and are incompressible and function normally at any depth, the gas-filled cavities are compressed by the increasing pressures. If the diver without any breathing apparatus takes a full breath at the surface his chest will be in full inspiration and contain say 6 litres. If then, holding his breath, he swims down to 99 ft (30 m) where the absolute pressure would be four atmospheres his chest volume will be decreased by three-quarters, down to $1\frac{1}{2}$ litres. This is the residual volume, and he has during the dive moved from a position of full inspiration to full expiration without breathing out. To go deeper than this would endanger the integrity of lung tissue and ultimately collapse the chest.

These physical limitations of pressure and volume are the reason why the pearl divers already mentioned cannot safely exceed depths in excess of about 100 feet (30 m). On return to the surface the lungs re-expanded to the state they were in before the dive.

To overcome this problem of pressure and volume change the simple expedient is to ensure that the air breathed by the diver is supplied to him at the exact pressure of the water which surrounds him. If he is at 66 ft (20 m) he will need air at a pressure of three atmospheres absolute (the atmospheric pressure $+2$) and at 132 ft (40 m) he will need it at five atmospheres absolute.

This is no problem. The older commercial standard diving suit with the metal helmet has air pumped down a pipe from the surface at the required pressure.

The present-day self-contained underwater breathing apparatus or aqualung is fitted with a demand valve which supplies air to the diver at the pressure of the surrounding water. This is actually controlled by the direct pressure of the sea water on a diaphragm attached to a valve controlling entry of air to the diver's mouthpiece.

Where air is compressed its density is also increased and this increase in density means an increase in effort required to breathe. More work is needed to move the air in and out of the lungs. This extra effort may surprise the beginner but, within the range of the conventional widely used underwater breathing apparatus, it presents no problem. Depths of 180–200 ft (55–60 m) should not be exceeded with this apparatus. At greater depths, the high density makes the use of air impracticable, and mixtures in which nitrogen is replaced with the lighter helium are necessary.

Professional very deep divers are also concerned that, if they breathed air, the excess pressure of nitrogen would incapacitate them with its pronounced narcotic effect and that the oxygen could also result in the convulsions of oxygen poisoning. Both these effects become critical if air is breathed at depths of 300 ft (90 m) or more.

The problem, however, is easily solved by using a mixture of a reduced percentage of oxygen in non-narcotic low density helium. There still remains a final major problem — that of decompression. On the way down, as the diver breathes air at increasing pressure, its nitrogen and oxygen (both soluble) pass in increasing amounts into the blood as it flows through the lungs, and thence diffuse throughout the tissues. When the time comes to return to the surface this process is reversed and the excess dissolved nitrogen, which is now in the tissues, passes back to the blood stream and to the lungs. In this case, however, since pressure is simultaneously reduced throughout the body, if the ascent is at all rapid there is a danger that bubbles of nitrogen may form in the tissues and produce the clinical picture of decompression sickness. This is the main concern in diving medicine today.

Decompression sickness

Much of present day knowledge on this subject has been obtained from painstaking experiments on animals and man largely from trial and error in carefully controlled pressure chambers.

It has been found that there is a scale of time and depth which may be used in diving without risk of bubble formation. It is possible to go to 30 ft (9 m), and remain at that depth indefinitely, and still surface directly in complete safety. At 60 ft (18 m) the safe time would be 60 minutes; at 100 ft (30 m), 20 minutes and at 300 ft (90 m) as little as 3 minutes.

Any dive which exceeds these figures in time and depth would result in bubble formation and decompression sickness if direct surfacing was undertaken. It has also been found that in these dives it is possible to ascend directly two-thirds of the way to the surface without any risk. At this level it is necessary to remain for a calculated period before ascending a little further, usually 10 ft. Thereafter the surface is eventually reached in steps by a series of 10 ft ascents with increasing periods of delay. This process is known as 'stage decompression' and a comprehensive series of diving tables has been worked out to cover all dives within the capacity of currently available diving apparatus.

Clinically the picture of decompression sickness is fairly typical. In its mildest form it presents with minor fleeting aches and itching or a rash known as 'niggles'. In more advanced cases severe pains develop in one or other joint at the end of or soon after completion of a dive. This can be quite incapacitating and is the typical 'bends'.

Respiratory symptoms occasionally develop due to bubble formation in the pulmonary circulation producing a cough, pain in the chest and evidence of pulmonary irritation—the 'chokes'.

More serious, however, is the condition which may occur after deeper and longer diving where something has gone wrong with the diving schedule. These are the spinal or cerebral 'bends' where bubbles have lodged within the central nervous system to produce a wide variety of clinical manifestations, commonly in the form of gross paralysis (e.g. paraplegia) or sensory disturbances. These are commonly known as the 'staggers'.

One more dangerous condition rightly included under decompression sickness is pulmonary barotrauma or burst lung. This was first encountered with men escaping or training for escape from sunken submarines but a parallel situation exists in diving. If for some reason the breathing apparatus of a diver fails under water he may have to abandon it and make a 'free' ascent without it. The correct procedure in such a case is to take a final breath from the apparatus if possible, shed weights and allow any buoyancy worn to carry one to the surface aided by swimming if necessary. During this ascent, air which occupied a given volume at depth would need to expand as the pressure fell at higher levels. The correct procedure is to relax with the mouth open, gently blowing out the expanding air. But in a moment of crisis when panic may not be far away the natural reaction is to hold on grimly to the breath with clenched jaws. In such a case expansion of the contained air is limited so that the surface is reached with air in the lungs at higher than atmospheric pressure. This may be released not only as forced expiration but also as expansion of the chest and lungs. The latter may easily rupture, in which case air may escape into the loose retrosternal tissues or those of the neck or, more seriously, actually enter the pulmonary circulation as bubbles which may be carried through the heart into the general arterial system. These may finally—and quite quickly—lodge as emboli in the small vessels of the cerebral or coronary circulations with localising cerebral symptoms, collapse and often early death.

Treatment of decompression sickness

Except for the very mild 'niggles', which usually disappear with rest and aspirin, the only effective treatment is prompt recompression. This is usually carried out in a chamber, but where none is available it is possible to reapply the breathing apparatus and return to the sea.

Once bubbles have formed it takes more than a simple return to the depth of the former dive to re-dissolve them and ensure a symptom free return. Experience and careful calculations have evolved a series of 'therapeutic tables' which cover all types of decompression sickness from the uncomplicated 'bend' to the serious central nervous system involvement and pulmonary barotrauma. Expert medical supervision is desirable, and this is to be found in the main naval bases in most countries. Most diving organisations issue their members with cards giving details of what action to take if decompression sickness is suspected, and advice can also be obtained from police headquarters.

Pulmonary barotrauma needs immediate recompression to save life and where training in free ascent techniques are taught a therapeutic chamber must be immediately available. If this is not the case and pulmonary barotrauma is suspected little more can be done than place the patient on his left side in a semi-prone position with the head low in hope that gravity will assist the bubbles in avoiding the cerebral and coronary arteries.

Safe diving

More than anything else, diving is an activity in which the diver should be trained to accept full responsibility for his own safety and so appreciate the need to care for others. He must look upon all his diving equipment as his life support system in the new environment. Regular inspection and careful maintenance is absolutely essential.

Diving itself can be a gentle pastime. The sea is supporting and gives a state of weightlessness so that energy consumption can be minimal. On the other hand, attempts at rapid movement are exhausting and unrewarding. There is no place underwater for competitive activities against the clock. It is a place for slow and purposeful movement, for contemplation and wonder.

Many organisations use diving as a means to an end in their operations. Thus an experienced diver is welcome in many fields. He would, however, do well to join a major diving organisation, accept its rules and—as he becomes more interested and experienced—progress steadily through its stages of competence, taking its proficiency tests and enjoying all that the vast underwater world has to offer.

14

Mountain Rescue and Ski Injuries

NEIL J MACDONALD

Risk is an inherent part of the challenge of the outdoors. The sense of adventure, together with a search for solitude, beauty and new experience entice the rambler, hill walker and rock climber to range further into remote and more demanding parts of the country.

Education Authorities, Duke of Edinburgh Award schemes and other youth organisations use the outdoors to channel the energies and interests of the young city dweller into more gainful use of leisure time. The armed forces have commitments in European defence and also use our mountains and moorlands for training in winter and mountain warfare, navigation and survival. The consequent increase in numbers causes a potential increase in casualties, with a corresponding load on local rescue services in geographically and medically remote areas.

The Mountain Rescue Committees of Scotland, England and Wales have no statutory functions, but do form a central point of contact for cooperation and coordination of other organisations with a statutory or voluntary interest in mountain rescue. Their aims are to assist in the setting up of rescue posts, the acquisition, maintenance and replacement of equipment; and also to promote the formation of rescue teams and to represent the interests of mountain rescue to other national bodies. Records of accidents involving mountain rescue teams are also collected and reported.

In this last connection the committees reported that in 1975 there were 236 mountaineering and caving accidents involving serious injury (Table I).

Enquiry into the causes of accidents showed many to be avoidable. The most common cause of summer mishaps was slipping on rock or steep grass because of unsuitable footwear. Winter causes were

TABLE I

Mountaineering and Caving Accidents

District	Total Accidents	Injured	Fatal
Wales	31	30	1
Pennines	64	55	9
Lake District	76	70	6
Scotland	57	50	7
Other areas	8	6	2

mainly slips on ice because of the absence, or improper use, of ice axe and crampons; poor navigation causing a party to become lost or benighted was also a prominent cause of accident both in summer and in winter; inadequate clothing contributed to the high numbers of cases of acute hypothermia.

Many other incidents involved more minor trauma, and acute medical emergencies. These included heart attacks, cerebrovascular accident and insulin coma.

Scotland is seen in a particularly bad light with regard to fatalities. Although the sparseness of population and remoteness of the areas are contributory causes, it must be remembered that above an elevation of 2500 ft (750 m) the climate of Scottish mountains is literally subarctic. In effect, this means that the ground can remain frozen for five months, precipitation may fall as snow on 273 days of the year, wind speed can exceed 130 mph (208 kph) and the daily range of temperature—night minimum to day maximum—can be as great as 28°C (50°F). Small wonder that along with head injury, the major cause of death is acute hypothermia. This condition also complicates other injuries, both in summer and in winter.

THE MOUNTAIN RESCUE SERVICE

The mountain rescue team is the basic unit of rescue. In the main, such teams are composed of civilian volunteers. The RAF also maintains rescue teams in areas especially dangerous to aircraft personnel. These teams are available for civilian incident when service requirements permit. In Scotland, the police maintain several teams in high risk areas.

Team members are all well trained and equipped. They have a vast local knowledge of the terrain and of the special hazards of their areas. Their skill, drill and team work allow the injured to be sought out and brought to medical care as rapidly as is practicable with as little risk of further deterioration of the victim's condition as possible.

Police have a special interest in any accident situation in which life is at stake. They will usually act as rescue coordinators, undertake the call out of teams and of individuals, provide transportation and liaise with other services such as helicopters, ambulance and doctors.

Search and rescue dog associations

Founded by Hamish MacInnes of the MRC of Scotland, this organisation trains dogs and their handlers to work in rescue situations. A good dog can cut search times, especially in bad visibility or when casualties are buried by avalanches. Used properly in search situations, a dog can cover the same area as 20 men.

Rescue posts

These are provided by the MRC in areas where accidents are prevalent. They are identified by the committee's sign (Fig. 14.1) and the position marked on Ordinance Survey maps. These posts have a comprehensive range of first-aid equipment contained in one or two rucksacks. Tubunic ampoules of morphine are included in this kit as well as a casualty bag and stretcher. Posts which are manned or associated with a local rescue team carry much more equipment. The list of the equipment and the location of the posts is contained in the Handbook of the Mountain Rescue Committee. Information about the rescue teams' methods of contact and call out are also listed in this most useful booklet.

St John Ambulance Brigade, St Andrew's Ambulance Association and the British Red Cross provide first aid boxes in many areas where mountain incidents frequently occur. They also provide very sound training for team members.

Finance

Mountain rescue services are expensive in manpower as well as hard

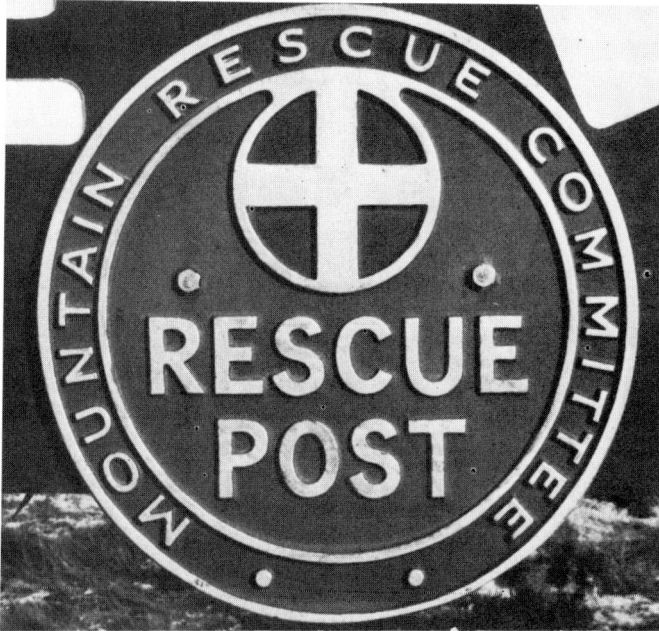

Fig. 14.1. Mountain Rescue Committee sign at rescue posts.

cash but are given free to the individual in Great Britain. Financing of the service is from government sources as well as public subscription.

Government spends money on mountain rescue through:

National Health Service

The cost of initial and replacement medical equipment at rescue posts is paid by the Department of Health, and in Scotland by the Home and Health Department.

Police

Provision is made for equipping police rescue teams and, in some instances, buildings for storage of equipment and for lectures, and drying and eating facilities.

Insurance covers civilian team members called out by the police, and loss of wages because of call out is reimbursed. In Scotland certain equipment, notably ropes and radios, is provided. Provision is also made for transport and, in some instances, for tracked vehicles.

RAF

Provision and equipping of RAF Mountain Rescue teams is arranged. It should be noted that the team members other than the leader and deputy are volunteers and train in their own time.

Service Helicopters

Direct cash grants

These are available occasionally through the Mountain Rescue Committee.

Voluntary subscriptions come from industry, individuals and charitable organisations.

The team members undertake many fund-raising ventures on their own behalf.

Equipment

Each team member is responsible for his own personal equipment which is kept at home at instant readiness for a call out. Equipment for support groups can be stored centrally and issued as required.

The team should be equipped as for mountaineering:

Clothing

Climbing boots with vibram soles
Woollen stockings
Good quality underwear
Climbing breeches
Woollen mitts; over-mitts in severe conditions
Nylon gloves, for fine work with metal in freezing conditions, to prevent contact freezing
Balaclava
Anorak and duvet jacket in severe conditions
Cagoule and overtrousers

The anorak, duvet jacket and cagoule should have a hood and be front opening to allow controlled ventilation of the body. Side zips on the overtrousers make for ease of putting on over boots and crampons.

Rucksack

Usually a medium to large frameless variety containing:
Map in polybag
Compass
Protractor
Head torch, spare batteries and bulbs
Personal first aid kit
Spare dry clothing in large polybag to act as emergency personal shelter
Food: day's rations and survival rations, plus extra sweets and chocolate
Whistle
Flares

In rescues involving rock climbing a helmet (conforming to British Standard 4423:1969) is carried as well as climbing hardwear such as slings, pitons etc. A waist line or harness is normally used.

Additional personal equipment for winter includes:

Gaiters
Ice axe
Crampons
Avalanche cord
Goggles—clear for wind protection, tinted for glare
Ultraviolet light barrier cream such as Uvistat

Team equipment

In rescue, away from roads, and involving the negotiation of rough and precipitous terrain, the mass of the equipment and its duplicity of function are very important considerations. Depending on the circumstances, a minimum of equipment might be required on a daylight search whereas a rock rescue at night might require a great deal of climbing hardwear, ropes, wires, winches, lights, etc.

Stretchers

For mountain rescue these should be robust to withstand rough usage and have runners to assist passage over snow and grass. The bed should be firm enough to support spinal injury and high enough to be clear of uneven ground. For evacuation over scree and steep ground a head guard is necessary to protect the casualty. Points for attachment of ropes are necessary for stretcher lowering and for allowing the maximum number of people to carry the stretcher. An adequate and comfortable system for securing the casualty to the bed is essential. If an under carriage with wheel and drum brake can be fitted, long carry outs—even over very rough terrain—are facilitated.

The, Thomas stretcher. Issued to rescue posts in England and Wales, is constructed of duralumin tubing with long extension handles making for ease of manipulation over rough terrain. It has a canvas bed and the frame is mounted on ski runners; total weight is about 40 lb (18·5 kg). There are two models available, a standard one-piece and a split two-piece. The latter makes an easier load, and can be quickly fastened together when the scene is reached.

The MacInnes stretcher. Issued to mountain rescue posts in Scotland, has also been adopted as standard equipment for RAF Mountain Rescue teams. It is constructed of continuous hiduminium tubing and has a folding frame for ease of transportation. Long extension handles, a head and back guard are standard. The bed is of prestretched terylene netting which reduces windage when carrying. Total weight is 33 lb (15·5 kg).

Many other types of stretcher exist, often designed for a specific task or for special terrain.

The Neil Robertson stretcher. This is standard helicopter equipment and particularly convenient for winching a casualty horizontally into a hovering helicopter and can also be used as a cradle to lift other makes of stretcher on which a casualty has been previously loaded.

The Duff stretcher. Used in very rugged cliff rescue in Scotland.

The Mariner stretcher. Fitted with a double leg traction splint, this is the standard stretcher for continental rescues.

Other stretchers. The **Paraguard, Stokes Litter, Perche Barnarde,** Norwegian **Hjelper** and the **Akja** from Austria are other designs in use in this country.

In an emergency, an ordinary climbing rope can be fashioned into various sorts of rope stretcher such as the rope basket and **Pigott** stretcher (Fig. 14.2 and 3). A coiled rope, with the coils divided into equal parts, can be used as a harness to aid a pick-a-back carry off or rock lower (Fig. 14.4(a) and (b)). The **Tragsitz** harness is specially designed for this purpose but a rucksack with leg holes cut in the sides is equally effective (Fig. 14.5).

Casualty bag

This is used in conjunction with a stretcher evacuation. In an emergency a 500 gauge polythene bag measuring 7 ft × 4 ft (2·2 × 1·25 m) can be used and is preferred for obvious reasons when evacuating a corpse. A good quality down filled sleeping bag is provided at mountain rescue posts. Many teams however are equipped with a specially designed combination bag incorporating a sleeping bag with hood, a canvas backed mattress with carrying handles and a waterproof cover. These bags afford maximum thermal insulation along with comfort for the patient and allow easy stretcher loading.

Lightweight bivouac

Although this is not standard equipment it can usefully be carried in severe conditions and could prove lifesaving to the severely exposed casualty where resuscitation is necessary before evacuation can take place. On wide scale searches each team must have some form of emergency bivouac gear.

Ropes

As a normal procedure, the team will be roped when traversing over snow slopes, rock climbing, and making river crossings. Similarly, ropes will be used for lowering the casualty on a stretcher down crag faces, steep snow and wet grassy slopes.

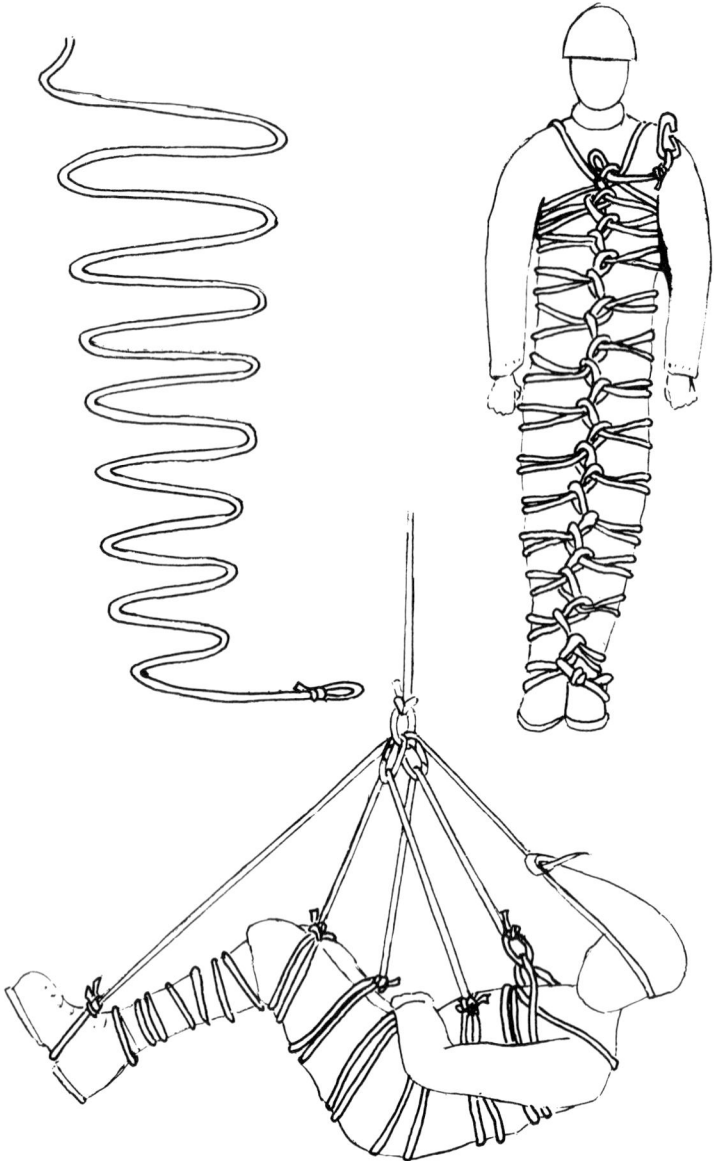

Fig. 14.2. Improvised stretcher. Rope basket, attached to lowering rope and rope slings by karabiners. The head is supported by a triangular bandage sling.

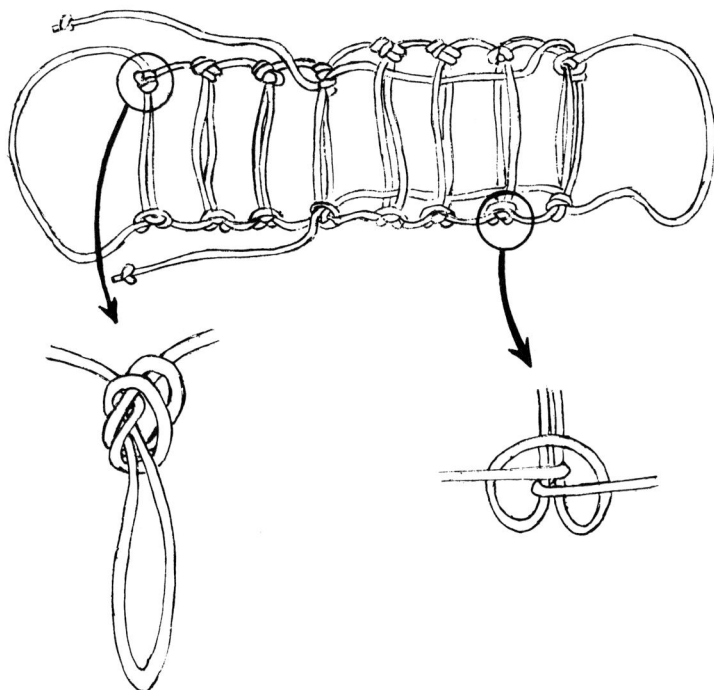

Fig. 14.3. Improvised stretcher. Pigott rope stretcher constructed from a normal climbing rope.

A minimum of two 120 ft (36 m) ropes are carried by a team for use in the many unforeseen difficulties of a rescue.

Nylon rope is preferred for climbing because of its strength and elasticity. This material resists rot and decay and does not absorb much water. It should be remembered that it is very susceptible to abrasion and, because of its low melting point, is weakened by friction.

Lowering ropes are of heavy-duty synthetic fibre with a circumference of about $1\frac{1}{4}$ in (3·1 cm). They are either hawser-laid prestretched terylene or braided terylene with a parallel core. These materials have low extensibility under load thus allowing precise control when lowering a casualty or stretcher. Lowering ropes are used in 500 ft (150 m) lengths and to avoid kinking are best managed on a reel. The complete equipment—rope, reel and carrying-frame—give a convenient load of about 30 lb (14·25 kg).

In use, the ropes should not be allowed to drag along the ground or run over sharp edges of rock. The rope should always be kept in neat coils and care should be taken not to stand on it. Good rope handling is the sign of a well drilled team.

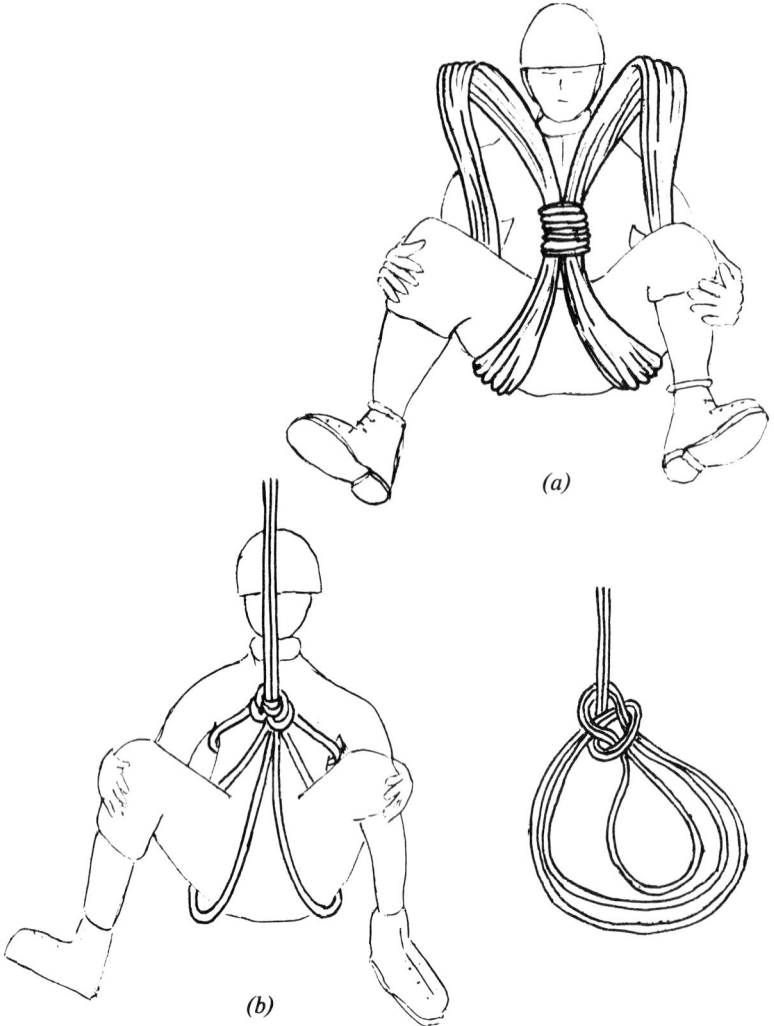

Fig. 14.4. (a) Coiled climbing rope used as a harness to aid pick-a-back carry. (b) Triple bowline knot used to lower casualty at rope end.

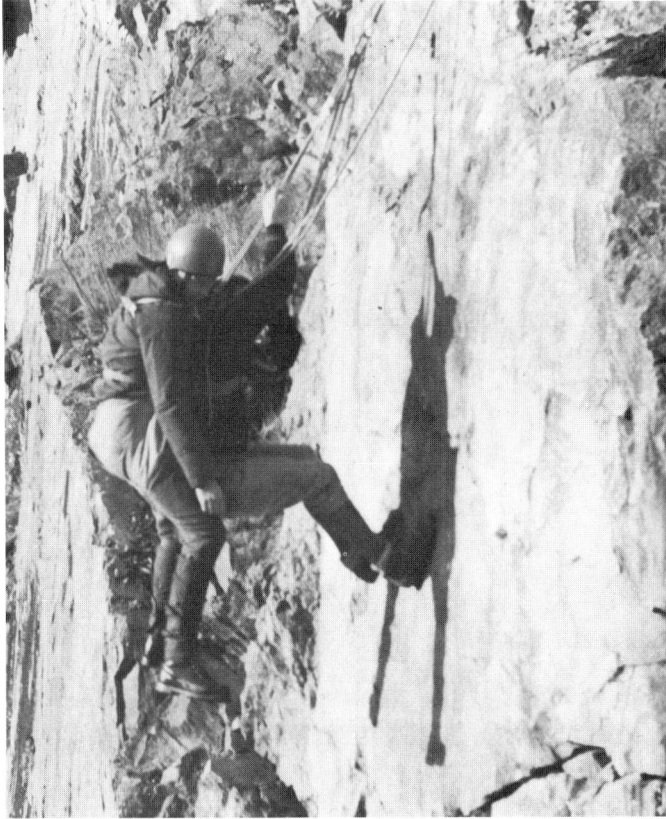

Fig. 14.5. Cliff lower using a harness for the patient.

After use the ropes are inspected for deterioration and fraying. Grit found within the lay is washed out as this can cause internal wear which is difficult to assess. Thereafter the rope should be dried and stored coiled, in a cool, dry, airy place away from strong light and chemicals such as creosote and battery acid.

Knots

The knots for use with sythetic ropes are shown in Fig. 14.6. It should be remembered that knots reduce the breaking load of the rope by 10–30 per cent.

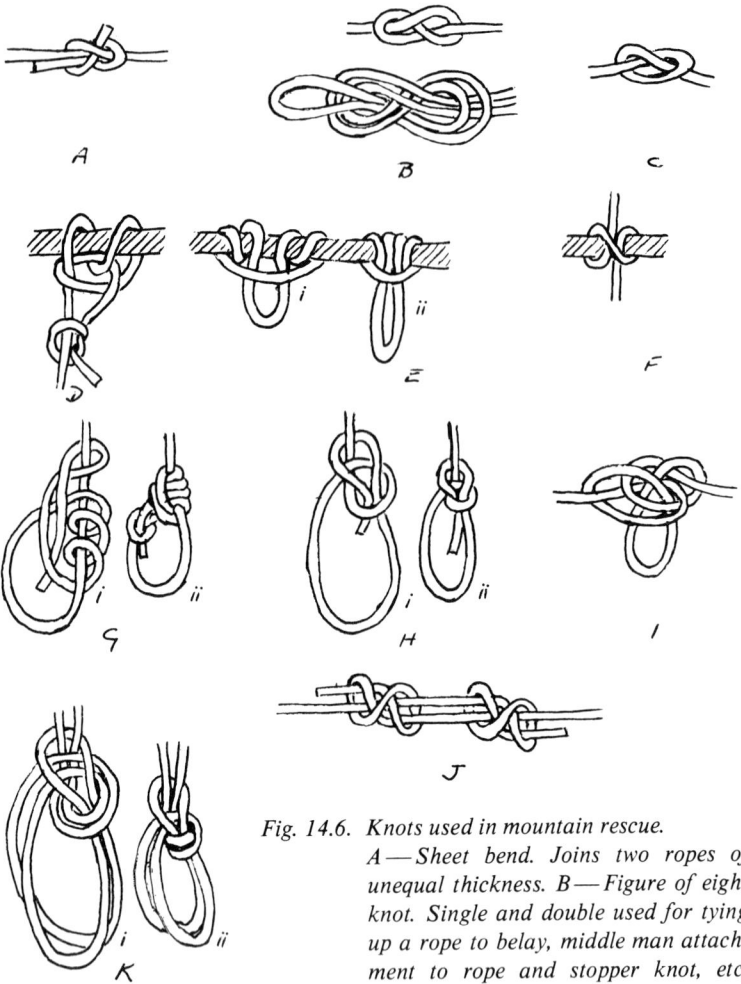

Fig. 14.6. Knots used in mountain rescue.
A — Sheet bend. Joins two ropes of unequal thickness. B — Figure of eight knot. Single and double used for tying up a rope to belay, middle man attachment to rope and stopper knot, etc. C — Thumb (or overhand) knot. Used to secure an end. D — Fisherman's bend. Used for tying rope to stretcher, tying off to another rope, etc. E — Prussik knot (i, ii). Used for making a sliding loop to aid climbing a thicker, static rope. F — Clove hitch. Used for tying off to a rope, ice axe belay or stretcher attachment. G — Tarbuck knot (i, ii). Attachment of rope to body sling karabiner. H — Bowline (i, ii). Making a loop. Tail should be secured with a thumb knot. I — Alpine butterfly knot. Middle man attachment to rope. J — Double fisherman's knot. Joining two ropes of equal thickness. Making body sling. N B Reef knot is not recommended for use with synthetic ropes. K — Bowline-on-a-bight (i, ii). Middle man attachment to a rope, securing double rope to a belay.

Communications

Radio

Many teams are now equipped with this valuable aid. A mountain rescue frequency has been allocated and police, RAF and civilian teams can now cooperate fully. As yet helicopters do not have this frequency.

Radio is of great value in the control of large scale search when many teams are involved in one rescue. It is also very useful in directing stretcher lowering when the stretcher is out of sight of the lowerers. Extra equipment and help can be summoned quickly, medical advice can be obtained, expected time of arrival at road head etc can be transmitted.

Mountains are notoriously bad terrain for radio communication; countless black spots exist, but the local teams have made radio maps showing these points. In difficult areas, permanent and temporary relay stations are set up. In the field, correct procedure and call signs must be strictly observed.

Visual, audible and pyrotechnic signalling can be used.

TABLE II

The Alpine Code

Message	Flare	Signal (light/sound)
I want help	Red	Alpine—six long flashes or notes in quick succession repeated after an interval of one minute.
Message understood	White	Alpine—a series of three long flashes or notes repeated after an interval of one minute.
Position of base	White or Yellow	Steady white or yellow light, e.g. car headlights or spotlights if possible pointing upwards.
Recall to base	Green	A succession of notes on bell, horn, siren or succession of yellow or white lights repeatedly switched on and off, or a succession of thunderflashes.

Thunderflashes or maroon flares can be used to attract attention before giving the message.

Smoke generators can also be used if a prearranged code is established. Smoke, however, is most commonly used to indicate wind direction when operating with helicopters or aircraft.

Illumination

Personal illumination is best achieved from some kind of head lamp which leaves both hands free. The power source has to be kept dry and is therefore carried in the pocket or rucksack. Ordinary dry batteries or rechargeable batteries such as Nife cells are satisfactory.

A search light with a quartz iodine bulb gives a good beam far in excess of the usual searching distance of 300 ft (90 m). The power source is a lead acid accumulator which must be carried in a spill-proof, well ventilated container incorporated in a carrying frame. The lamp can be hand held or attached to the frame.

The more portable Police Search and Rescue light has a good beam but a limited charge, giving only four hours illumination.

Floodlighting can be achieved by a portable gas lantern. Propane is less affected by low temperatures. These and pressurised paraffin lamps give mantle trouble in wind and must be protected.

Illuminating flares, especially the parachute variety, are very useful when searching in corries etc. They burn for 30–50 seconds at a height of some 1200 ft (360 m). Care must be exercised, however, to ensure that the smoke generated does not interfere with the search.

Organisation of search

An efficient rescue operation is run to a set pattern which experience has shown to be the most efficient for that area. No two areas are alike, just as no two incidents are identical. Good organisation is essential because it allows the various rescue facilities to be used in whole or in part with a minimum of delay, thereby giving the best chance of a satisfactory result.

The incident starts when the person bringing news of an accident is interviewed by the police and the coordinator who will take charge of the rescue. It is very important to establish as much information as possible at this interview, e.g. the time, location, numbers involved, equipment and food available, injuries sustained and amount of self-help available.

On this information a plan of operation can be drawn up, and a log started. Teams can be put on standby or called out and leaders briefed. Transport can be organised, radio call-signs allocated, equipment checked and special equipment issued. A base control is established whose functions include communication, press communiques, liason with the doctor, and organisation of food. Base control remains on duty until the end of the rescue and until all the teams return and are debriefed.

Frequently the accident is reported at the end of the day when darkness is falling. In such circumstances unless the exact location is known, it is both hazardous and a waste of man power to start a comprehensive night search. Likely shelter spots such as refuge huts can be checked, and teams assembled for a dawn start.

If the precise location is known, a small party can be sent immediately to render first aid and establish radio communications. This is followed up by a larger stretcher party for evacuation.

If the locality is unknown but the general area fairly well defined, an advance base can be set up in the hours of darkness and heavy equipment left there. The teams can then move to the start line of their prescribed search sector ready for an early start.

Depending on the area to be searched, the number of teams available, the ground to be covered and the prevailing weather conditions, a controller has three recognised methods of search available to him:

Reconnaisance search

The search is made by small units of highly mobile, skilled rescuers in an effort to locate a victim or party rapidly. Dogs and helicopters are particularly useful for this form of search and can save many man hours.

Block search

This is a more detailed search of a fairly large area which is allocated to a team. It is usually bounded by easily defined natural features.

In the more incident-prone areas, special maps exist with pre-determined sectors marked and coded for identification. The team leader will decide the exact method of covering the ground, depending on the numbers of men, overhead conditions and the terrain involved. It is usually a kind of sweep search employing the men in line abreast.

Contact search

As the term implies, this is a very detailed, precise search of highly probable places, e.g. at the foot of cliffs. This type of search must be conclusive so that when finished, that area can be excluded from further thought.

Use of dogs in search and rescue

In many countries, dogs are used principally to locate victims buried by avalanche. In Britain their use is of particular value in searching out a victim lying on open moorland perhaps hidden by undergrowth or lying covered by snow.

To be of maximum use, the dog should work well away from its handler and into the wind. It should be employed in the initial stages of a search preferably in advance of a full search before the area is filled with conflicting scent. Dogs can work well at night and in bad visibility when other forms of search are difficult or impossible. Some dogs can find bodies even when partly frozen.

Any dog with a good nose, natural aptitude, and large and strong enough to travel over rough terrain and through snow, can be trained as a rescue dog. The alsatian is said to be the best breed but collies, labradors and large terriers have been successfully trained.

The Search and Rescue Dog Association organises annual training and grading courses. The dogs are graded as in other countries as A, B, or C. The A grade is subdivided 1–10, A1 being the highest grade. Any A grade dog can undertake summer and winter search of moorland and easy mountain terrain.

The handler is also classified, the letter M denoting a competent mountaineer. The certificates last for two years before reassessment is required.

Evacuation

The evacuation might be merely an assisted walk off for the patient, a full stretcher carry to a road head, taking many hours, or a helicopter rescue.

Initial assessment and first-aid treatment must be meticulous, because further work on the casualty is very difficult once stretcher loading has taken place. Particular attention must be given to the maintenance of airways and adequacy of splintage.

A stretcher evacuation may have to be delayed until the casualty is in a fit state to be moved, e.g. in extreme cases of exposure. It may also be quicker and safer to evacuate to a good landing site and then await removal by helicopter when overhead conditions allow.

Night evacuations must be adequately illuminated and an experienced navigator should be sent ahead to act as pathfinder. Normally a stretcher party consists of 16–20 people working as two teams and carrying for 10 min shifts. In long carry-outs the greater the manpower available, the more easily and effectively the job is done.

Helicopters in search and rescue

These machines are of maximum value for reconnaisance, search, evacuation, and transportation of heavy equipment, teams and dogs to an advanced base. Their advantages are speed and comfort of evacuation.

The RAF Search and Rescue helicopter squadrons are equipped with the Whirlwind Mark 10. When not committed to Service use, they can be made available for civilian incidents when life is at stake. Requests for assistance are made via the police to the Rescue Control Centre at Mountbatten in England and Wales, and at Pitreavie in Scotland. This type of helicopter has a range of three hours flying time depending on load. Strategic fuel bases are established throughout the area of operation of each of the squadron flights.

The helicopter pilot will decide to land or hover according to his own judgement. Help can be provided on the ground by clearing a space of 20 yd × 20 yd (18 × 18 m) to act as a landing zone. There must be no loose stones, sticks, blankets, polythene sheeting, etc. lying around which might get blown about or even sucked into the air intake of the engines. The wind direction can be indicated by the ignition of a smoke cannister placed so that it will be on the pilot's right hand side when approaching the landing zone head into wind. If smoke is not available the wind direction can be indicated by standing with outstretched arms, back to wind, facing the approach path.

The utmost care must be exercised in approaching the helicopter as the rotor blades can come to within 3 ft of the ground in gusting winds. The aircraft should only be approached from 45° from in front, on the pilot's side (right), when the pilot has given the clear indication to approach by giving the thumbs up sign. On no account should the aircraft be approached from the rear near the tail rotor.

The pilot may decide to hover and pick up or lower by winch. In a single lift, care should be taken to allow the winch hook to reach the ground so that any static charge can be earthed. The more usual double lift is made with the assistance of the winch man being lowered on the hook.

The helicopter has a nose down attitude in flight. The shocked or unconscious casualty should therefore be loaded head towards the nose of the aircraft.

Avalanche

This is an ever present danger in the mountains during winter and spring. They occur surprisingly frequently in Scottish mountains. Public awareness of this risk is poor and accidents from avalanches increase yearly.

Wet snow loosened from its attachment by melt water and unstable wind-driven slab snow are the most frequent types of avalanche. Some avalanches can involve the movement of up to 100 000 tons of snow which even by continental standards is quite large.

Death is caused immediately by severe multiple injury, in a few minutes by asphyxia from airway obstruction and rib cage compression, and in a matter of hours by heat loss and slow asphyxia. The chance of survival decreases greatly as the depth and the length of time of burial increase. The longest reported incarceration with survival in a Scottish avalanche is 22 hours.

Speed is the essence of success in this type of rescue (Fig. 14.7). Information required from survivors includes the position of the victims when the avalanche struck, the position where the victim was last seen in the debris and the position of any equipment or survivor when the avalanche came to rest. From this information it is possible to work out the positions where victims are most likely to be buried.

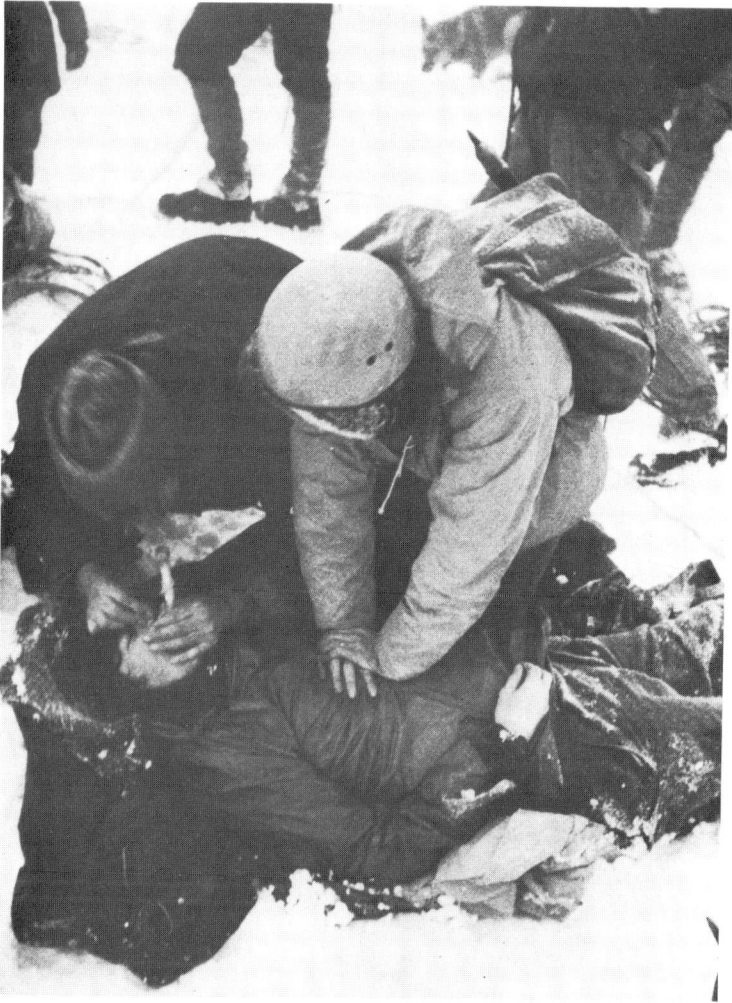

Fig. 14.7. Attempted resuscitation after recovery from a wet snow avalanche. (Reproduced with permission of Hamish MacInnes.)

An immediate search by survivors and witnesses using ski sticks, ice axes, etc. as probes is instituted while help is summoned.

Trained dogs are of immense value in accurate, speedy search of avalanche debris and every effort should be made to get them and their handlers into the area quickly. The area should be cleared for 10–15 min to allow the dog to have the best chance of success.

A probe search using 12 ft (3·6 m) metal probes, even with a line of 20–30 searchers takes a very long time, and its accuracy is in no way greater than the nose of a dog.

SKIING AND SKI ACCIDENT

Unlike mountaineering and hill walking, downhill skiing in this country takes place in fairly well-defined locations. A few suitable snowfields have been developed and, as the popularity of the sport has increased, more uphill transport has been provided. There are three such areas in the central highlands of Scotland which, although unable to compare with the gigantic runs of the Alps and Rocky Mountains, compare very favourably with skiing in Scandinavia and the Eastern Coast of North America.

The average accident rate of downhill skiing, at 5 per 1000 ski-man days, is high compared with other sports. Various accident studies from the Scottish resorts show that skiing in this country is just as hazardous.

The popularity of the sport is such that there can be as many as 6000 active participants at the largest Scottish resort on Cairngorm on a busy day. Uphill transport can cope with a maximum 7800 persons per hour. During a season some $2\frac{1}{2}$ million runs will be made on skis and 450–550 accidents are expected to occur.

Although almost any injury can occur from this sport, skiing typically results in a single twisting injury to the leg.

Nature of injury

TABLE III

Skiing injuries

Torsion injury of leg	65%
Injury to finger	5·5%
Other fractures	3·5%
Other strains	1%
Laceration	12·5%
Contusion and abrasion	8%
Dislocated shoulder	1%
Others	2%
Concussion	1%

TABLE IV

Torsion injury to leg

Strain of medial collateral ligament of knee	36·8%
Strained lateral ligament of ankle	18·1%
Fracture of tibial shaft	15·6%
Crush sinovitis of anterior tendons of ankle	7·3%
Fracture of lateral malleolus	6·4%
Other fractures	3·9%
Other strains	9·4%

The injury of skiing is a strain of the medial collateral ligament of knee. The novice skier is particularly prone to this injury. As he loses balance at low speed and topples over, his reaction involves straightening the leg, which prevents any rotation at the knee, making injury to the ligament inevitable.

Injury to the lateral side of the ankle is numerically next in importance. Although relatively minor it still requires evacuation by the ski patrol and will cause the holiday skier considerable trouble in getting about in his resort and in getting home. The tendency is for the patient to treat such an injury as 'just a sprain' and to allow insufficient time for the damaged ligaments to heal properly.

The third and most important injury is fracture of the tibial shaft, with or without associated fracture of the fibula. Most commonly it is an oblique or long spiral fracture of the bone, sometimes involving half the bone length. Compound fractures are very rare. The mechanism of injury is a sudden rotational force caused by catching the ski tip when travelling at speed.

The less common transverse 'boot top' fracture of tibia and fibula occurs when the ski digs into the snow and is suddenly arrested. The momentum of the skier passing on in the same axis as the ski results in this injury.

Cause of injury

Viewed simply, injury occurs from skiing when the participant loses balance and falls. Loss of balance is caused by many factors such as experience, technique, control of speed, fitness, snow conditions, concentration and fatigue. The type of injury is dependent on the numerous consequences of the fall and to a large extent is modified by whether the ski release binding has time to work, or indeed can work.

The novice tends to fall frequently and is in the group most at risk. Some 65 per cent of all injuries reported from the Cairngorm resort occur in those with less than two seasons.experience.

Release bindings should be looked on as an automatic device which will release under certain predetermined conditions, provided the binding is set and maintained correctly. Unless these conditions are fulfilled the binding will not release and injury is to be expected. The binding must be set to open in response to an injurious force and not to a torque or shock involved in normal skiing. The speed of application of the shock is important, for if applied slowly, the mechanism tends not to work or to work too slowly to prevent injury. This is the reason for the many knee injuries sustained by novices. Design changes and improves yearly, but is still far from being perfect.

Rescue

Specialist rescue services have evolved in the busier ski areas because of the sheer volume of accidents. On Cairngorm some 300 casualties will be seen by the ski patrol in a season and two-thirds of these will require evacuation by stretcher. The techniques of rescue vary from area to area depending on the numbers involved, the distance from a road head and the suitability of the chairlift for stretcher evacuation. In smaller ski areas rescue is effected by volunteers manning a rescue post at weekends. The basic unit of rescue in Cairngorm is the full time ski patrol. These men are experienced in mountains and mountain craft as well as being expert skiers and competent first aiders. First aid training has been by the normal Red Cross instruction to advanced level, augmented by courses in accident units and courses in mountain, avalanche and ski rescue at home and abroad. Like mountain rescue first aiders, the ski patrolmen have high patient responsibility, because of the distance from medical aid.

Apart from managing the first aid post and effecting rescue a patrol-man has many duties. These relate particularly to the safety of the slopes. Ski trails are marked to show their degree of difficulty, danger areas are marked off. T-bar tracks are checked for snow cover. The runs are regularly patrolled for rapid identification of accidents and to promote courtesy on the slopes and discourage the 'ski bomber' who is a danger both to himself and everyone else. Checks are held on the use of safety straps which prevent loose skis from running off down hill and causing severe injury.

In sudden weather changes involving increase in chill factor, the patrolman specifically looks out for cases suffering from acute hypothermia. These casualties have to be removed to the ski patrol hut for rewarming. 'White out' causes particular problems. In this, wind and driven snow reduce visibility to nil. All sense of direction and inclination are lost with the result that navigation becomes very difficult and completely dependent on a compass and previous known bearings. When 'white out' occurs the evacuation of the hill becomes the patrolman's immediate concern. Even in good conditions all runs are checked before closure to ensure that nobody is left behind.

When a call comes in, the patrolman takes his sledge and prepacked rucksack from the rescue post, and takes the nearest uphill transport to above the accident site. He skis down to the accident, marks it by setting up crossed skis, and leaves the sledge on the uphill side of the casualty. He examines the casualty and if necessary splints the limb, the casualty is then placed in a casualty bag inside a box on the sledge and skied down to the rescue post. Here the diagnosis and splintage is checked and the casualty given time to warm up and compose himself before being evacuated off the hill.

Equipment

Much of the equipment, such as casualty bags, etc. is the same as used in normal mountain rescue.

The box however is the brain child of the Cairngorm Ski Patrol. It is simply a 7 ft $\times$ 2 ft 9 in (2·15 $\times$ 0·85 m) plywood box with a 6 in (15 cm) wall. It offers protection against wind, and will be the stretcher for the patient until he reaches hospital. It also allows the patient to be brought down horizontally on the chairlift.

Sledges

Two rescue sledges are in use in this country.

Canadian. This is a fibre glass 'boat' with long shafts at the front end. It has twin ribs on the underside ending in fins to give directional stability when traversing, especially in spring snow. Hooks are provided for attachment of a rope to secure the casualty. A chain when positioned acts as a brake when evacuation is over ice.

Akja. This is a fibre glass 'boat' with long handles both at the front and rear. It is used by two patrol men and is very suitable for long evacuations.

Splintage

The ski patrol usually prefer a padded Kramer wire splint for leg injuries. It gives good control of the injured limb without the necessity of removing a 5 lb ski boot. Domette bandage strips or home made Velcro fastened ties secure the limb to the splint. Padding is made from polythene sheet crumpled into polythene bags. The water repellent nature of polythene is a great advantage. Long leg inflatable splints are also used.

Analgesia

Although the ski patrol carry morphine it is very seldom used. Virtually all leg fractures settle down to a dull ache when adequately splinted and remain so if evacuation is smooth and unhurried.

Perhaps the most painful injury from skiing is the dislocated shoulder. This injury becomes increasingly painful with time, as well as more difficult to reduce. It is well within the scope of a well trained first aider to attempt a reduction by the Hippocratic method when the injury is new and relatively easy to reduce.

MOUNTAIN ACCIDENT PREVENTION

Accurate statistical assessment of accidents is essential if changing patterns of injury are to be monitored and accidents prevented. Too much reliance is placed on data from serious incidents, when *all* accidents should be investigated, whether serious or trivial. Once the train of events leading to the accident situation is initiated, sheer chance often dictates a serious outcome, requiring spectacular rescue, or a trivial outcome with no injury worth reporting.

There is general agreement that the major cause of accident in mountains and to a lesser extent skiing, is the fault of the individual. In ignorance he exposes himself to potentially dangerous environmental conditions and when caught out, lacks the knowledge and experience to cope with the situation. Only promotion of public awareness of the dangers, and thereafter education in the safe use of the outdoors will reduce the accidents from this cause.

Film shows, poster campaigns, public lectures by mountaineers and team members all help to advertise the dangers. The travelling Duff Memorial Exhibition 'Adventure in Safety' organised by the MRC of Scotland is particularly successful in this field.

'First teach the teacher' is the approach made to the problem by Education Authorities and the Mountain Leadership Training Boards of Great Britain. Physical Education students and other Youth Leaders are trained to the Board's Certificate standard of competence both in summer and winter mountaineering. These people in due course will pass on their knowledge and experience to the youth of the country.

The British Association of Ski Instructors run training and grading courses for ski teachers thus ensuring a high standard of instruction on the ski slopes. A recent survey from Cairngorm showed the rate of injury to be almost halved when skiing under instruction.

Although obvious headway is being made in the field of prevention of accidents, the various methods tend to the long term. Complacency is intolerable when the numbers of people exposed to risk rise so rapidly each year.

FURTHER READING

Avalanche

Fraser (1966), *Avalanche Enigma*, London: Murray.
La Chapelle E R (1970), *Avalanche safety*. Denver: Outdoor Sports Industries.

Mountaineering

Blackshaw A (1970), *Mountaineering: from hill walking to alpine climbing*. London: Penguin.
British Mountaineering Council (1975), *Safety on mountains*.
Langmuir (1976), *Mountain leadership*. Sports Council.

MacInnes (1972), *International mountain rescue handbook*. London: Constable.
Mountain Rescue Committee (1974), *Mountain rescue and cave rescue*.

Skiing

British Association of Ski Instructors (1973), Ski Technique and Instruction Manual BASI.

15

Radio Communications for Accident and Rescue Services

NEVILLE SILVERSTON

If it is accepted that the medical management of the injured should begin at the accident site, it must quickly become apparent that the realisation of this ideal will depend as much on the communication system as on any other single factor. Only frustration will result if the doctor arrives too late to render effective resuscitation, and even more frustration will result if he fails to locate the accident at all.

The development of emergency after care schemes has awakened the interest of many doctors in the problems of radio communication and the place this holds in the organisation of emergency services. It is vitally important to understand the range of radio equipment available and some of the factors which limit its usefulness in various situations. In the flush of initial enthusiasm, it is remarkably easy to spend large sums of money setting up a radio scheme that, for various reasons, will not achieve its object and may have to be modified at a later date at considerable extra cost.

SOME BASIC FACTS ABOUT RADIO COMMUNICATIONS

This is a vast and complex subject which, for the purpose of this chapter, can be narrowed down to radiotelephones operating on very high frequencies (VHF) as it is in this band that the Home Office has made available a number of wavelengths (known as 'channels') to mobile radio systems. It is important to bear in mind that wavelengths are a natural resource, there being only a finite number of them and that very strict regulations must govern their allocation. As the maximum permitted power of a transmitter is limited to 25 watts, these radio systems have a relatively short range of 30 to 40 miles, so that the same channels can be allocated to users in different parts of the country without fear of interference. However, it is possible to extend the range of a system by the use of repeater stations, radio links or Post Office landlines.

For practical purposes, VHF waves should be considered as travelling in straight lines, the so-called 'line of sight', and radio shadows tend to be created in valleys and on the other side of high ground. For these reasons, aerials should be positioned on the highest ground in the neighbourhood with the transmitter situated immediately adjacent because the 'feeder cables' that connect the aerial to the transmitter are particularly expensive. In rural areas, there may be the added problem of bringing in an electricity supply and the Post Office landlines to connect the transmitter to the (remote) control room. The annual rental on these can be a major recurring cost. However, there is no substitute for aerial height if a reliable radio system is to result. VHF waves do have a certain ability to penetrate into vehicles but, for effective reception and transmission, one of the various types of external aerials should be fitted. In towns, VHF waves do penetrate into buildings and they also 'bounce' from surfaces such as the walls of buildings but not to the same extent as ultra high frequency (UHF).

Two-way radio systems operate on the method known as 'two frequency simplex' which means that the **control transmitter** and the **mobile receiver** are tuned to one frequency, while the **mobile transmitter** and the **control receiver** are tuned to a second frequency. As a result, all the mobiles in the system hear the controller speaking but they cannot hear each other. If it is necessary for the two mobiles to speak to each other directly, the controller can put the transmitter on to the facility known as 'talk through' so that the incoming message on the second frequency is transmitted out again on the first frequency.

Selective calling

Radio paging or 'bleeping' is a well-tried method of contacting personnel within buildings and on large sites and most doctors have personal experience of its use in hospitals. However, it is only in recent years that long-range radio paging equipment, sufficiently small, sensitive and with a long battery life, has been developed. Systems are now available which can accommodate thousands of paging units operating on one radio frequency and each responding to its own 'code'. When this operating frequency is the same as that being used for transmitting voice on a mobile radiotelephone system, it is known as 'overlay paging'. The Post Office has plans to develop a national radio paging service operated through the public telephone system.

Car radiotelephones can be fitted with an accessory module which permits the central control operator to call a particular mobile selectively. This obviates the driver having to listen for his own call sign amid considerable, distracting radio 'chatter'. Should he be away from his vehicle at the time he is called, a light comes up on the radio so that he is aware, on his return, that there is a message for him.

One-way speech facility can be introduced into a pocket pager but the applications of this are strictly limited except, for example, on a building site where it it known that reception is 100 per cent. Out in the field with its inevitable radio shadows, there is no means by which the base operator has feedback that a message has been received.

Radiotelephones

There is a bewildering range of radiotelephones available in this country manufactured by British, European and American companies. For reasons that will be mentioned later, doctors should only concern themselves with very high frequency/frequency modulated (VHF/FM) equipment and this can be divided basically into portable and fixed car models.

Portable radios are battery operated and are ideal when the need rescue work. Groups of doctors working on a rota can also find them useful as the instrument can be passed to the doctor on duty for the day. When used in a vehicle, it can be slipped into a special adaptor on the dashboard which not only connects it to an external aerial but also to the car battery. The main disadvantage of these small sets is the limited range of the 1·5−2 watt transmitter which, even under ideal conditions, rarely exceeds 10 miles.

The fixed car radiotelephone is now a very compact piece of equipment and models can be obtained with transmitters of 5, 10 and 25 watts. Furthermore, they are 'multi-channel' which means that they can be tuned into a number of different transmitters. Most manufacturers make both dashboard and boot mounted models and it is important to ensure that radiotelephones are not installed in a position that would guarantee a fractured patella in the event of an accident! If space in the passenger compartment is really limited, the radio should be fitted in the car boot as then only the control switches and the microphones need to be fitted on the dashboard. Boot mounted sets are also useful where the radio is shared between a number of users as the aerial and power supply can be unplugged very easily.

Aerials are a most important feature of the car radiotelephone system. There are many types and sizes but the radio manufacturer will recommend the correct one for the particular radio fitted. The position of the aerial on the vehicle is also important. Ideally it should be mounted on the roof in order to give the greatest height but this may lead to a problem in bringing the cable down within the fabric lining and, also, many household garages are too low to accommodate the aerial in this position. Radiotelephones are particularly sensitive to emissions from the car electrical system even though these may be adequately suppressed for the ordinary car radio. For this reason, aerials are often sited at the furthest point on the vehicle away from the engine but, here again, the radio manufacturer who usually installs the set will give advice.

AMBULANCE RADIO NETWORK

Prior to the reorganisation of the National Health Service in 1974, each ambulance authority negotiated its radio frequency with the Ministry of Posts and Telecommunications. It was a chaotic situation which made it almost impossible for an ambulance passing into an adjacent county to communicate with that county's ambulance control. Following discussions between the Department of Health and Social Security and the Radio Regulatory Department of the Home Office, it was agreed to reserve 25 VHF/FM frequencies in the 166 megaHertz band for the sole use of the ambulance services in the United Kingdom and to allocate these to various Authorities in such a way that there would be no overlap in the areas of reception. For example, the identical channel has been allocated to Cambridgeshire, Derbyshire, Devonshire, London (emergency), West Sussex, Anglesey and

Montgomery. One frequency, known as the emergency reserve channel (ERC) is common to all ambulance systems and is reserved for use in the event of a major accident. It is now possible for an ambulance to communicate with its neighbouring control room on entering their territory, and this facility has led to considerably increased efficiency in the use of ambulances.

Radio communications in relation to GP accident services

There is such great variation in the size of the many schemes in the UK and also in local conditions and administrative attitudes that it is impossible to lay down hard and fast rules applicable overall. Certain principles have come out of a recent survey of radio schemes of GP accident services throughout the country. First and foremost is the facility to speak to the local ambulance control as this provides the following benefits:

(i) It confirms to the ambulance control and also to the crew of the ambulance en route to the emergency that the doctor is also on his way.

(ii) As the initial information regarding the geographical location of the accident is frequently incorrect, further incoming details can be passed to the doctor by the ambulance control.

(iii) Should the doctor's services not be required, his call out can be cancelled without his wasting further time.

(iv) The doctor may be able to pass back valuable information to the ambulance control as he may be the first at the scene of the accident and, in rural areas, his local knowledge can be extremely useful.

(v) Many ambulance controls have extensions of their radio system into the accident department of the local district general hospital and, therefore, the GP can speak from his vehicle directly to the medical and nursing staff. For example, he can pass on details of the number of casualties being sent to hospital, their injuries, the treatment given and recommendations that certain specialists should be called to the accident department in order to deal with particular injuries. On occasions, the GP needs to give blood and he can instruct the hospital staff to make this ready and then despatch a police patrol car to bring it to the accident scene.

(vi) The place of the GP in the renal transplant service is only just being recognised. In the event of a fatality, it is usually the GP who certifies death, in which case the body should be sent to a hospital with renal transplant facilities. The GP can inform the hospital over the radio that the cadaver might provide suitable kidneys and that the transplant team should be assembled. The GP, together with the police, should obtain as many details as possible regarding the exact time of death and the deceased's personal particulars, all of which could be transmitted to the hospital.

The department of Health and Social Security, in contrast to the Scottish Home and Health Department, has not viewed the extension of ambulance radio facilities to GPs with any enthusiasm. It is to the credit of many senior ambulance officers that they have had the foresight to cooperate with accident after care schemes, especially with regard to radio communications. Clearly, conditions and pressures of work vary considerably from one geographical area to another but most area ambulance officers do have a fear that unlimited access of radio facilities to GPs, say for the passing of domestic or practice messages, would be quite unacceptable and they lay down strict conditions which will prevent this type of 'abuse'. Ambulance control staff appreciate the doctor using his radio in accordance with accepted radiotelephone 'jargon' and all GPs should be encouraged to spend an hour or two in the ambulance control room being instructed in this discipline. For example, a typical conversation between a doctor and an ambulance control officer would sound something like this:

'**Medic 4 to CAM 1, over**'. The control will reply '**CAM 1 receiving Medic 4**' whereupon the doctor, after identifying himself again, will give his message quickly and smoothly—much more like a telegram than a telephone conversation. All details given are usually repeated back by the controller and, if correct, the exchange would terminate by the doctor saying '**Roger, Medic 4 over and out**'.

Hospital based schemes

It is much easier to consider the place of radio communications in accident and emergency departments of hospitals which are staffed throughout the day and which are often connected to the local ambulance station by both telephone and radio links. Additionally, some departments have multi-channel transmitter/receivers in their departments so that they can not only tune in to the frequencies of all the local ambulance service networks, but also communicate with their own flying squads when these are called out. In some instances, hospitals, especially near motorways, have cooperated to link their radio systems so that, in the event of a major accident, they can coordinate their efforts.

SETTING UP A RADIO COMMUNICATION SYSTEM

Initially it must be determined exactly what is required from the system, how many doctors will use the facilities, how much it will cost and how the money should be raised. It is a prerequisite that both the area ambulance officer and the sales representative of the radio manufacturing company shall be involved from the start. It is also important to consider in what way the radiotelephone system can be used for practice work in the absence of this facility being offered by the ambulance service. It really is a waste of the radio communication facilities if the expensive equipment can only be used for accident work for, however much the GP may be involved in this field, his involvement in practice work must be very much greater. In the smaller schemes, which may only consist of one partnership of doctors, the GPs can purchase their own transmitter on which practice messages can be relayed. In the event of an accident, they can change channels and communicate with ambulance control. For this reason, it is essential when applying for a radio frequency, to have one allocated within 'switchable' distance of the ambulance VHF/FM network.

Some of the larger schemes have devised methods of utilising their radio systems for practice purposes without involving themselves in the financially unrealistic problem of having to man their own base stations. The Somerset and Avon Voluntary Emergency Service (SAVES) has an arrangement whereby they contribute to the salary of one of the ambulance staff who operates the radio paging and radiotelephone transmitter during officer hours with the main ambulance control centre taking over during the night. The North East Essex Doctors' Emergency Service (NEEDS) makes use of the switchboard operator of a small local hospital for a similar purpose. The Doctors' Accident Rescue Service (DART) of Doncaster make use of the staff of a doctors' surgery during the daytime to operate the transmitter, the police taking over this function during the night. On the other hand, the Lincolnshire Integrated Voluntary Emergency Service (LIVES) has developed its radio scheme in a similar manner but covering a much larger area and the ambulance service takes over the call out function after surgery hours. It is of interest that the LIVES scheme originally equipped over 80 of their doctor participants with portable radiotelephones intending that these instruments would serve the dual function of call out **and** voice communication but experience has proved that, in many cases, they failed on both counts. Some doctors found the instruments too large to carry around with them all the time and, in the absence of a selective call mechanism, others found it tedious to keep listening for their own call sign. Furthermore, some doctors have found that they have needed to replace the portable sets by the more powerful car models in order to obtain reliable transmission and reception.

In Scotland, both the Highland Regional Health Board and the Dumfries and Galloway Health Board have allocated funds to GPs in their areas for the purchase of radio and medical resuscitation equipment. Neither service has been going long enough to determine the efficiency of these pilot schemes, but, clearly, if successful, they should set a precedent which must be emulated elsewhere in the UK.

The Mid Anglia General Practitioner Accident Service (MAGPAS) has linked up with a medical radio paging service operating from Addenbrooke's Hospital, Cambridge. This organisation, Cambridge Medical Answering Services Ltd (CMAS), was set up in 1968 to determine the applications of radio paging in a medical community and Fig. 15.1 indicates the medical and para-medical personnel who currently make use of its facilities. The radiotelephone and radio paging service now cover the new county of Cambridgeshire, about 2000 square miles, and operates from three transmitters with UHF radio links. When an accident is reported to the police or ambulance service, details are usually passed to the CMAS radio control room and the operator on duty 'bleeps' the doctor who has agreed to cover the area in which the accident has occurred. He can ask for details on his car radiotelephone and then change his channel to that of the ambulance frequency.

It can be seen that, to be efficient, two separate items of radio

HOSPITAL DOCTORS ⟶   ⟶ FAMILY DOCTORS

   Renal Transplant Team   Locum Register
   Obstetric Flying Squad
   Coronary Care Unit
   Neurosurgery
   Orthopaedics
   Renal Dialysis Unit
   Anaesthetist
   Geriatric Hospital
   E N T Department

   Theatre Sister
   Biochemistry Technician
   Haematology Technician

DISTRICT NURSES

CONSULTANTS

MIDWIVES   M A G P A S

SENIOR AMBULANCE PERSONNEL

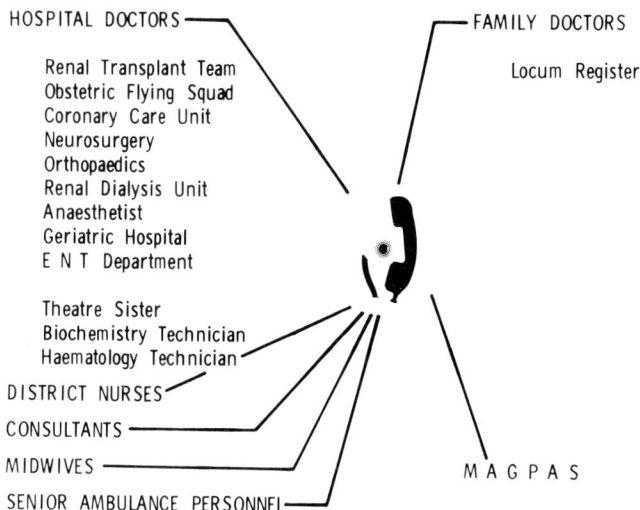

Fig. 15.1. Diagram to show the medical and para-medical personnel using the medical radio paging service of the Cambridge Medical Answering Services Ltd.

equipment are essential. The first is a selective call pocket bleeper, which bypasses the Post Office telephone system with all its inherent delays and frustrations and contacts the doctor wherever he may be. The second item is the portable or car radiotelephone, which confers all the communication advantages outlined above.

Radio equipment is expensive and can account for 80 per cent of the cost of the equipment for each doctor. The items can be obtained either by capital purchase, leasing or rental maintenance. It is important to go into the financial aspects very carefully for maintenance can be expensive and it is equally important to negotiate with a firm who can offer a truly reliable back-up service. While transmitters and car equipment are extremely reliable, portable radiotelephones and pocket pagers are much more vulnerable to being dropped and are likely to need repairing more frequently.

THE FUTURE

The place of radio communications in the accident and rescue services is still in its infancy and GP accident after care schemes are still pioneer organisations without official recognition. It is certain that, in the years to come, this attitude will change and will lead to far better cooperation between GPs, ambulance services and hospitals. One of the prime areas of integration will be in the field of radio communications.

16

The Police Role in Emergency Care Schemes

F W SHAKESBY

THE TASK

It is fair to say that the civilian police are the accepted guardians of public safety and are usually the first of the emergency services to be called when an emergency arises. In 1970, during a debate in the House of Commons about a proposal for a National Emergency Organisation, it was said: 'It is to the Police Service that the public always turn first when in distress. With their communications they are able to assemble their forces rapidly and to call on other services to assist . . . the police will also establish where necessary, traffic control points and information posts, and direct the removal of casualties to places where they can be dealt with expeditiously.'

This chapter is concerned with the day-to-day road accidents to which police patrols are called rather than with major incidents. The extract quoted from the debate, however, clearly indicates the role of the police officer in emergencies and defines his role as co-ordinator until such time as the injured have been removed into care and the situation restored, more or less, to normal. He can then revert to his professional role of investigator into the cause of the accident.

When a road accident occurs there may be, and usually are, many interests to consider—parties to the accident who may be dead, injured to a greater or lesser degree, or uninjured; vehicles, which may be beyond repair, or superficially damaged; private property, such as walls, fences, gardens or structures, which may be damaged and unsafe; public utilities such as electricity supplies, water, gas, telephones, which may be hazardous; highway and street furniture or even the highway itself that may be damaged.

Any one or a combination of these adds to the problem of controlling the incident and it is here that the policeman not only assumes but accepts his responsibility for control and coordination of the different interests.

No individual can take on such a task without assistance and this is readily obtained through the control information room which is the nerve centre of the force.

Here is kept a veritable mine of information which is indexed, cross-referenced and immediately available to each operator. A bank of consoles each equipped with incoming and outgoing facilities provide telephones and radio links on VHF and UHF channels. These are supported by a teleprinter network throughout the force and telex connections outside. In order that priorities are maintained basic procedures must be laid down and followed. These are contained in standing orders which are circulated throughout the force to every regular member. They can be summarised as:

Priorities

(a) To save life and relieve suffering;
(b) To protect property;
(c) To liaise with all involved—communications;
(d) To get things back to normal as soon as possible.

Method

(a) To alert other essential services, i.e. ambulance, fire, post office, public utilities, etc.
(b) To ensure that these services can operate. This entails traffic control, protection of the scene of the incident and site discipline.

For many years, until the introduction of emergency care schemes, persons injured in road accidents received first aid from the police officer until the arrival of the ambulance.

The police officer carried almost all the immediate responsibility, and due to devoting his attention to the casualties was often unable to give full attention to his basic function.

The introduction in 1967 of the Road Accident After Care Scheme in North Yorkshire cleared the way for the police officer to carry out his responsibilities more efficiently. The arrival of a qualified medical practitioner within a very short time of the accident being reported to the police enables each of the emergency services to get on with its specialist work. The task of dealing with road accidents takes a basic pattern:

(i) The police officer protects the scene by putting out emergency traffic control signs and warnings.

   The doctor attends to the casualties and works with the ambulance crew.

(ii) The fire brigade, when called upon, rescues those casualties that are trapped in the wreckage and takes fire preventive measures. The severely injured are accompanied by the doctor to the hospital when necessary.

(iii) The police ensure that the fire brigade, ambulance service, and doctors can reach and depart from the scene smoothly and speedily. The detailed investigation into the cause of the accident can then commence.

(iv) Contact is also made with local police forces to keep relatives of casualties informed of what is happening.

   During the whole operation the police officer at the scene maintains contact with the control room, which has opened up a communications link with the other emergency services, control rooms, hospital and other organisations that are involved.

A picture should now have emerged of the police responsibility and the extent to which individual officers become involved. This raises the question of training and equipment.

THE TOOLS

The old adage 'Jack of all trades and master of none' could, quite unfairly, be applied to a policeman. He is expected to meet and respond to all manner of problems affecting the community. By the application of his training and use of plain common sense, he can usually bring most situations to a satisfactory conclusion, or control it until assistance is forthcoming.

His chief tools of trade are, therefore, knowledge and training to which he applies such human qualities as courage, sympathy and tact.

Unwittingly he becomes a student of human nature. His professional knowledge starts with basic recruit training, followed by other specialist and refresher courses as his career develops. To this is added whatever knowledge he acquires through private study for qualifying examinations for promotion or external qualifications. Most professional courses include practical application of the specific subject; but his real training must develop from experience when doing the job.

First aid is an essential part of his training and is included in every recruit's training syllabus. During this time he will acquire the First aid Certificate of the St John, Red Cross and St Andrew's Standard Course. On joining his parent force from the training establishment, he is then expected to requalify in first-aid every three years until he has at least ten years service. This emphasis on first aid is marked in most police forces by inter-divisional and regional competitions, perhaps leading to an appearance at the National 'PIM' Trophy Competition, held annually in London. Many chief officers encourage their members to enter local and national first aid competitions where they can compete against outside bodies such as miners, public utility and factory teams.

Equipment

In the North Yorkshire Police, as a result of the introduction of the pioneer pilot after care scheme in 1967, training in the use of specialist first aid equipment was given to selected police officers engaged on traffic patrol duties by local medical practitioners involved in the scheme.

In the light of experience and with the extension of emergency care schemes to other areas, it was necessary to consider which vehicles should be equipped and what scale of emergency care equipment should be carried. A discussion took place between the police and the doctors which resulted in an agreed policy that special equipment (Fig. 16.1) would be carried in all traffic patrol vehicles to the following scale:

1 Spinal board
1 Cervical collar

1 'Space' blanket
1 Standard resuscitation pack
1 Portex Resusciade for mouth-to-mouth resuscitation
1 'Urias' pack of leg and arm splints (one of each)
2 Extra large wound dressings 8 in × 7 in

In a modern society, knowledge, training and a study of human nature alone are not enough to cope with its needs and problems. Our policemen should have available to them also, not only the means of transport, but reliable transport and communications.

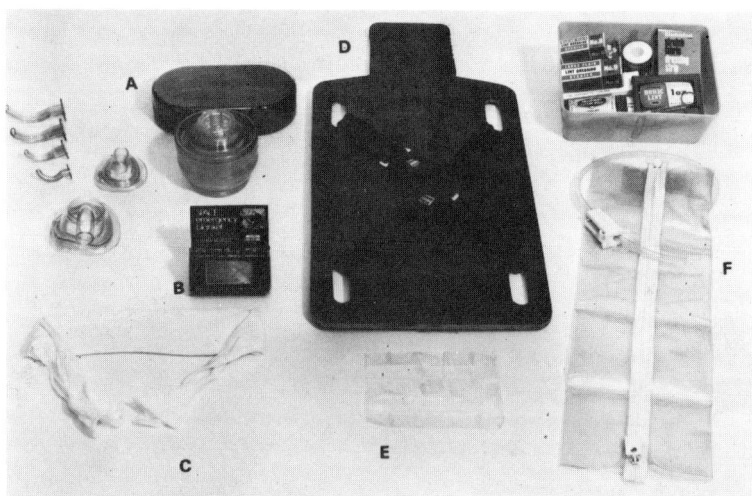

Fig. 16.1. Special equipment carried in all traffic patrol vehicles: standard resuscitation pack. A. space blanket. B. cervical collar. C. spinal board. D. Portex Resusciaide. E. 'Urias' leg and arm splints. F. wound dressings (top right). (Copyright Chief Constable, North Yorks Police.)

Police transport is normally required to meet four needs:

(i) Divisional transport. For day-to-day service to the community and for law enforcement.
(ii) Traffic patrols. Supervision of all road users, and law enforcement, accident prevention and attention to road accidents.

(iii) Specialist vehicles: CID, dogs, mounted, etc.

(iv) General transport.

Although divisional transport carries a limited amount of emergency equipment, it is the traffic patrol vehicles which are equipped to an agreed scale.

As traffic patrol vehicles operate on all major roads and highways in the force area and are superimposed over divisional and specialist vehicle availability, it is reasonable for doctors engaged in emergency care schemes to expect assistance from a trained policeman carrying the necessary equipment and within an acceptable response time.

The three types of traffic patrol vehicle in use are:

Range Rover fitted with 'Stemlite' (Fig. 16.2)

These vehicles are deployed throughout the area so that emergency lighting (Fig. 16.3) is available quickly.

Ford Consul 3000 GT patrol car

This vehicle is in general use and is shown (Fig. 16.4) with complement of equipment; this car comprises the bulk of the patrol fleet.

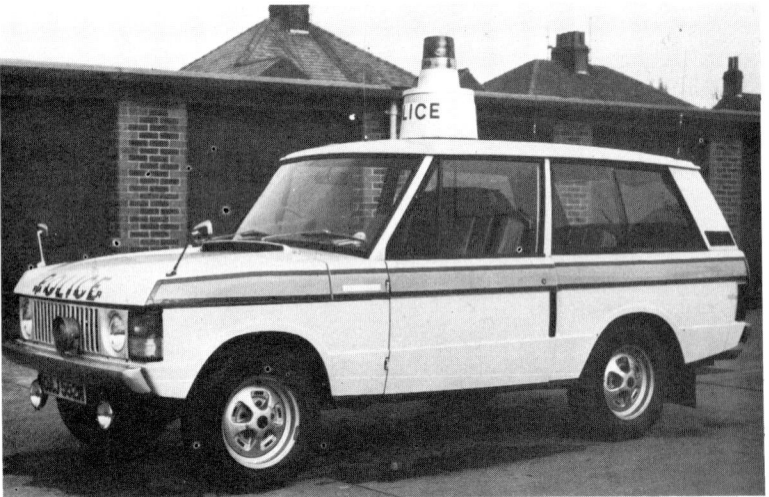

Fig. 16.2. Range Rover fitted with 'Stemlite'. (Copyright Chief Constable, North Yorks Police.)

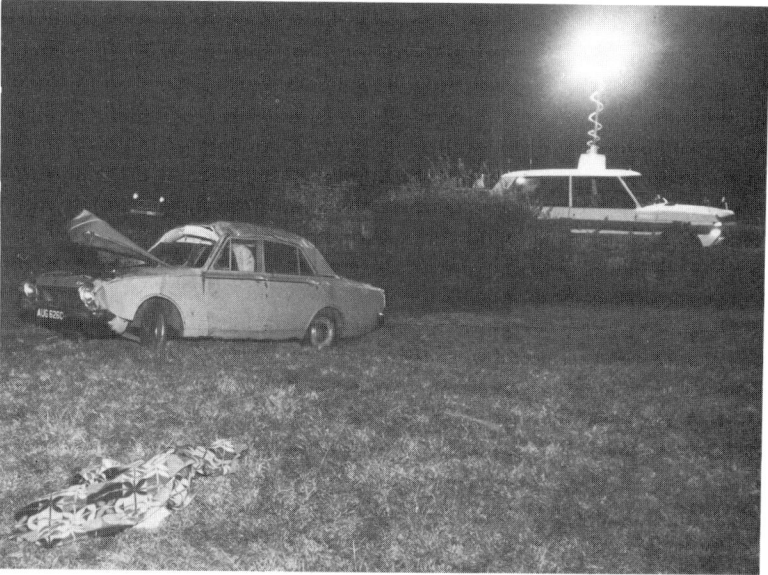

Fig. 16.3. 'Stemlite' operating at scene of actual incident. (Copyright Chief Constable, North Yorks Police.)

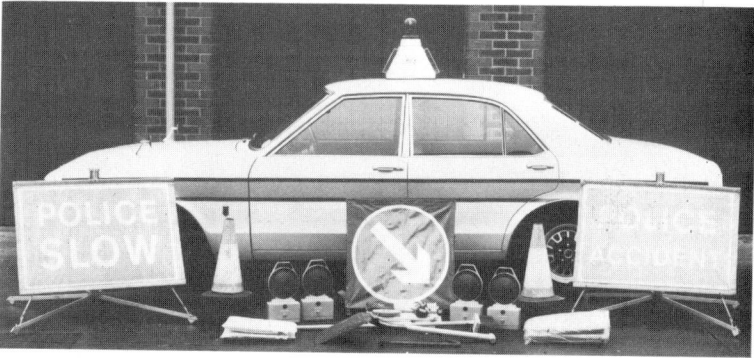

Fig. 16.4. 3000 GT Patrol Car. (Copyright Chief Constable, North Yorks Police.)

Ford Transit van accident unit

These operate only on the major through roads such as the A1, and carry twice the complement of emergency signs and equipment

(Fig. 16.5). Their purpose is to supplement patrol cars on motorways, dual carriageways and busy high speed roads where advanced warning to road users is essential to prevent multi-vehicle accidents. Once the scene has been properly signed and protected, the van is free to continue as a patrol or to supplement another patrol car which might be involved with a separate incident.

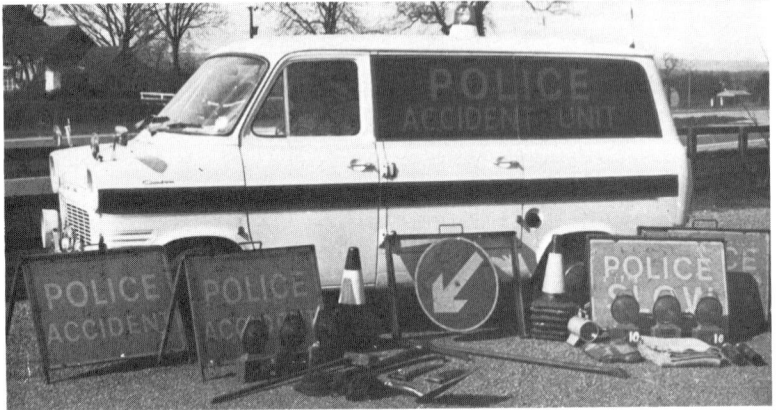

Fig. 16.5. Ford Transit type van with equipment. (Copyright Chief Constable, North Yorks Police.)

Communications

The communications department is centred in the control room at headquarters and supported by a teleprinter room and records office. The main function of the control room is to collect and disseminate information received from all sources, comply with requests for assistance and record action taken. Its aim is to give a continued and efficient service to the public and to police personnel alike. It also provides communications between the various specialised departments of the force engaged in major incidents and other emergencies.

When the occasion arises, control room personnel direct radio vehicles to incidents and maintain communication, not only with the vehicles but with their divisional headquarters. It is, therefore, essential that in order to operate with maximal efficiency the full cooperation of all members of the force is necessary and accurate transmission of information is essential.

The control room is equipped with two-way radio communications with all mobiles and divisional stations within the force area; and links exist with adjoining forces.

Each operator in the control room, in addition to the radio channels, has access to telephone connections not only to Post Office exchange lines, but to private lines linking divisional and sub-divisional stations. The 999 emergency system in North Yorkshire is decentralised to divisional headquarters by arrangement with the Post Office. Teleprinter facilities are also available.

The records office coordinates all incoming information and in addition keeps permanent records which could be of assistance in dealing with incidents of all kinds. Maps are kept for plotting services at serious incidents etc; details of coroners' districts, parish boundaries, traffic zones, garages where assistance and equipment is available, to mention but a few, are all contained in a comprehensive filing system, which also includes other useful information.

Divisional vehicles are normally deployed at the discretion of the divisional commander, but they can, in cases of emergency, be placed under headquarters' control and the authority of the officer-in-charge of the control room. The specialised road traffic vehicles are under the direction of control at all times when on duty and are available instantly to be directed to any incident that is reported. It is possible through the control room systems for vehicles to be given 'talk through' facilities. Whenever more than one vehicle is directed to a major incident, one mobile remains on radio watch, maintaining communication between the scene and the control room until a mobile control can be established at the scene.

A command vehicle for emergency operations is kept at headquarters and equipped with a ten channel VHF radio with channel selection capabilities on all force radio channels and inter-post communications. This vehicle also carries a portable VHF system with pocket phones which is readily available at the scene of an emergency (Fig. 16.6).

It will be seen, therefore, that the police service has instant communication facilities available to deal with almost every kind of incident that might arise.

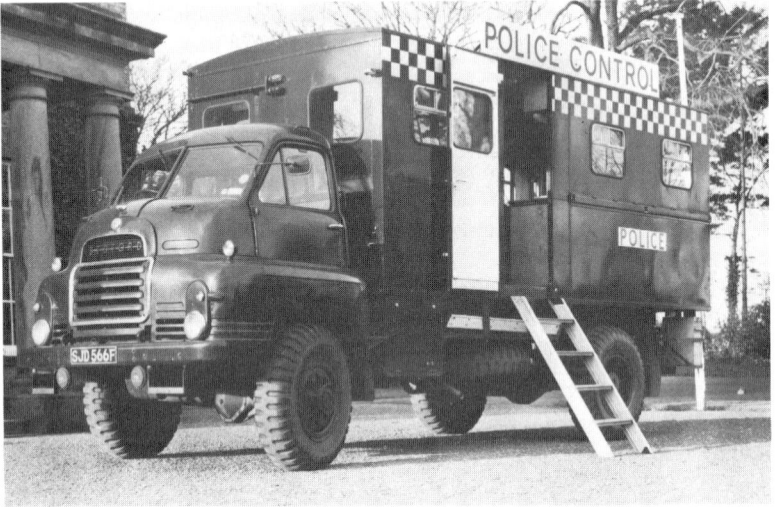

Fig. 16.6. Police Mobile Control Vehicle used for emergencies and serious accidents. (Copyright Chief Constable, North Yorks Police.)

THE LAW

Road accidents

It is not only difficult but dangerous to condense any law, and the purpose of this section is to outline those parts of the law which may affect the action of the police when dealing with road accidents. The reader should, therefore, refer to statutes if he wishes to pursue this aspect in more detail. The law is under constant review and amended in the light of changing social and economic conditions.

Reporting of accidents

The statutory requirements (Road Traffic Act 1972, section 25(1) (2)) for the driver of a motor vehicle who is involved in an accident are:

(i)   that he shall stop;
(ii)   give his name and address;
(iii) the name and address of the owner of the vehicle;

(iv) the identification marks of the vehicle—to any parties having reasonable grounds to require same.

Provision is also made for the driver who does not give the particulars at the time and allows him to report the accident at a police station or to a constable as soon as reasonably practicable, and in any case within 24 hours.

The law requires production of insurance in the case of injury accidents and places the onus on the driver to report the accident within 24 hours (Road Traffic Act 1972, section 166).

Notification to hospitals

Under section 156 (5) of the Road Traffic Act 1972, a Chief Officer of Police is required to furnish particulars of vehicles and drivers on the request of a person who claims that he is entitled to a payment for emergency treatment resulting from an accident.

Testing and examination of vehicles involved in road accidents

Any authorised examiner or any constable authorised in writing by the Chief Constable, has the power to test and inspect any motor vehicle or trailer in respect of: brakes, steering, lighting equipment, reflectors, tyres, silencers and smoke and fume vapour. The driver may elect for the test to be deferred and carried out a time and place fixed in accordance with the Third Schedule to the Road Traffic Act 1972, section 53.

When it appears to a constable that an accident has occurred, he may test the vehicle forthwith and may detain the vehicle until the test has been carried out. It is an offence to obstruct any authorised examiner acting under this section.

Regulations (Motor Vehicles (Construction and Use) Regs. 1973, reg. 137) provide for any police officer in uniform to test and inspect the brakes, silencer, steering gear, tyres, lighting equipment and reflectors of any motor vehicle or trailer on any premises provided the consent of the owner of the premises and the owner of the vehicle is given.

Refusal of consent by the owner can be nullified by serving him with a notice of the proposed examination, either personally or leaving it at his address at least 48 hours before, or sending it by recorded delivery at least 72 hours before the examination.

When the vehicle has been involved in an accident, the serving of the written notice is unnecessary (even if the owner objects) if the examination takes place within 48 hours of the accident.

Weighing of vehicles

A constable may require the person in charge of a motor vehicle or trailer to proceed to a weighbridge to allow the vehicle to be weighed. He may not, however, order the unloading of a laden vehicle simply to ascertain its unladen weight. Section 57 of the Road Traffic Act provides for a constable (authorised in writing) to prevent the driving of a vehicle after an offence in the relevant Section of the Act is disclosed.

Drinking and driving

The law on drink and driving is contained in the Road Traffic Act 1972. The main features are outlined in the following summary.

A constable may arrest any person who is driving or attempting to drive a motor vehicle, or being in charge of a motor vehicle on a road or other public place when unfit to drive through drink or drugs (section 5).

Driving or being in charge of a motor vehicle with a blood/alcohol concentration above the prescribed limit, i.e. 80 mg of alcohol in 100 ml of blood (section 6).

A constable in uniform may require a person driving or attempting to drive a motor vehicle to provide a specimen of breath if the constable has reasonable cause: (a) to suspect him of having alcohol in his body, or (b) to suspect him of having committed a moving traffic offence while the vehicle was in motion (section 8).

After an accident has occurred, a constable in uniform may require a driver to provide a breath test if he has reasonable cause to believe that the person was driving or attempting to drive the vehicle at the time, except whilst the person is at a hospital as a patient.

Refusal to provide a breath test is an offence (power of arrest). After being arrested under section 8, or section 5, the offender is taken to a police station where a further breath test is given.

Should both tests prove positive, the offender is then required to provide a specimen of either blood (taken by a doctor) or urine. These specimens are sealed and taken for analysis to determine the amount of alcohol. The offender is always offered a sample for his own analysis. In most cases the offender is released from custody pending the result of the analysis.

In the case of a person who is a patient at a hospital, the permission of a doctor is always required before any specimen is obtained.

The offence is proved not by the breath test being positive, but on the forensic evidence of the alcohol content in the blood/urine samples.

Whenever persons are detained under the drinking and driving laws they are taken to the nearest police station. Each police station has a list of doctors who are willing to be called upon for the purpose of taking blood or urine specimens. These police surgeons do not respond to emergency case call out: nor do the police ask the volunteer rescue doctors to take blood/urine specimens, as having subsequently to appear in court proceedings would mean a waste of valuable time and availability.

MOTORWAYS

Motorways are patrolled at all times by the police because it is most important to deal promptly with the slightest interference with traffic flows. If this was not so, the obstruction could rapidly escalate into a multi-vehicle pile-up. To this end police officers are specially trained and equipped to deal with such incidents. These often occur in conditions of fog and poor visibility or by a broken down vehicle on the carriageway and in some cases, bad driving behaviour.

Despite training and having the necessary equipment available it is an alarming experience for the emergency services who are called to deal with these emergencies, until the scene is protected and under control. Only those services that are essential will be allowed at the scene and will be subject to a strict code of discipline. Basic advice to doctors called upon to work in these conditions is summarised as follows:

The law contained in the Road Traffic Acts, in the Motor Vehicles (Construction and Use) Regulations and in the Motorway Traffic

Regulations (Statutory Instrument No 1147 (1959), London: HMSO) must be complied with at all times.

It should be noted that all access/exit link roads are part of motorways. Doctors and others attending a motorway incident, should:

NOT drive on to or across central reservations.

NOT reverse, except as permitted by regulations.

ALWAYS carry some authoritative form of identification. This will enable the police to facilitate attendance at the scene.

Care should be taken not to approach the scene of an accident at too fast a speed—a fast approach may endanger the lives of persons already at the scene. The road surface may be affected by ice or by spillage being the original cause or an effect of the accident.

Upon arrival at the scene, look out for directions from the police as to the most suitable place to stop.

If a directive is not received, stop on the hard shoulder beyond (in front of) the police vehicle or within the protection of traffic cones.

Leave room for and do not obstruct other emergency service vehicles.

Never stop on the carriageway.

You may be directed to an assembly point, in the event of a serious multiple accident, to await instructions. The assembly point may be on the access link to the main carriage of the motorway.

Be prepared to extinguish any emergency identification lamps if this should be a distraction.

Control will be exercised by the police at all times.

THE EFFECT

Having looked at the task, the tools and those who use them, it is perhaps appropriate to consider the benefits from the police point of view.

When notification is received that an injury accident has occurred in an area where an emergency scheme is operating, the control room immediately despatch a patrol car to the scene and notify the nearest available doctor. Each of the emergency services cross check with each other when calls for assistance are required. If the call is first received by the ambulance service it is possible, and frequently happens, that the doctor will be at the scene before the arrival of the police.

Even though police patrols are trained to deal with injured persons it is a great help to find that medical assistance is readily available, not only to the casualties but also to advise in the event of toxic substances or drugs being involved. Apart from the obvious benefit to the injured, an after care scheme relieves the police of much responsibility in the immediate care and treatment of badly injured casualties and enables them to concentrate on other aspects of the accident. In more tragic circumstances there is an added benefit in that death can be certified at the scene in fatal accidents, thus reducing the administrative complications if casualties are moved and death certified in another coroner's district.

From a police point of view, emergency care schemes work well and have done much to cement a sound working relationship between the emergency services. They promote respect for each other's enterprise and each service enjoys a spin-off in the good image which is presented to the public.

This close working relationship was put on record on the 16th August 1970, in North Yorkshire, when a film was made to demonstrate the after care scheme in action. It depicted a road accident involving a two car-crash with seven passengers. (Produced by Rock Humphries Television and Film Productions, 72, Lombard Street, London, EC3; Producer/Director—Rock Humphries. Running Time—20 minutes; Optical: sound. Available by arrangement with Roche Products Ltd, Manchester Square, London W1.)

Overseas visitors studying the scheme are invited to visit the North Yorkshire Police Headquarters, Racecourse Lane, Northallerton, where they are shown the control room and see the vehicles and equipment used. Most have been favourably impressed by, and ask questions about, the training in the use of spinal boards, application of cervical collars and resuscitation equipment. They express deep interest in the adaptation made to the accident unit vehicles and the equipment carried. Without exception they are particularly impressed by the emergency 'Sparlite'/'Stemlite' lighting equipment. ('Sparlite'/'Stemlite' is a product of Neeco Industries, Ltd, 307, Mainway Drive, Burlington, Ontario, Canada. Sole United Kingdom Distributors: Dale Electric of Great Britain, Ltd, Electricity Buildings, Filey, Yorkshire.) This has proved to be the most significant and effective acquisition in recent years for dealing with accidents in darkness and medics have not hesitated to express their appreciation of it when called out at night. In practice it is possible to read a book at 25–30 m distance and there have been many instances of casualties treated at the roadside under this lighting. Doctors engaged in treating casualties at the scenes of cave rescues in the Yorkshire Dales have also praised the efficiency of this equipment. By fitting to the Range Rover/Land Rover type vehicles it enables emergency lighting to be available in the most difficult surroundings.

THE FUTURE

Ideally, it would be of benefit to the whole community if emergency care schemes were a requisite part of the National Health Service. It is not easy to convince everyone that they work and achieve the savings in life and limb attributed to them; and until such times as they can be financed other than by charitable schemes, it will fall to local interest and enthusiasm for them to be introduced. If there is sufficient interest at local level perhaps the best method is to invite all those who would be involved to a meeting. It is, however, important that the local general practitioners are favourably disposed towards a scheme. Without their support, no scheme will get off the ground. Once this support is forthcoming then the ambulance service, police, fire brigade and representatives from the District Health Authority should be called in to discuss the implications.

Senior police officers from North Yorkshire are frequently invited to seminars and to speak at meetings where emergency schemes are being considered. A frank exchange of views and listening to those with first hand experience is to be recommended.

17

Fire Services

P J BRENNAN and A STOW

The British Fire Service as we know it today had its conception in the Fire Brigades Act of 1938. Unfortunately, the gathering clouds of World War II overshadowed the effect of many of its provisions and it was not until the passing of the Fire Services Act in 1947 that these were truly realised. However, the 1938 Act for the first time laid a statutory duty on each district council (except the London County Council) to make provision for an official fire service in its area. At the outbreak of war there existed 1440 separate fire brigades in England and Wales and 228 in Scotland. These continued until August 1941 when, as a wartime expedient and in consequence of experience of air raid conditions, it was decided to nationalise the Fire Service. Thirty-nine fire areas were created, each commanded by a Fire Force Commander, and subsequently divided into divisions, columns and companies. Rapidly on the heels of nationalisation there followed standardisation of conditions of service, ranks, equipment and training—achieving a nationwide advance in fire service efficiency. After the war, the Fire Service reverted to local authority control, under the Fire Services Act of 1947 except that control was handed over to Councils of County Boroughs and Counties, not District Councils as was formerly the case. This had the effect of reducing the number of brigades to 148.

STATUTORY OBLIGATIONS

The 1947 Act required the new fire authorities to maintain efficient fire brigades, capable of dealing with all normal demands, and also providing:

(i)   Efficient training of the members of its brigade.
(ii) Efficient arrangements for dealing with fire calls and the summoning of personnel.
(iii) Efficient arrangements for obtaining information required for firefighting purposes, i.e. with regard to the character of buildings and other property in its area; availability of water supplies, means of access thereto and other material circumstances.
(iv) Efficient arrangements for giving, when asked, advice in respect of buildings and property as to fire prevention measures, restricting the spread of fire and means of escape.
(v)   The provision of an adequate water supply for use in the event of fire.

Furthermore each fire authority had to make arrangements for reinforcement schemes with either another fire authority or a private fire brigade. Provision was also made for a fire authority should it so wish to cede all or any of its functions in all or any part of its area to another fire authority. Any such scheme could contain provisions for apportioning expenses.

ORGANISATION

On 1 April 1974, as a result of local government reorganisation, the number of brigades in England and Wales (excluding London) was reduced to 54 in much larger units than had existed previously. In order of seniority, the ranks are: Chief Fire Officer, Assistant Chief Officer, Senior Divisional Officer, Divisional Officer, Assistant Divisional Officer, Station Officer, Sub Officer, Leading Fireman and Fireman.

In the North Yorkshire brigade a simple three tier command structure was adopted. This consists of brigade headquarters controlling four divisions. Each division (commanded by a Divisional Officer) is made up of a varying number of fire stations, manned by either whole-time or part-time firemen, each in command of an officer of suitable rank.

Brigade Headquarters is responsible for carrying out a number of specialist functions such as planning and technical support services; recruitment, training and promotion procedures; staff administration; fire prevention policy; communications and mobilising.

The Divisional Commander is responsible for the efficient day-to-day running of his command. He is also responsible for the fire prevention function which has been decentralised to divisions because of the large geographical area of the County of North Yorkshire and the necessity to maintain contact with district councils and members of the public at local level.

All 999 emergency fire calls are received in the control room situated at brigade headquarters and the appropriate fire appliances accordingly despatched from the nearest fire station(s) to the incident. This is achieved by using a private wire network which links all fire stations to brigade control. The duty mobilising officer is therefore fully aware at all times of the availability of all fire appliances in the brigade.

FINANCE

The fire service is financed from the rates, and the cost of the service is one of the factors taken into account by central government in assessing the rate support grant to individual local authorities. It is the normal practice for salaries, cost of uniform, operational equipment, training, communications equipment and even in some instances fire appliances and ancillary vehicles to be financed from revenue expenditure. The replacement of a substandard fire station or the building of a new additional fire station, however, is borne out of capital expenditure.

The Chief Fire Officer is required annually to prepare the budget estimates for the brigade and in so doing he considers the policy which has been adopted by the particular committee to which the Council, as Fire Authority, has delegated its functions. This is usually in accordance with improvements which the committee has decided to effect over a 5 to 10 year programme.

TRAINING

The recruit fireman has to undergo a three month training course at a recognised training school. The course consists of 450 hours of training, of which 272 hours are spent in practical training of one type or another. This is designed to give him confidence in his ability to use the tools of his trade—pumps, ladders, hose, breathing apparatus, cordage and 'small gear', i.e. breaking in tools, door openers, cutting away apparatus, rescue gear, jacks, etc. This is combined with the necessary technical instruction which complements the practical aspects of his work.

Methods of rescue are also gone into in detail, i.e. rescue at fires using fire brigade equipment as well as the techniques necessary in releasing people trapped in or under vehicles, in lifts, sewers, machinery, railings, etc. The trainee is also taught first aid and given practical training in the handling of casualties.

Following completion of his recruit training, the fireman receives regular training at fire station and divisional levels within his own brigade. In the main this consists of instruction in the use of breathing apparatus, driving, and the operation of special appliances. Practical exercises are held at intervals. These are designed to be as realistic as possible and the cooperation is sought, particularly in large scale exercises, of other emergency services. This is supplemented by participation in an integrated and progressive training programme at the Fire Service Technical College, Moreton in Marsh, which is designed to meet the training needs of the ranks Leading Fireman to Station Officer, including fire prevention. Training for intermediate and senior command is carried out at the Fire Service Staff College at Dorking.

EQUIPMENT

The bulk of equipment carried on fire appliances is designed to enable the fireman to carry out his job efficiently and quickly. But it is a sad fact of modern life that the fireman is increasingly called to road accidents, some comparatively simple to deal with, others very complicated—particularly the multiple crash that happens in bad weather on motorways. Although there is no specific obligation laid on the fire authority to provide the specialised equipment necessary for this type of incident, nearly all fire brigades provide power-operated cutting equipment (such as pneumatically operated chisels and cengar saws), hydraulic equipment (comprising a small pump and armoured connecting hose, a ram or spreader), jacks, and Tirfor hauling and lifting equipment (see Figs.).

ADVICE ON FIRE FIGHTING

To be successful in fighting fire, and this is an additional hazard

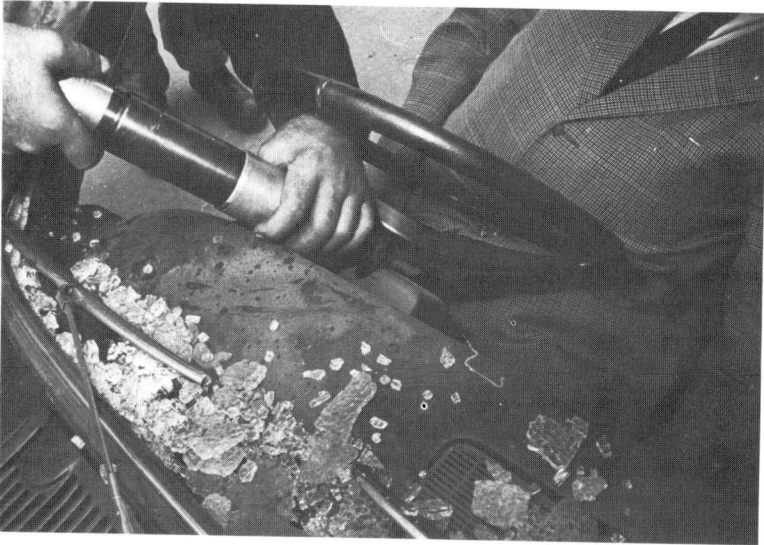

Fig. 17.1. *Reciprocating saw being used to cut steering column of motor vehicle to remove steering wheel.*

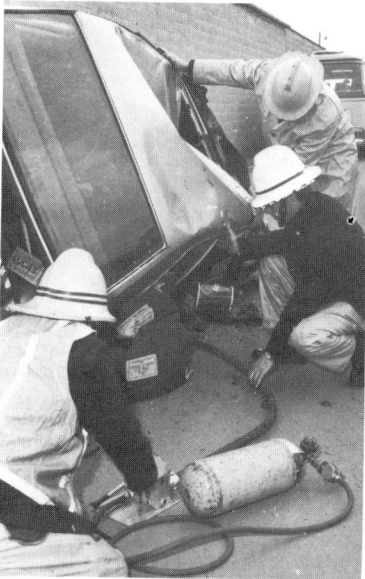

(a)

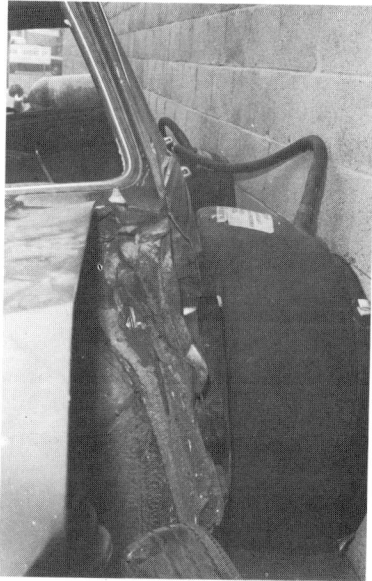

(b)

Fig. 17.2. *(a) Inflatable air bag in position (shown semi-inflated) to raise vehicle. The picture clearly shows the compressed air breathing apparatus cylinder and control valve used to inflate the equipment. (b) A pair of semi-inflated air bags in position.*

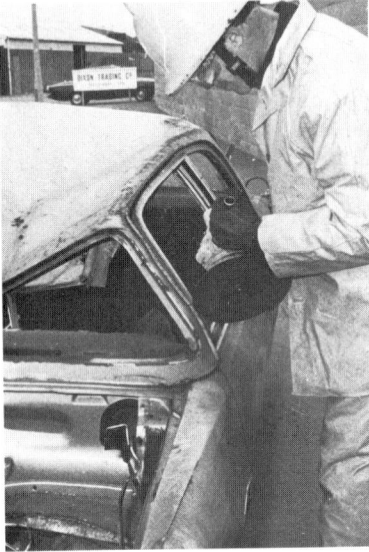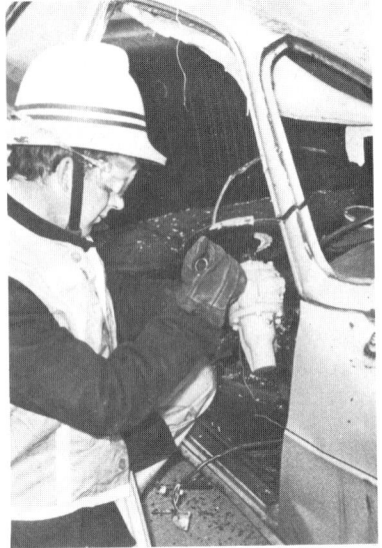

(a)   *(b)*

Fig. 17.3. (a) and (b) A power-operated abrasive cutting disc being used to cut through a structural member. Note the hand and eye protection afforded to the operator to supplement his normal operational uniform.

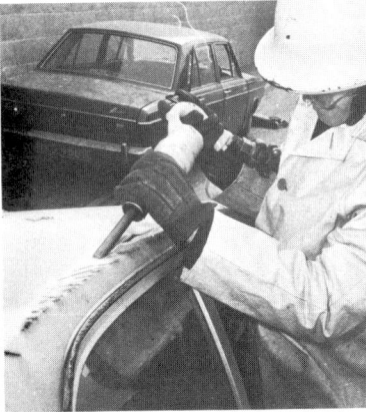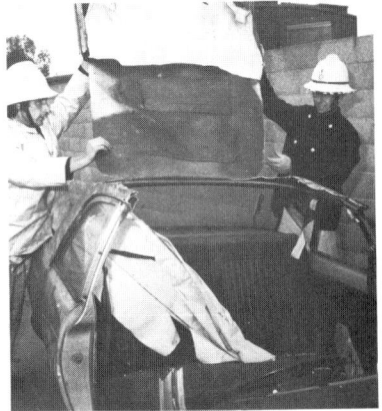

(a)   *(b)*

Fig. 17.4. (a) A compressed air operated cutting tool removing a section of roof. (b) A roof section being removed after cutting.

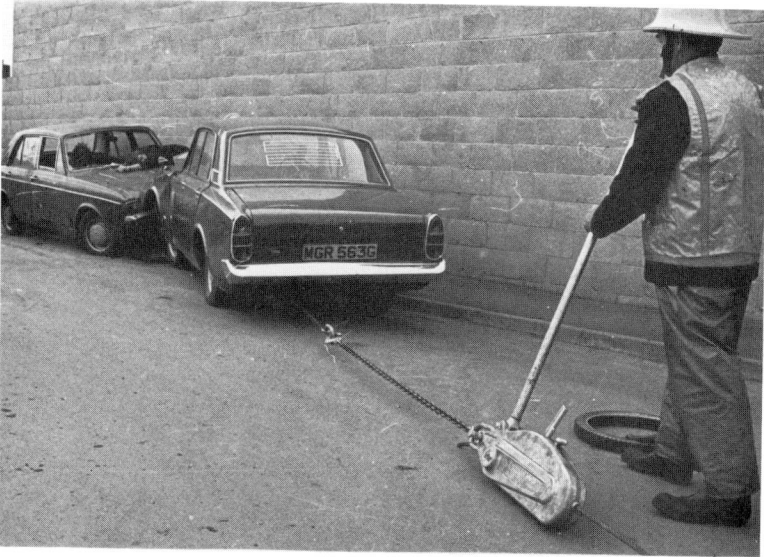

Fig. 17.5. A manually-operated winch being used to separate two vehicles.

in some road accidents, it is necessary to know how it is caused. Before any fire will start three factors must be present:

(i) Fuel—gaseous, liquid, or solid.
(ii) Oxygen—usually in the air.
(iii) Heat.

Extinguishing the fire therefore consists of removing one or more of these factors.

A fireman achieves this by using the techniques of starvation (i.e. limiting the supply of fuel), smothering (by reducing the supply of oxygen) and cooling the burning materials.

Smothering is usually effected by the use of foam, discharged from a hand extinguisher or foam generating equipment, which forms a blanket over the burning material—thereby limiting the supply of air and preventing the formation of flammable vapour. Cooling is effected by the application of water either in jet or spray form. In the process, some water is converted into steam which has the additional effect of smothering. It must be remembered that while the theory of

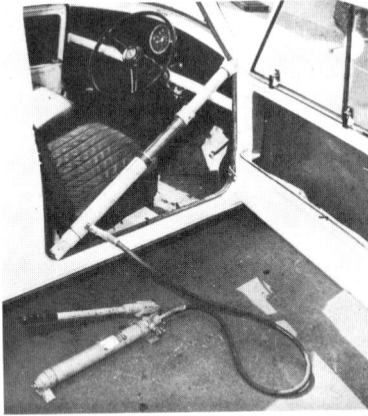
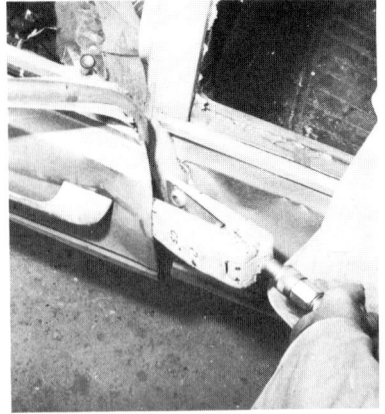

(a)   *(b)*

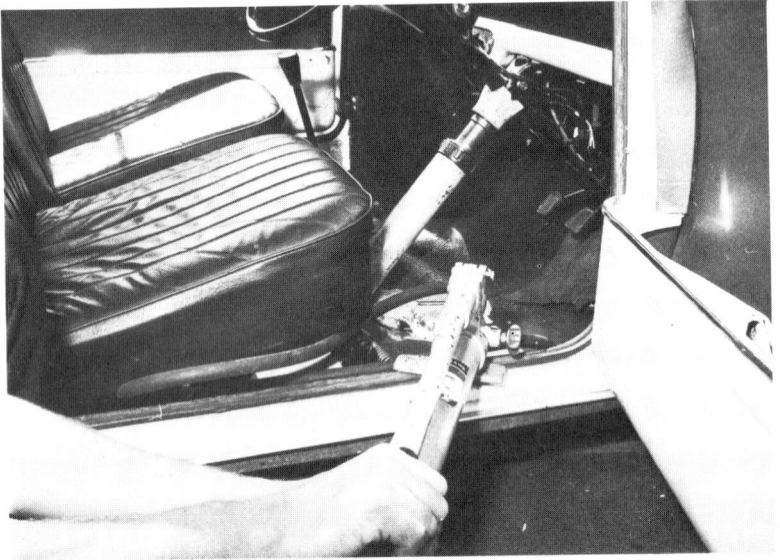

(c)

Fig. 17.6. *(a) A partially extended hydraulic ram in position. (b) A hydraulic attachment ideal for use in small openings. (c) A hydraulic ram in position against a steering column.*

fire fighting is relatively simple the practical application of this knowledge when dealing with large fires can at times prove most difficult and demanding both physically and mentally.

Fires have been classified into four groups, which are indicated below together with the most common extinguishing methods.

Organic materials

That is—carbon compounds in solid form. Generally these are the most common and are extinguished by water applied either in jet or spray form.

Flammable liquids

These are divided into two groups; those which mix with water and those which do not. Dependent upon their properties they may be extinguished by water spray, foam, carbon dioxide or dry powder (e.g. petroleum spirit   does not mix with water—use foam.)

Gases or liquefied gases

These may be in the form of a jet or spray emerging from a gas cylinder or from fractured pipework. Water in the form of a spray should be used to cool the cylinder or container and if the control valve is operable the gas supply should be turned off. With shallow liquid spills, foam should be applied until an effective seal has formed over the liquid.

Metals

Water is not to be used as an extinguishing agent as alkali metals react with the water to form hydroxides and the release of hydrogen. Dry powders of a special type are normally used as extinguishing agents; these form a crust over the burning metal.

Practical fire-fighting measures fall into two broad categories: for small fires and for large outbreaks.

Portable fire extinguishers, handled correctly, can usually deal efficiently with the small fire. The extinguisher provided should be suitable for the type of fire: e.g. water gas extinguishers for the domestic or office risk; foam or dry powder for flammable liquids of the immiscible type; CO_2 or vapourising liquids for fires in electrical or laboratory equipment.

The potential operator should always familiarise himself with the method of operating the extinguisher so that when the time comes he is capable of using it efficiently. The contents of extinguishers should always be directed at the seat of the fire.

Car fires are usually caused either by electrical or by fuel system faults. The electrical fault is the most common and generally caused by a short circuit. The condition which caused the short circuit will remain until the current is switched off, and it may be necessary to disconnect one of the car battery leads. A fuel fire can be caused through petrol leaking from a flooding carburettor or a loose union connection in the fuel line, the petrol being ignited by falling onto a hot exhaust manifold or by the ignition. In road accidents, fuel may escape from damaged tanks or pipes and be ignited by sparks. Where appropriate, the fire should be fought by discharging a suitable vapourising liquid extinguisher under the partially opened bonnet on completing the discharge. If a vapourising liquid extinguisher is not available, a foam extinguisher may be used or alternatively the fire may be smothered with a mat or rug.

When dealing with large outbreaks of fire, water is still the main weapon. Jets are placed to contain or prevent the fire spreading and then to attack the seat of the fire until it is extinguished. In preventing the fire spreading regard must always be paid to the protection of any adjoining premises, ensuring that the fire is confined and not driven before the attacking jets.

In view of the vast and growing number of chemicals in daily use it is not possible here to detail the firefighting measures necessary to deal with them individually. It is necessary for the firefighter to know their chemical properties, for example whether they are toxic, corrosive, or spontaneously inflammable on exposure to air. The advice of the fire prevention staff of any fire brigade should be sought particularly in the planning stages of any industrial process involving hazardous chemicals so that the requisite firefighting provisions, whether fixed or mobile, can be considered. Furthermore, the fire brigade will always be pleased to advise and demonstrate the way in which firefighting appliances should be used, whether they be portable extinguishers or water hoses and jets.

THE NEEDS FOR THE NEXT FIVE YEARS

The needs for the Fire Service over the next five years arise quite simply from ever increasing involvement in rescue work of all kinds and in the field of fire prevention. A degree of rescue work is always associated with firefighting, and in work where fire is not present there may be a greater need for certain members of every fire appliance crew to receive more intensive training on practical first aid measures and casualty handling, so as to increase the casualty's chances of recovery. There is no intention to encroach on the recognised skills and practices of the Ambulance Service, but the Fire Service is always on standby and the fire appliance is therefore often the first to arrive at an accident site. Expertise should be available to reduce the effects of trauma until the doctor or ambulance arrives. In this context it is worth noting the formation, on an experimental basis, of a heart rescue unit by the Los Angeles Fire Department. Manpower is so valuable in the emergency services today that there is every need to ensure its maximum use. There should not be lines of demarcation; such luxuries can no longer be afforded.

As regards prevention, it is regrettable that the majority of deaths by fire occur in the home. Apparently, the 'it couldn't happen to me' attitude takes over in the adult when he or she steps across that familiar threshold and closes the door. Although fire prevention campaigns have been mounted at various times in recent years, one cannot help wondering if this is enough and whether such propaganda should not be embarked on earlier, as part of a school curriculum.

18

Ambulance Services

ROBERT F LEA

That the ambulanceman has an important part to play in the care and treatment of the seriously ill and injured patient has not yet received universal acceptance by the medical profession. Perhaps the reason for this is the mistaken concept that the Ambulance Service is merely a means of transporting the sick and injured and the ambulanceman can offer little more than basic first aid skills and the physical ability to load and off-load patients.

With the development of hospital accident flying squads, the involvement of general practitioners in accident after care schemes in various parts of the country, and the increase in incidents where members of the medical profession are being called to the scene of accidents or sudden illness, this misconception about the role and function of the Ambulance Service is slowly being changed.

Unfortunately such schemes are as yet thin on the ground and in many parts of the country the immediate care and early management of the acutely ill and injured is still the responsibility of the Ambulance Service. This chapter is an attempt to reach a wider medical audience in order that they will have a better awareness of the organisation, function and expertise of the Ambulance Service.

HISTORY

In considering the Ambulance Service, one needs to look back at its development. Before 1948, local authorities had powers, but not a duty, to provide ambulance services. Many local authorities made some use of these powers, and voluntary bodies—notably the St John Ambulance and the British Red Cross—also provided services, either independently or as agents of local authorities. During the 1939–45 War, local authorities had the duty to provide a Civil Defence ambulance service, and this gave them an impetus after the war, as many authorities retained some of these ambulances for peacetime purposes, though they still did not have a statutory duty to provide a service. The standards of service varied considerably, some authorities providing a free service whilst others provided no service whatsoever, leaving patients in need to find their own means of transport.

From the appointed day of 5th July 1948, Section 27 (i) of the National Health Service Act 1946 imposed a duty on local authorities to provide free ambulance transport. They discharged this responsibility not only by providing a service themselves, but also by appointing agents such as the St John Ambulance and the British Red Cross, or by some combination of these two methods.

No one in 1948 had any idea of the truly colossal demand on the service that was to develop, but it was not long after the introduction of the Act that hospital authorities began to make demands on the service to transport patients to and from out-patients departments. It is interesting to note that prior to 1948 requests for sitting case transport were almost negligible. However, from that time the demand rapidly overtook that for stretcher patients and the ratio today is in the order of 5: 1. This demand for out-patient transport began almost immediately, with a steady but positive rise until, in 1974, a total of about 23 million patients were carried over a distance of about 140 million miles. Of this total, approximately 9 per cent were emergencies, with the bulk of the remainder being out-patients.

TRAINING

In the early years of the service, the possession of a valid first aid certificate issued by the voluntary aid societies was the only qualification required and this covered the right to extra pay. It was not until the early 1960s that any concentrated attempt was made to improve the standard of training and equipment, and in 1963 the Minister of Health set up a working party to report and make recommendations on ambulance training and equipment. Their report on training was issued in 1966 and this was followed in 1967 by their report on equipment (HMSO, 1966 and 1967).

Among the recommendations were:

(i)   A six week course for all new entrants to the service.
(ii) A suitably modified course for those with 2–5 years experience.
(iii) A refresher course every three years for all members.
(iv) A period of detachment to accident and emergency hospitals.

The Minister then requested nine local authorities that were already undertaking training to arrange experimental courses in conformity with the recommendations. The working party also recommended that a central Ambulance Service Council be set up, and in 1969 the Minister appointed the Ambulance Services Advisory Committee. This committee concerned itself principally with training, equipment and organisation. Shortly after it was set up, the experimental courses were confirmed and extended to 12 centres, which accept trainees from designated catchment areas providing national cover.

The object of the training is to extend the range of knowledge and skills well beyond the state of elementary first aid and by so doing improve the standard of the initial management of the seriously ill or injured patient. Included in the training are:

Care and management of the unconscious patient.
Care of the airway and emergency resuscitation measures.
Control of bleeding.
Assessment of priorities in the single and multiple casualty situation.

Other matters, such as relationships with other emergency services are also part of the training programme, as well as the less spectacular aspects of the job i.e. special problems of the geriatric, psychiatric, maternity and other types of patient.

In addition to the basic training now fully implemented nationally, many ambulance authorities have arranged organised training in accident and emergency hospitals in accordance with the DHSS circular (LHAL 9 / 1972). The purpose of this training, in addition to improving skills, is to give ambulancemen a greater insight into the wider aspects of patient care. It also results in the cross-fertilisation of ideas between medical, nursing and ambulance staff.

Advanced training

The 1966 report had also considered the need for advanced training in para-medical skills with particular emphasis on the two principal practices in the early management of the severely ill and injured patient: maintenance of respiration and circulation.

The idea that ambulancemen could and should be taught the more advanced techniques such as intubation, infusion, interpretation of ECG tracings, and the use of the defibrillator has received a lot of attention and a number of pilot schemes have been carried out in Bournemouth, Brighton and Nottingham and other parts of the country. These controlled schemes have been well documented and the DHSS have intimated that evaluation is now progressing; as a result of this a decision will be taken on whether these skills should be taught in the ambulance scheme of training. The medicolegal aspects of such training will require detailed consideration.

EQUIPMENT

The working party was fairly precise in its recommendations for equipment that should be carried, but accepted that local conditions varied enough to make it necessary for certain special items to be provided for local hazards. The Advisory Committee were responsible for bringing about a greater conformity in equipment, and today the majority of emergency vehicles carry the following items:

Wheeled lightweight stretcher trolleys which can be raised to various heights and allow the patient to be placed in varying positions.
Bag/mask resuscitation unit.
Suction apparatus.
Oxygen supply.
Entonox.
Oropharangeal airways.
Spinal boards and cervical collar.
Orthopaedic scoop stretcher.
Rescue equipment, crowbar, hacksaw, bolt cutters, etc.
Canvas sheet and poles.
Carrying chair.
Inflatable splints.
Frac immobiliser and straps.
A wide range of dressings.

COMMUNICATIONS

Invariably every report on a major accident contains some form of criticism regarding lack of communication. Communication can be lacking due to the failure of people to communicate or to an inefficient or ineffective communication system.

In considering communications we need to study the points between which there is a need to communicate. These can be broken down into three main headings:

Static to static points (generally best served by telephone).
Static to mobile points (which lend themselves to radiotelephone).
On-site communications (portable radiotelephone).

In the early days of radio within the Ambulance Service, each authority was allocated its own frequency and these were such as to prevent interference between neighbouring authorities. This was ideal for day-to-day operations. However, in the case of a major incident where vehicles from different authorities were in attendance, it prevented efficient control in that the control in the area of the incident could only contact the vehicles on its own frequency. A recent development has been the introduction of an emergency rescue channel which will enable vehicles to communicate with controls outside their own area (DHSS circulars LHAL 9/1972 and HSC (IS) 186). This system should be fully operational in the near future. It is also anticipated that the majority of accident and emergency hospitals will be equipped with radio on the emergency channel, thus allowing communication with any major incident.

REORGANISATION

The transfer of functions from local authorities to the National Health Service in April 1974 was a traumatic experience, probably more so within the ambulance service than anywhere else. This changeover created many problems, the principle ones being:

(i) The amalgamation of different services, each with different terms and conditions.
(ii) The putting aside of long-established loyalties and pride in their own services.

(iii) The variations in rank structures and pay of officers.

These problems have not yet been fully resolved. However, the creation of larger services under the reorganised National Health Service presents an excellent opportunity for closer collaboration with the medical services. The service is now an integral part of the NHS, giving the opportunity for the ambulance man to be recognised as an important member of the patient care team. The rank structure for the reorganised service has recently been agreed, from Metropolitan or Area Ambulance Officer, down through Assistant, Divisional, and Assistant Divisional Ambulance Officers to Superintendents, Station Officers, and Sub Officers.

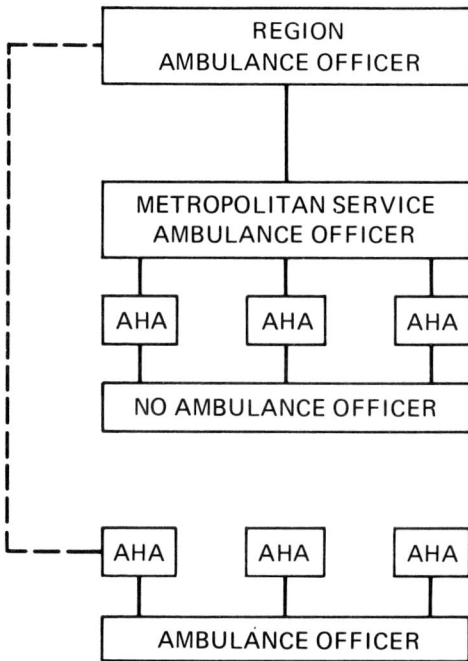

FUTURE DEVELOPMENTS

In considering the future it will be useful to look at the work the Ambulance Service has to do and then consider if it is appropriately organised.

The primary function of the Service is to care for people who, by reason of accident, illness, mental illness, childbirth, etc. can no longer care for themselves and are in need of specialised transport. Patients range from those in need of a great deal of skill and care— ideally the skill of a doctor trained to work in the accident and emergency situation—to those whose prime need is transport and who could be conveyed by public transport if it were able to call at the patient's home and then assist the patient aboard.

At the top of the scale, the degree of skill required has been increasingly influenced by:

(i) Growing medical opinion that earlier and better patient care, such as earlier replacement of fluid loss and intubation would reduce mortality and morbidity.

(ii) The concentration of accident and emergency facilities in District General Hospitals and the consequent lengthening of ambulance journeys.

(iii) The increase in the number of incidents of collapse in the home where relatives are unable to contact a doctor, and the need in such cases for ambulance staff to make appropriate decisions.

(iv) The tendency for motorway accidents to produce casualties with injuries of greater severity and complexity.

The majority of services currently operate a dual purpose service, that is to say all vehicles are fully equipped and manned by fully qualified crews. This means that trained staff can go for long periods without being called upon to deal with an emergency.

With the possible development of advanced training in para-medical skills for ambulancemen and the introduction into the service of more sophisticated equipment, the question may well be raised as to whether this is the most efficient way to operate the Service. To raise the standard of training and equipment will be a costly exercise. Can we, therefore, afford to engage these men and vehicles on work which could be adequately carried out by lower grade staff in less costly vehicles? In the rural situation it may be necessary to retain the flexibility of a dual purpose vehicle, though in urban areas it may be worth considering a tiered system, with fully equipped ambulances and highly trained crews being used only for stretcher cases. Multi-seat vehicles would probably be a safer and more economical way of transporting routine out-patients.

REFERENCES

Adgey (1971), *Lancet*, **ii**, 201.

DHSS (1972), Circular. LHAL 9 /1972 DHSS.

DHSS (1975), *Radiotelephone emergency link between ambulances and hospitals.* Circular. HSC (IS) 186 DHSS.

Hayle (1971), Medical Commission on Accident Prevention.

Local Government Training Board (1972), *Memo 14.* Local Government Training Board.

Report by Working Party on Ambulance Training (1966), London: HMSO.

Report by Working Party on Ambulance Training (1967), London: HMSO.

Walsh (1972), *British Heart Journal*, **34**, 701.

White (1973), *British Medical Journal*, **3**, 618.

19

Special Aspects of Voluntary Service

PETER BUSH

In Australia where disastrous bushfires (Fig. 19.1) take their toll of life and property, it is essential that emergency services should be effective, efficient and mobile. The nature of the terrain, the vast distances, the fierceness of the elements, all contribute to the creation of a situation demanding well organised and highly trained emergency forces.

Under these conditions, it is not possible to rely entirely upon the statutory government or local relief forces. The military are thinly spread throughout the continent and cannot provide sufficient additional manpower to meet all needs. It is for this reason that, in addition to the statutory forces, the voluntary agencies—St John Ambulance Brigade, Red Cross, Civil Defence and others—have to provide the backbone of the emergency services. One of their greatest difficulties in this is that these voluntary agencies frequently have to rely upon public support for funds to produce the equipment and materials required for efficient management of emergencies. Natural disasters such as hurricanes and floods, as well as industrial accidents, road traffic collisions, searches for missing persons in overgrown bush country in summer and in winter all create situations which test the emergency rescue services. They must therefore be effective and efficient.

ORGANISATION OF RELIEF WORK

For all relief work involving the treatment of injured persons, the four important steps for their care are:

418

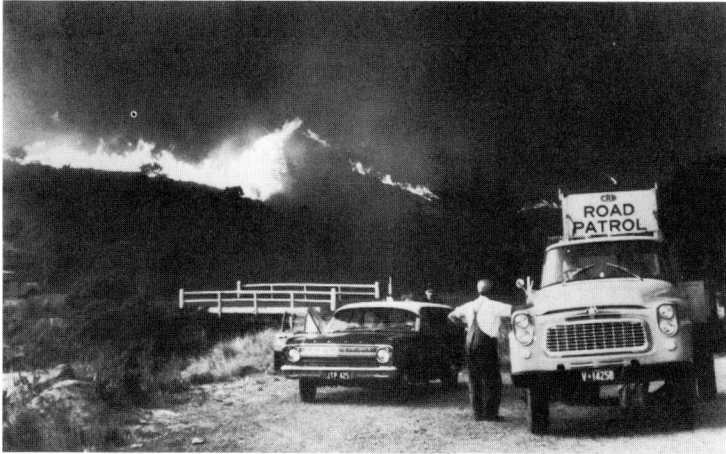

Fig. 19.1. The threat of a bushfire: in this situation the immediate availability of voluntary help is invaluable.

C   Communications
A   Assessment
R   Resuscitation
E   Emergency treatment

To be effective, all four steps must be efficient.

Communication (as referred to below) includes interpersonal communication, i.e. adequate history-taking of the incident producing injury, inter-service communication, and intra-service communication (Fig. 19.2).

Assessment of the injuries requires a knowledge of first aid and especially a recognition of priorities, and an ability adequately to differentiate between life-threatening situations and less serious injuries.

Resuscitation   ⎫   These require training and preparedness
Emergency treatment ⎭   as detailed below.

The ingredients of success for counteracting the effects of these disastrous situations can be summarised as follows:

(i)   Communications.

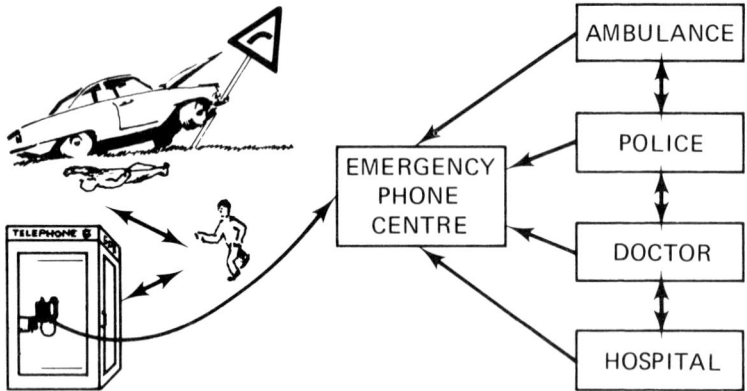

Fig. 19.2. Communication: in an emergency, all these lines of communication are required. The first person on the scene is the key.

(ii) Complete cooperation and compatibility of the personnel making up the different forces.
(iii) Preparedness which requires training, skill and provision of adequate equipment.
(iv) Availability.

Communications

In many respects, communications are most important. The principles of good communication apply equally to major and minor incidents. It is as important that an emergency call to the doctor in the early hours of the morning should give adequate information about the nature of the emergency and the address of the patient, as it is that information passed to an ambulance service should accurately pinpoint the site of a disaster. Many of the incidents producing these emergency situations cause severe interference with normal communications. The St John Ambulance Brigade in Victoria has its own radio channel which has, on several occasions, been used by the police and other services as a communications network. It is therefore important that adequate facilities for radio or radiotelephone operations should be available.

Personnel

Complete harmony between the executive officers as well as the operative members of all the different forces involved in a major disaster is essential. It is important that rights and privileges should be subordinated to the needs of the individuals for whom the relief is required. There is no place in a disaster situation for any individual or service to consider its own personal or service interest before the interests of those affected by the disaster. It is important that all organisations involved in rescue should have a well-organised, disciplined and well controlled body. It is equally important that all organisations should have a mutual respect and knowledge of each other's capabilities and responsibilities. It is quite unthinkable that two organisations should meet at the scene of a disaster without prior recognition of the duties, responsibilities and capabilities of each other. In Victoria, for this reason, joint training exercises have been held. Each individual organisation conducts its own training, including large scale exercises where appropriate, but in addition at regular intervals, joint exercises are planned enabling individuals from separate organisations to meet and learn of each others' capabilities and responsibilities. On the declaration of a 'State Major Disaster', overall coordination of all these bodies rests with the Chief Commissioner of Police in Victoria.

Equipment and availability

The usefulness of any organisation in its rescue capability depends upon immediate availability and equipment. Statutory authorities, i.e. police, ambulance, fire brigade, etc. as a general rule have an organisation providing immediate availability. In major towns and cities these are radio controlled and have a constant service availability. However, these statutory authorities in major disasters, and at times in smaller scale situations of major gravity, frequently need to be augmented by voluntary organisations.

RESCUE SQUADS IN VICTORIA

In the early 1960s, through the inspiration and leadership of an ex-policeman, Max Phelan, then a Divisional Superintendent, now District Superintendent, the first St John Ambulance Brigade Rescue Squad was formed. The motivation grew from the idea that a highly-trained brigade must be mobile to reach the site of an incident in order to be able to carry out its functions, and similarly that existing services able to reach the scene of an isolated accident are ineffective unless they are trained and equipped to perform useful and at times, life saving first aid.

Training was intensive and included various methods of rescue techniques; cliff climbing, map reading, navigation, bushfire survival, radio communications, as well as the normal St John training in first aid. Today the Rescue Squads within the St John Ambulance Brigade in Victoria comprise over 650 men in more than 50 squads with over 60 vehicles ready at a moment's notice to answer emergency calls for major disasters as well as less spectacular incidents, such as freeing trapped occupants of vehicles, searching for lost persons, etc.

It is perhaps difficult for people living in a highly urbanised modern community to appreciate that a light aircraft carrying four passengers can disappear completely without trace less than 50 miles from the centre of Melbourne, a city of two million inhabitants, and fail to be located despite intensive search over a week by 120–150 St John Ambulance Brigade volunteer Rescue Squad members, as well as other organisations, police, Country Fire Authority, bush walkers, etc. Such is a recent major incident covered by the Rescue Squads in Victoria.

The Rescue Squad organisation—available night and day, 365 days of the year—due to the remarkable and commendable cooperation and support of the employers of the members, has answered many calls. An alert is usually initiated by a call from D24, the Victorian Police Headquarters radio network, to the District Superintendent of the Brigade. Squads are then contacted and within minutes, if necessary, the first unit is on the road. Specialised services are available, and within the organisation are men experienced in bush walking, cave rescue, cliff climbing, underwater rescue, handling of industrial chemicals, etc.

Training

Training is undertaken within the Divisions of the Brigade; two weekend training camps are held annually with large scale exercises. Recently, because of the increasing numbers in the Rescue Squads, training has been reorganised on a group basis, certain squads being grouped together for training and operational purposes. A weekend training course of lectures has been held annually at Monash University,

Melbourne, at which over 400 members of the Brigade attend. Lectures have been given on specific types of injuries and other subjects. These have included resuscitation and intensive care, injuries to the spine, head, eyes, face and chest, the psychiatric aspects of disaster, emergency childbirth, incident control and road accidents.

These weekend training courses have proved invaluable for introducing specialists in different fields of practice to the members of the Rescue Squads and 'Mobile Nursing' (see below). Personnel involved in the more advanced first aid must be conversant with modern techniques and advances in the treatment and management of patients with severe trauma. Much of the material in the specialised lectures is perhaps too technical for all members of a voluntary lay organisation fully to comprehend. A careful choice of lecturer who is able to deliver his message of specialised care in an interesting manner, however, overcomes this difficulty for the required information is eagerly and completely absorbed by many of the members and 'rubs off' on most of the others.

Mobile nursing

The Nursing members of the Brigade soon followed the example of their male colleagues by forming 'Mobile Nursing'. This organisation has now grown and comprises over 100 nursing members with nearly 30 state registered nurses, formed into teams which, complete with Mobile Nursing vans, are available for call to an emergency situation. Their prime function is to set up a Mobile first aid post where resuscitation can be given, emergency first aid already carried out by Rescue Squads at the disaster scene can be reviewed, and if necessary complemented, and the condition of casualties reassessed before onward transfer to an emergency or base hospital.

The equipment available includes provision for oxygen administration and suction, fluid infusions, as well as the accepted first aid materials. In view of the fact that doctors are now making themselves available for call out with these teams, provision is being made for the nursing vans to be equipped with an emergency drug supply.

Mobile Nursing training involves a deeper appreciation of the effects of severe injury, and is designed to train the members of these teams to a level of competence at which they can safely and efficiently care for injured people under field conditions for extended periods in the absence of trained medical or nursing personnel.

Treatment

The initial treatment given to victims of disasters at the scene of the incident is of prime importance. When diagnosis has been made and emergency treatment carried out, the transport of the patient for further treatment at a first aid post, clearing station, field or base hospital is required. Such an aid post, catering primarily for a transitional stage in the care of casualties may yet be an area where resuscitative measures can be initiated which will make the difference between life and death for the patient. It is imperative, therefore, that such facilities as are available at the forward first aid post be as highly organised and as efficient as conditions allow (Fig. 19.3).

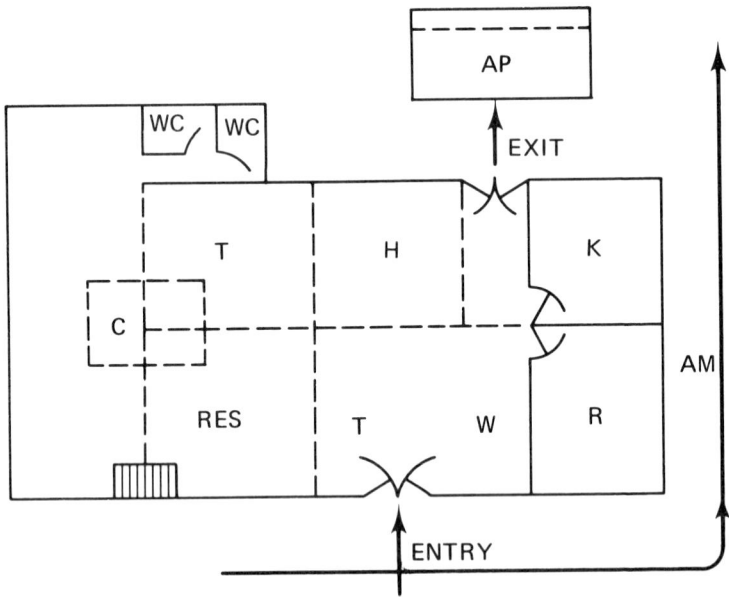

Fig. 19.3. *A typical hall adapted for emergency use. A–ambulances. AM– movement. AP–parking. C–control centre for Medical Officer and Officer Nursing. Table on stage for overall supervision, and clear area on floor. H–holding area. K–kitchen, for use as staff rooms. R–radio control, also police. RES–resuscitation area. W–walking wounded and uninjured if no other accommodation available in separate building. WC–toilets.*

Facilities

The circumstances of the disaster will determine the exact nature of the facilities which are available for the reception of the casualties. It is unlikely that premises suitable in all respects will always be available at or sufficiently close to the scene of the disaster. Under these circumstances, the use of imagination and ingenuity will be required to improvise from the most suitable accommodation available.

Selecting suitable premises

The following factors should be taken into consideration:

- (i) Ready and easy access for foot parties and ambulance transport.
- (ii) Standing and parking areas for motor transport.
- (iii) Separate entrance and exit to working areas to facilitate free flow of casualties.
- (iv) Administrative control area readily accessible to all treatment areas.
- (v) Adequate space for the number of casualties anticipated.
- (vi) Main services, e.g. water, electricity, gas.

The extent of the facilities required for a field hospital of this type will inevitably depend upon the nature of the incident, number of casualties involved, situation, distance from nearest major hospital, availability of supporting medical or surgical teams.

The involvement of the medically trained

Brigade surgeons, general practitioners, consultants and house officers are also involved in the Rescue Squad and Mobile Nursing activities, assisting both in training and also being available for duty on 'call out' with the squads. The additional experience and service they can bring has already shown itself in the training sessions (Fig. 19.4), but has yet to be fully measured in terms of lives saved and morbidity reduced.

In the early days of the Rescue Squads, doctors attended the weekend training camps, primarily in the role of observer, critic and adjudicator in the exercises which were conducted in a competitive spirit between

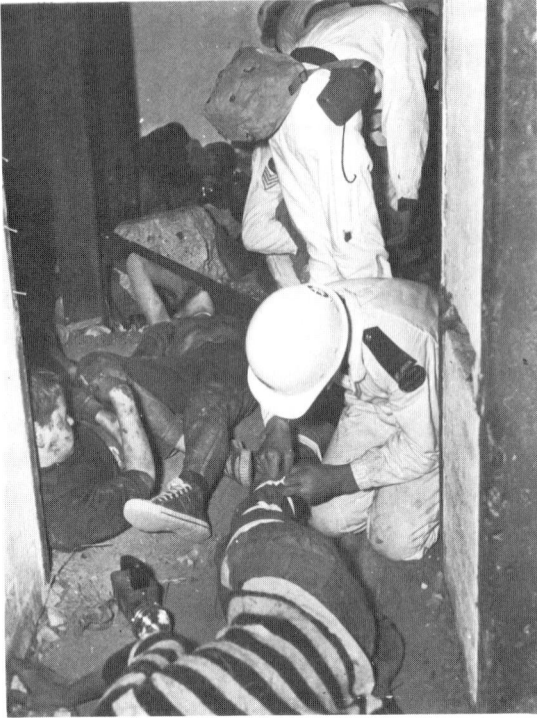

Fig. 19.4. An exercise with simulated casualties.

the squads. After a while it became apparent that the criticisms, comments and exhortations offered at the 'debriefing session' at the conclusion of each weekend camp were repetitive.

Discrimination and 'triage' was obviously difficult for even the more experienced and senior first aiders. It was therefore decided that the doctors (Brigade Surgeons) should participate actively in the exercises, and that training should continue by example and encouragement, rather than observation and subsequent criticism.

THE SUNBURY POP FESTIVAL

There is no substitute for practical training and this is not easy to arrange on demand. However, an annual pop festival held on a farm at Sunbury, 25 miles from Melbourne, has provided an opportunity for practical training in mass casualty first aid under near-disaster conditions.

A report made following the first 'Sunbury Happening' in 1972 continues the story . . .

'The St John Ambulance Brigade in Victoria was asked to provide first aid and medical cover for a three-day music festival to be held on a farm 25 miles from Melbourne. Little did we know what this was to mean. Prior to the event, we endeavoured to get some information on the numbers expected; to get some help from the State Health Department and other statutory authorities. We began to plan.

A visit to the site was certainly informative. A dusty farm strewn with rough, volcanic rocks, a narrow creek with at least one hole 30 ft deep, little covering vegetation and no snakes. The situation for the field hospital was selected, ideal in all respects except possibly access. With little to guide us, we determined that we must plan for any eventuality and any or every type of injury. Later experience confirmed the wisdom of this decision. The points at which Brigade vehicles would be placed as static first aid posts were decided. The roster, eight hours on, eight hours off, was worked out. The doctors, nurses, and Brigade members who were to be involved then continued their scrounging. We asked medical representatives for samples which might be useful. The nurses collected dressings and other equipment. Divisions stocked their vehicles.

The Festival was due to commence at 10 am on Saturday, 29 January. By Friday evening the crowds were gathering and by dark a tented city had already sprung up. The sound of music from transistors and guitars came across the field.

The Brigade vehicles and tents (Fig. 19.5) were arranged, a communications radio base was established, the two tents to serve as field hospital were erected and emergency lighting was provided by a generator. Before these preparations were complete, the casualties started to arrive. Cut hands, cut feet, scalp wounds, splinters, foreign bodies in the eyes, etc. These were attended to in one of the Brigade first aid vehicles.

It had been agreed that we would have to suture all but the major wounds ourselves—distances were too great and communications too difficult for transfer of all wounds to Melbourne for suture. A sixteen-year-old girl was brought into us as the night progressed, and it

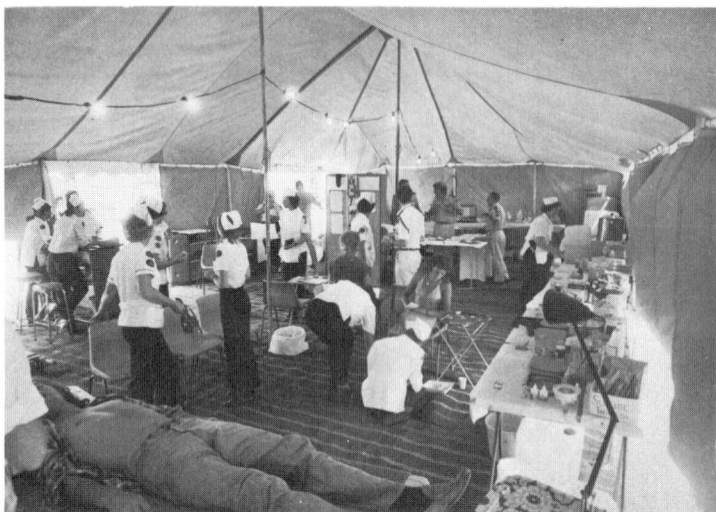

Fig. 19.5. The marquee, staffed entirely by St John Ambulance Brigade volunteers, in use at the Sunbury pop festival.

was claimed that she had consumed a bottle of gin. She was examined and then slept it off under our observation. The pattern of that first night was to continue throughout the three days. Twelve Brigade vehicles were stationed at various points throughout the farm to act as static first aid posts. The first aid personnel at these points were able to deal with all minor casualties and were in constant radio contact with the mobile base headquarters situated next to the hospital tents. During the 72 hours of the festival, nearly 3000 casualties were treated, approximately 1200 at the field hospital and of these many were sutured and a few (1 per cent) were transferred to hospital in Melbourne.

Cases of poisoning involved alcohol, drugs of various sorts, and some probably a mixture. Situated close to our field hospital was a tent set up by the Buoyancy Foundation, a voluntary organisation whose aim is to provide support and assistance for the drug-dependent young. This is an organisation which retains its original character of informality and flexibility. Our close proximity was a mutual advantage. The drug and alcohol problem at this festival was significant but seen in perspective against the numbers attending it was small.

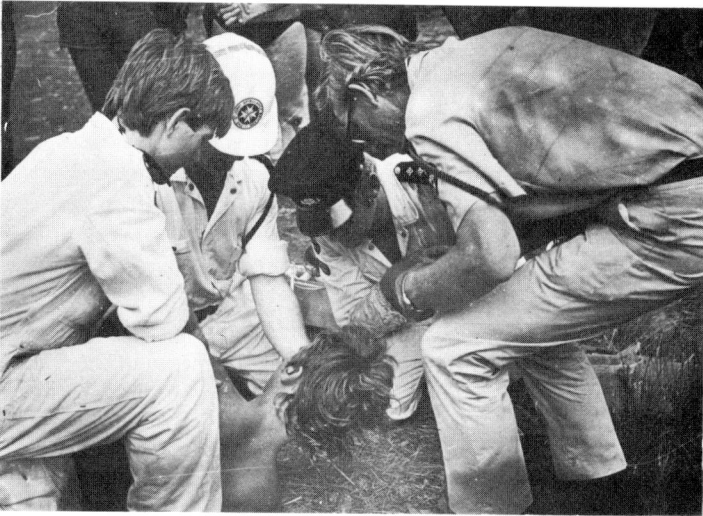

Fig. 19.6. A St John Ambulance Brigade surgeon and other volunteers assist in a resuscitation at the Sunbury pop festival.

The administration of the Brigade at this festival was excellent, the morale of the volunteers was tremendous and the degree of physical effort by every single member was superb. No one could be singled out for special mention. They all gave their all.

Lessons were learned. It was realised, and senior police officers had no hesitation in saying, that without the help provided by the volunteers of the St John Ambulance Brigade, this festival could have been a state disaster (Fig.19.6). That such was the case did not surprise. This was the sort of situation for which the Brigade had been trained for years, but it seems unreasonable to me that such a situation should have to rely on a voluntary organisation dependent on public support for its finances. The equipment and supplies could have been improved. The men and women could not. The facilities could have been better, the dedication of the personnel could not.

For the future and for possible future pop festivals, we could make improvements. There were a number of things which we learned about our own administration. For example, we had for years been aware of the necessity to maintain a record of patients when they were discharged from the field hospital. In fact this was done, but because of the peculiarities of the situation with the statutory ambulance authority who had the responsibility of transporting patients referred to hospital, we had no control over the hospital to which patients were admitted. Subsequent enquiries by relatives of a person admitted to hospital showed the defect of this system, for we were unable to give information as to which hospital the patient had been referred.

The total banning of glass bottles and containers on the festival site would undoubtedly reduce very considerably the number of lacerations. Strict control of the introduction of alcohol is desirable, and close supervision to control or eradicate the use of drugs and particularly hallucinogenic drugs at this type of gathering is equally helpful. The control exercised on this occasion by the members of the Victorian police force and their restraint despite considerable provocation was very commendable.

In conclusion perhaps it would not be out of place to make some reference to the financial implications in the setting up of an organisation such as the Brigade provided for this festival. Seven doctors were involved, putting in a total of 296 hours. Ten nursing sisters played a part. One hundred and thirty-six lay Brigade personnel attended, and if these were assessed on a time basis, the wage bill alone would come to nearly \$A15 000 (£11 000). Perhaps \$A500 (£360) or more was used in equipment and supplies. The capital cost of medical consumable equipment, divisional equipment, would be in the region of \$A1500 (£1080). The civil Ambulance Service charges \$A200 (£140) per day for a vehicle and two men. On this basis, the Brigade provided ten vehicles for the equivalent of nine days, a total of \$A18 000 (£13 000). With these figures alone, the total is approaching \$A35 000 (£25 000), and this does not take into account the capital cost of the vehicles, the communications equipment, etc.'

For this festival, as at all functions attended by the St John Ambulance Brigade, personnel gave their services freely and in a voluntary capacity.

Lessons for the future

In future planning for this type of event, as well as for major disasters, there are three essentials:

  (i)   The right personnel welded together as a team and suitably trained.

(ii) Adequate equipment and support.

(iii) The finance to provide both of these.

It may well be that highly trained mobile teams of this type could be used to meet the situations created by natural civil disasters, transcending state and national boundaries. Then availability, mobility, and preparedness would be vital.

At the second pop festival held at Sunbury the following year, the experience already gained was of great value, and was added to. Over 4000 casualties throughout that weekend still produced a steady average of around 1 per cent who required referral to a major hospital. In 1974, the Brigade system of recording was much more efficient, although the total numbers were lower than on the previous occasions, the Brigade was functioning much more effectively and the principles used at this festival involving the establishment of field first aid posts and the field hospital were fully justified. On this occasion, patients were seen in the field hospital only after referral from the field first aid post. This reduced the overlap between first aid post and hospital, which occurred on previous occasions, and also reduced the congestion in the field hospital.

The complete analysis of the records of the cases seen for the three years' festivals is being prepared for publication.

It may seem unlikely that voluntary organisations would be able to use an event such as a pop festival as a training exercise; however, the experience gained is of inestimable value in training members of the organisation involved. One defect of this particular exercise was that not all other organisations involved in major disaster relief work in Australia were involved in this festival. It has, however, given further opportunities for working in close liaison with the Victoria Police Force, Salvation Army and Country Fire Authority. A pop festival could easily provide the ingredients of a major disaster if not adequately controlled and catered for in every sphere.

In other states—South Australia and Western Australia—the St John Ambulance Brigade provides the full-time ambulance service in addition to the voluntary service. This makes integration and co-ordination easier, but does not necessarily entirely resolve the 'industrial' problems which unfortunately still pervade the Ambulance industry.

Hospital medical teams

At times the Brigade Surgeons—doctors engaged in active practice who are willing to assist in an emergency—may not be immediately available because of their other commitments. It may be possible, however for a doctor to make himself available at a later time. This arrangement has proved very valuable in long term disaster situations, for example bushfires, and prolonged searches when a roster of medical personnel can be arranged.

However to meet the immediate requirements of an impending or actual disaster, for example a plane or train crash, it may be desirable for a medical team to be immediately available at the scene of the disaster. For this reason medical teams from some of the major hospitals in Melbourne have been mobilised. The training of these teams requires as much preparation and organisation as any other part of the rescue services. It is not sufficient for a group of persons, medical and nursing who have had no previous experience of working together or under the exacting and very different conditions in the field to arrive at the scene and attempt to provide cohesive medical support.

FOOTBALL

The Brigade provides full first aid coverage for many sporting events and other public functions and occasions. Adequate care of the 110 000 people who attend the final series of football matches in Melbourne requires an organisation of military precision. Five first aid posts are manned around the ground. In addition, two or more resuscitation teams are available, comprising one doctor, a Brigade Surgeon (preferably a resuscitationist or anaesthetist), a trained nurse, two stretcher bearers and a radio operator. Upon the alert from a member of the Brigade on duty in the crowd that a collapse has occurred, the team springs into action. Immediate cardiopulmonary resuscitation is initiated if necessary and continued until the collapsed patient is conveyed to the major first aid post. Here, facilities for cardiac monitoring, defibrillation and telemetry are available.

Training for disaster work is arduous and must be conscientiously undertaken. There is no room for inefficiency.

Close attention to every detail in planning is necessary, but the unpredictable nature of disasters requires that all concerned in the management of the situation must have a flexible approach, and all planning must be adaptable to the peculiar conditions of the incident at the time.

SUPERVISION

Finally it is essential that at the scene of a disaster, large or small—a car crash, train crash or major hotel fire—one person must assume command. He must be given authority which must be respected. In most instances, this command will be the responsibility of the senior police officer present, but any member of any rescue service must be prepared to assume that command until a more senior officer is present.

THE FUTURE

Improvements in the services provided for the victims of emergency situations, medical, surgical, or traumatic, require a deeper and clearer recognition by all concerned of the importance of emergency medicine in all its aspects as a speciality in its own right. Emergencies can no longer be allowed to be attended by the least experienced or most newly qualified and only partly trained physicians and nurses.

Disaster preparedness is not postponable. The preparations for emergency care must be adequate and complete.

Emergency care requires a team approach. This involves:

(i)   Public education in first aid; the first person present at the scene of a disaster or emergency frequently carries the greatest responsibility and opportunity to avert a fatal outcome.

(ii) Improved ambulance care—involving more advanced ambulance officer training, better equipment and more modern vehicles.

(iii) Increased support, financial and personal to the voluntary services which have to provide such a valuable portion of the emergency services under many conditions.

(iv) Improved training for medical students, physicians and surgeons and nurses in emergency care. The development of a speciality of emergency medical and nursing will improve these factors.

(v)   The administrative structure within hospitals and organisations responsible for disaster work must be such that any situation can be attended to immediately and efficiently.

(vi) Hospital reception of severely injured patients must be improved.

(vii)   The development of highly sophisticated trauma shock centres (as in University of Maryland, Baltimore) for the research into and treatment of severely injured patients.

(viii) The involvement of doctors, both from hospital staff and general practitioners (family physicians) in emergency care outside hospitals, surgeries and clinics. There are many occasions when the presence of a doctor at the roadside, in the factory, at the beach or swimming pool, can be of incalculable value in preserving life, preventing further injury and promoting recovery—the three vital principles of first aid.

20

Ambulances of the Past, Present and Future

ROGER SNOOK

Originally an ambulance was defined as a mobile field hospital following an army. Although the word is now taken to mean a vehicle for the conveyance of the sick or injured it is interesting to note that there is a return to the mobile hospital concept in the recent development of specialist intensive care vehicles.

HISTORY

According to Encyclopaedia Britannica, the organisation of military ambulance services only dates from the end of the eighteenth century. Before that time the surgical treatment of wartime casualties was often delayed for several days. In 1872 the French army introduced a system of 'ambulances volantes' or flying field hospitals and at about the same time corps of 'brancardiers' or stretcher bearers were also introduced. The next major development came with the Geneva Convention of 1864 which declared that wounded soldiers, ambulance staff and equipment were to be given the protection of neutrality. With this convention was born the Red Cross and the international respect for the symbol of rescue in time of hostilities.

In 1865 Great Britain acceded to the Geneva Convention and in 1870 a National Society for Aid to the Sick and Wounded in War was formed in response to the needs of the casualties of the Franco-Prussian war. Florence Nightingale, drawing on the wealth of experience gained in the Crimean War, was able to lend powerful support in an advisory capacity and medical supplies, personnel and ambulances were sent to the scene of hostilities.

One such detachment was the Woolwich Ambulance Unit which consisted of 8 ambulance wagons and 12 stores wagons, together with 12 medical officers and 27 men. The unit was able to provide hospital accommodation for 200 casualties complete with all the necessary equipment. The Unit was fitted out under the supervision of the Director General of the Army Medical Department, and with the assistance of the Professor of Surgery at Netley. Professor Longmore was to have taken command of the unit, but at the last minute was taken ill and so Dr Guy, the Deputy Inspector General of Hospitals took his place.

The ambulances (Figs. 20.1 and 2) were divided into three parts; the front, the central area and the rear. Each ambulance was equipped with two permanent stretchers and in addition could carry 7 lightly wounded.

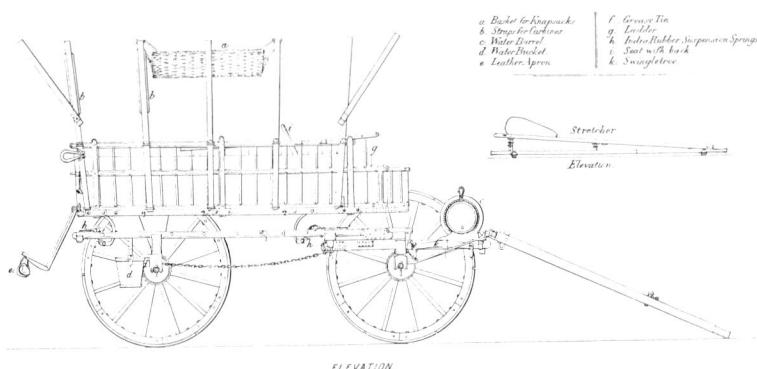

Fig. 20.1. Diagram of Woolwich Ambulance Unit horsedrawn ambulance. (By courtesy of The British Red Cross Society.)

From examining old documents it is evident that, even in those days, a variety of suspension units were employed, including the familiar leaf springs and special 'India Rubber Suspension Springs'.

The official archives of the Red Cross contain several letters from officers working on the ambulances giving their 'considered criticisms' of the structure of the vehicles. The ambulances were found to be very difficult to turn sharply, the roofs being made only of canvas did not wear well and the permanent stretchers were found to be difficult in use. As an improvement it was recommended that these stretchers should have longer handles and should not be permanent fixtures. This would allow the problem of moving the wounded from field stretcher to the ambulance stretchers to be avoided. Instead the same stretcher could be used in the field and then put straight into the ambulance. It is interesting to note that 100 years later we still encounter problems with the transfer of patients from ambulance to hospital equipment.

At the beginning of the 1914–18 First World War the British Red Cross Society joined in partnership with the Order of St John of Jerusalem under a Joint War Committee and built up a network of services in France and the United Kingdom for the sick and wounded.

Ambulances, equipment, Voluntary Ambulance Detachments,

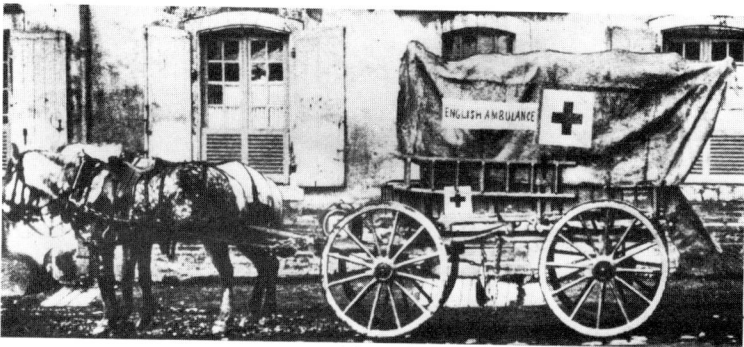

Fig. 20.2. 1870 (Franco–Prussian War). One of the ambulances of the 'Woolwich Ambulance Unit', sent out by the 'English National Society', later to become the British Red Cross. (By courtesy of the British Red Cross Society.)

hospital trains, hospitals, convalescent homes, relief parcels and casualty lists were all organised and supplemented the Medical Corps of the regular armed services.

By now the horsedrawn ambulances had given way to motor ambulances but the latter showed their ancestry in the horse and cart by still retaining such features as the open driver's cab and the canvas covering of the rear. As can be seen from Fig. 20.3 the two permanent stretchers of the horsedrawn ambulance had been replaced by four removable stretchers with no central gangway, making attention during transit very difficult.

After the First World War the Home Ambulance Service was organised and operated jointly by the Red Cross and St John, starting with the vehicles left over from the war which were distributed among the county branches.

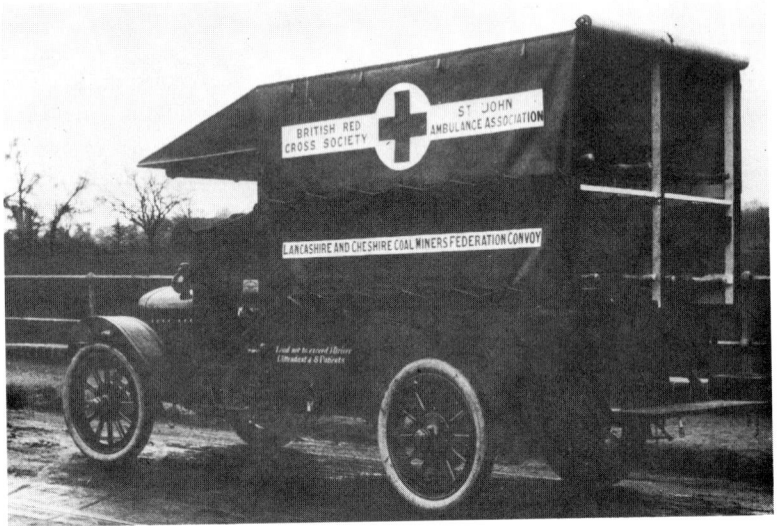

Fig. 20.3. 1914–18 (First World War): Ford Ambulance in France. (By courtesy of the British Red Cross Society.)

By 1927 ambulances were beginning to take on a more conventional shape and were coachbuilt with an enclosed cab and windows in the patient compartment. Two radical changes in design could be noted in the physical separation of cab and patient areas and the provision for only one stretcher patient. By way of digression it is interesting to note that the road accident casualty list in Great Britain for 1927 was already very high with 5329 fatalities and 148 575 injuries, and it is surprising that even in those days one stretcher was considered adequate.

Developments continued between the World Wars and then again in 1939 ambulances and other medical services for treating the injured combatants were organised and supplied by the Red Cross and St John Joint War Organisation. After the Second World War the next major change in the ambulance field followed the introduction of the National Health Service in 1948. City and county authorities were then required to provide an ambulance service either directly or on an agency basis. In many areas the voluntary aid societies maintained

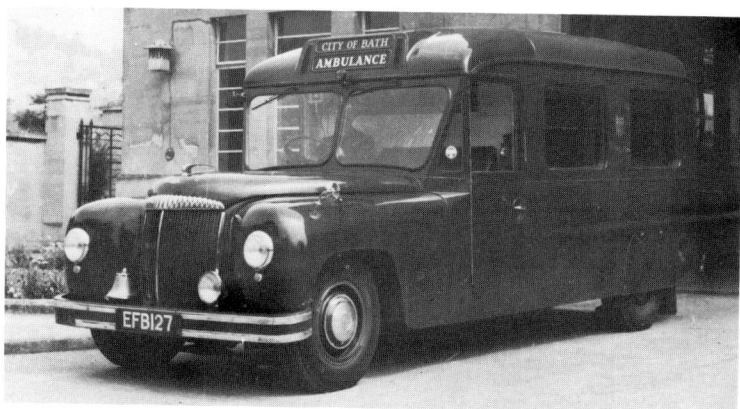

Fig. 20.4. A Daimler ambulance of the City of Bath Ambulance Service, 1950. (Photograph L Roberts.)

the ambulance service for the Local Authorities on an agency agreement but in England and Wales the amount of voluntary aid involvement in the day to day running of the local authority ambulance service gradually declined with the passage of time.

In the 1950s the ambulance of note was without doubt the Daimler (Fig. 20.4). Built on a solid chassis with a 12 ft 6 in wheelbase it had a spacious patient compartment 9 ft long, 6 ft wide and 5 ft high with room for two stretchers. The loading platform was 1 ft 10 in from the ground and with the weight, large engine and preselector gearbox the ride was very acceptable in the rear compartment. Disadvantages centred around the length of bonnet (5 ft 4 in), the low interior height and solid bulkhead between cab and patient area. The bell and an orange emergency light were by this time a standard external fitting but the interior of the ambulance reflected how even in these recent times ambulance aid was still in a comparatively early stage of development; basic stretcher equipment together with dressings, splints and blankets still formed the mainstay of patient care in the ambulance.

AMBULANCE DESIGN

In the 1960s ambulance design largely centred around the commercial van chassis with the exception of the Austin Princess ambulance. This last mentioned had many features in common with the Daimler, which it outlived by many years before finally being taken out of production as well.

The quiet revolution of the 1960s was the upsurge in interest in the training of ambulancemen, and with this the beginning of an awareness in medical circles of what could be done for emergency patients before arrival at hospital. Training will always force the pace of equipment as the latter is of little consequence without the former.

In 1967 the Millar Report made recommendations on the improvement of ambulance training and equipment. A survey of ambulance equipment by the working party that prepared the Millar Report revealed that of 142 authorities in the UK only 107 had oxygen and only 27 had aspirators available on all their vehicles used for emergencies. The same working party recommended that a committee should be set up to review training and equipment in the ambulance service continuously.

The Ambulance Service Advisory Committee held its inaugural meeting in April 1969 and then held regular meetings to advise the Secretary of State for Social Services, the Secretary of State for Wales and the Secretary of State for Scotland on the training of ambulance staff, and to advise on the vehicles, equipment, organisation and operation of ambulance services.

The committee consisted of 26 members, including representatives of local authorities, the ambulance service associations and unions, and the hospital and general medical practitioner services. In addition there were 12 co-opted members representing the National Research and Development Corporation and the voluntary aid societies.

Three sub-committees were appointed to consider 'organisation and operations', 'equipment', and 'training'; and in addition working parties to the sub-committees considered particular subjects such as ambulance interior design.

Since 1974 the Advisory Committee has been replaced by the

DHSS Ambulance Service Advisory Group to advise on ambulances and equipment and the NHS National Staff Committee for Ambulance Staff to advise on recruitment, training and development of ambulance staffing. Both committees include ambulance service personnel, doctors and health authority representatives.

The years following the Millar Report have seen rapid expansion in the fields of training and equipment with the exception of the most important item of all, the vehicle itself, which has progressed little beyond the conversion of standard commercial vans.

In the subject of ambulance design one factor is found to be missing —the minimum standards of the various parameters affecting patient comfort and treatment. Once defined these would both show up a poor ambulance and allow a better one to be designed. Reports such as that of the Millar working party recommended the equipment that should be carried and others such as the NRDC Ogle Report recommended how this equipment should be presented and how some of the tasks performed in the patient compartment could be made easier. Even so the scientific data of actual measurement was still missing.

In 1968 the University of Bristol approved a research project into medical aspects of ambulance design and a little more evidence started to emerge (Snook, 1972b). For long enough ambulancemen had given voice to the problems of noise, vibration and other difficulties encountered in the back of the ambulance, but once actual figures could be quoted then it became easier to convince those not actively involved of the problems encountered in patient transport.

Lighting

Nine ambulances, representative of those commercially available, were used to take measurements of lighting intensity in the stretcher area. The measurements ranged from 1 to 12 lumens with artificial light compared with an average daylight value of 70 lumens. Even with the best of the interior lighting a marked reduction to 8 lumens was associated with the shadowing effect of the attendant bending over the stretcher. The lighting intensity advised for accurate colour discrimination of shades such as healthy pink, the pallor of shock or the blue tinge of early cyanosis is 28 lumens. This was confirmed with tests using a simple finger tourniquet, as well as in at least one clinical case. In the last mentioned case the facial pallor of traumatic shock was not evident in the dim glow of 1 lumen in the back of an ambulance!

In providing an acceptable level of interior illumination, point sources of intense light which cause glare and cast shadows must be avoided and similarly matt neutral colours should be used for the interior trim to avoid specular reflection and colour distortion. Should the artistic protest at the lack of colourful decor the defence must be that the patient spends little time in the vehicle, and that clinical needs cannot be subordinated to aesthetic appeal in the emergency situation.

Increasing the intensity of the interior light to those levels readily accepted in a public transport vehicle will obviously make the dark glass of the ambulance less effective at night. To counter this the glass may have to be more deeply tinted, partially frosted or obscured with blinds, but care must be taken not to screen completely the patient's and attendant's ability to monitor external reference points. Once the eyes and the balance organs start to feed conflicting stimuli the response of motion sickness will soon become evident.

Noise

Measurement of sound levels were taken in the patient compartments of three ambulances using a meter weighted to equal the sensitivity of the human ear. Readings taken in town at 30 mph gave levels of 70 dBA: going uphill at 40 mph gave readings of 80 dBA and at 50 mph on an open road with sirens going, levels of 91–97 dBA were obtained. When it is realised that levels of 60 dBA are considered acceptable in a hospital and 70 dBA in a coach then levels approaching 100 dBA in an ambulance are clearly unacceptable. An increase of 10 dB represents a doubling of loudness and at 100 dB communication between patient and attendant, attendant and driver, and driver and control becomes difficult if not impossible.

Efforts to reduce noise levels must include consideration of such factors as engine size, bulkhead soundproofing, siting of emergency horns on the roof and specifying sound insulating material in the roof cavity beneath.

Heating

Other research investigations (Stoors, 1970) have shown that the effect of temperature variations in an ambulance could be potentially serious for babies in an incubator, as well as being uncomfortable for adults. To provide a powerful heat source is an expensive way of dealing with a problem that would be best solved by reducing heat loss. Whether this is achieved with an interior physical barrier or a less tangible but equally effective 'hot air curtain' is immaterial. What is required is avoidance of major temperature variation. The latter system is quite capable of maintaining a temperature differential of 20°C between external and internal conditions.

Vehicle progress in traffic

In an emergency most people will accept that the emergency vehicle should arrive at the scene with the minimum delay that is compatible with public safety. Of necessity therefore the fire, police, or ambulance emergency vehicle must travel more quickly than the prevailing traffic flow. In order that this may be achieved with safety, vehicle identification should be positive and effective. This requires a clearly recognisable symbol which is visible at maximum distance. In addition an audible warning will be required to focus attention on the visual identification under certain conditions. Use of a standard vehicle colour and lettering may be helpful in identifying emergency vehicles under certain conditions, but on its own achieves little without some immediately identifiable symbol that is effective by day and by night.

The blue beacon is the symbol, and with attention to design and placing could be made to be much more effective. Investigations (Snook, 1972c) have shown that the most important factors are the light transmission ratios of the various colours together with a combination of reflector size, apparent area illuminated, and width of the more intense part of the beam, which in summation gives the effect of a large sustained image. The alternating horns are the most directional of the audible warning devices and those who complain of the occasional 20 second exposure from a passing emergency vehicle would do better to consider the statements of people trapped by fire for instance. These people are often reported as having deferred a dangerous jump from a multi-storey building on hearing the approach of a fire engine.

Effective identification of an ambulance in traffic will mean a smoother journey to hospital for the patient on the stretcher. Automatic identification of the ambulance by a miniature transmitter–receiver system attached to traffic lights will ensure that the vehicle is not held up on the journey to or from an emergency. Such a device will also eliminate the braking deceleration effect on the patient and attendant when the lights change to red, as well as solving the problem of whether to cross red lights or not. Such a system was installed in Bath in June, 1971 and has proved safe and effective, but still awaits implementation nationally (Snook, 1972a).

Within the cab of the ambulance the driving position in particular requires attention to detail. Postural support provided by cab seating would help to reduce the occupational 'backache' endemic amongst ambulance staff. A poorly contoured seat can be avoided whilst a certain amount of strain from lifting patients is inevitable. At least the strain of the latter could be aided by the prophylaxis of the former.

From the driving position the ambulanceman should be able to reach the normal controls, emergency switches and radiotelephone. In addition the driver should be able to wear a seat belt which is an integral part of the seat, and the area in front of him should be padded for safety and free from obstructions. If this can be achieved in a car then it can only be a question of attention to detail to provide the same facilities in an ambulance.

The patient compartment

Enough space to stand, sit and work are the basic requirements. Interior height will not be a problem on a low chassis, and the requirements of length and breadth are already met by most larger ambulances.

The entry to the patient compartment should be wide enough to accept a hospital bed for emergency purposes—such as evacuating a hospital following fire. The rear loading height should preferably allow a ramp to avoid lifting. Failing this it should be designed to accept the wheels of the trolley at a height which ambulancemen can achieve without strain. In noting this it should be recognised that too low a platform may be as problematical as one that is too high. The trolley itself should be provided with large wheels, effective side rails, provision for 15° head down tilt, a vertical arm for infusion apparatus, a means of holding other resuscitation equipment, and should be marked with reflectors for safety at night.

Within the vehicle provision should be made for attaching the trolley to one side wall or diagonally across the patient compartment. Only in this latter position can access to both sides of the trolley be ensured with the second trolley still in place.

The attendant is best seated at the head of the patient and if facing forwards will be able to anticipate changes in vehicle progress. This means placing the patient in the ambulance feet first. In most ambulances engine size ensures that the forces of deceleration will be greater than those of acceleration, so such a position will be dynamically more physiological.

The interior design of the ambulance should ensure that the seated attendant can reach the equipment from that position without leaving the patient. This may be achieved by either displaying the equipment on special 'clip-boards' or by mounting the various items in cut-out recesses on pull-out trays.

With a modular design featuring equipment, cupboards and trolleys held by the 'clip-on rail' principle the interior of an ambulance would then be flexible enough to allow use of the same vehicle for different purposes.

Vehicle ride

The effect of linear and angular motion on the supine ill and injured has received scant attention in the past. The effects may be both direct and indirect: influencing the comfort or condition of the patient or the performance of life support tasks by the attendant.

Motion in the longitudinal axis is a function of such factors as vehicle identification in traffic, engine size for overtaking and automatic gear change for smoothness. Roll is a function of chassis height, centre of gravity and suspension travel. Linear movement in the lateral axis is a function of speed and radius of cornering, and in the vertical axis is a function of road surface, tyre pressure and construction, suspension characteristics, stretcher mounting and vehicle speed.

There is now sufficient evidence (Cullen, 1967; Pichard, 1970; Snook, 1972b, 1974) to suggest that vertical motion can affect the seriously ill and injured. Measurable differences can be demonstrated between standard ambulances on a commercial chassis, a specially designed ambulance and a private car. Taken together these results indicate that efforts must be made to insulate the patient from the harmful effects of vehicle motion (Snook, 1976).

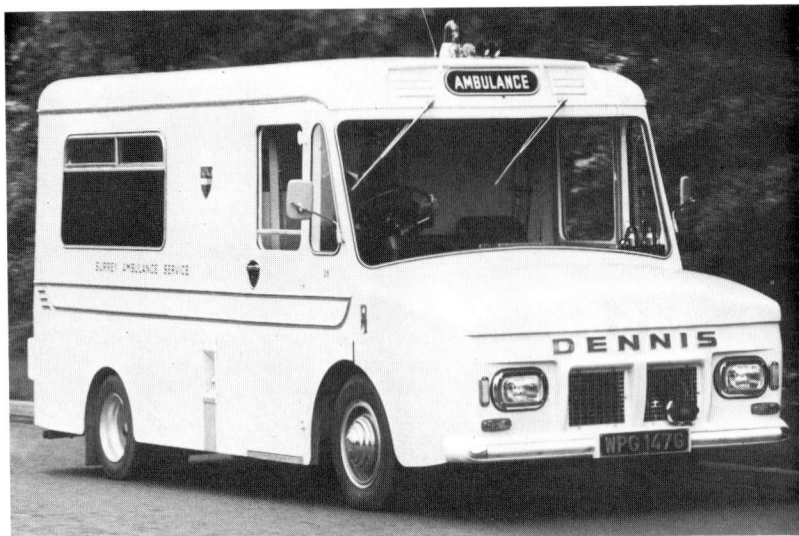

Fig. 20.5. The Dennis FD4 prototype ambulance. (By courtesy of 'Commercial Motor' and Dennis Motors Ltd.)

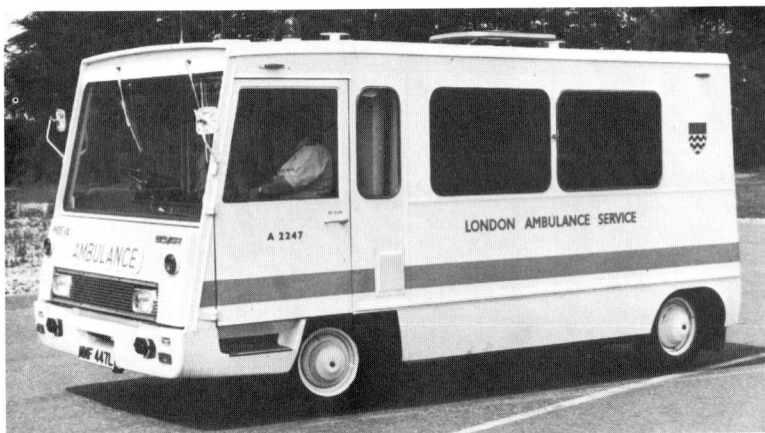

Fig. 20.6. The Reeves–Sovam prototype ambulance. (By courtesy of the London Ambulance Service.)

This may be achieved in one of two ways: designing a complete vehicle with the optimum characteristics or using a standard vehicle and insulating the patient on an active or semi-active stretcher suspension system. The first approach has the advantage of completeness, the second the drawback of applying only to the patient, but both represent such an obvious subjective improvement that their respective contributions to patient transport must be utilised.

Both the purpose-designed ambulance (Figs. 20.5 and 6: see also Table I) and the semi-active stretcher suspension system (Fig. 20.7) already exist in more than one form and the subjective assessment of ride in or on them is noticeably better than in a standard commercial chassis conversion.

TABLE I

Ambulance	Dennis FD4 (Fig. 20.5)	Reeves–Sovam (Fig. 20.6)
External dimensions		
Length	18 ft	17 ft
Width	6 ft 7 in	7 ft 4 in
Height	7 ft 6 in	8 ft 4 in
Wheelbase	10 ft	10 ft 8 in
Patient compartment		
Length	10 ft	8 ft 3 in
Width	6 ft 2 in	6 ft 8 in
Height	6 ft	6 ft 4 in
Drive	Front wheel	Front wheel
Driving position	Semi-forward control	Forward control
Suspension	Independent front and rear	Independent front and rear
Engine	6-cylinder Jaguar	4-cylinder Peugeot petrol injection

TABLE I—cont.

Ambulance	Dennis FD4 (Fig. 20.5)	Reeves–Sovam (Fig. 20.6)
Rating	2·8 litre 140 bhp	2-litre 110 bhp
Gearbox	Borg Warner 35 Automatic	4-speed syncromesh manual
Wheels	16 × 600 front 14 × 165 rear	19 × 400
Turning circle	39·5 ft left 41·7 ft right	56 ft
Weight	2 ton 14 cwt	2 ton 1 cwt
Loading height	18 in	10 in

The final hurdle therefore in the race for ambulance improvement is not a technological one but rather one of cost effectiveness. Does the cost of the vehicle match the effectiveness of providing sophisticated transport? The argument that only 15 per cent of the work load of an ambulance concerns emergency cases is one that should be countered by another argument. Why do we use specialised vehicles for carrying patients who do not require these facilities? The needs of the emergency patient must not be prejudiced by the statistics of those who least need transport in an ambulance.

The seriously ill or injured patient is probably one of the most valuable commodities to be transported by road.

The evidence now exists to show that patient care can be related to ambulance design and that this can be measured. The future must see a continuing process of research to identify, regulation to define and design to comply with the needs of the sick and injured. As the standards of ambulance aid increase so must the standard of the most basic of equipment, the ambulance.

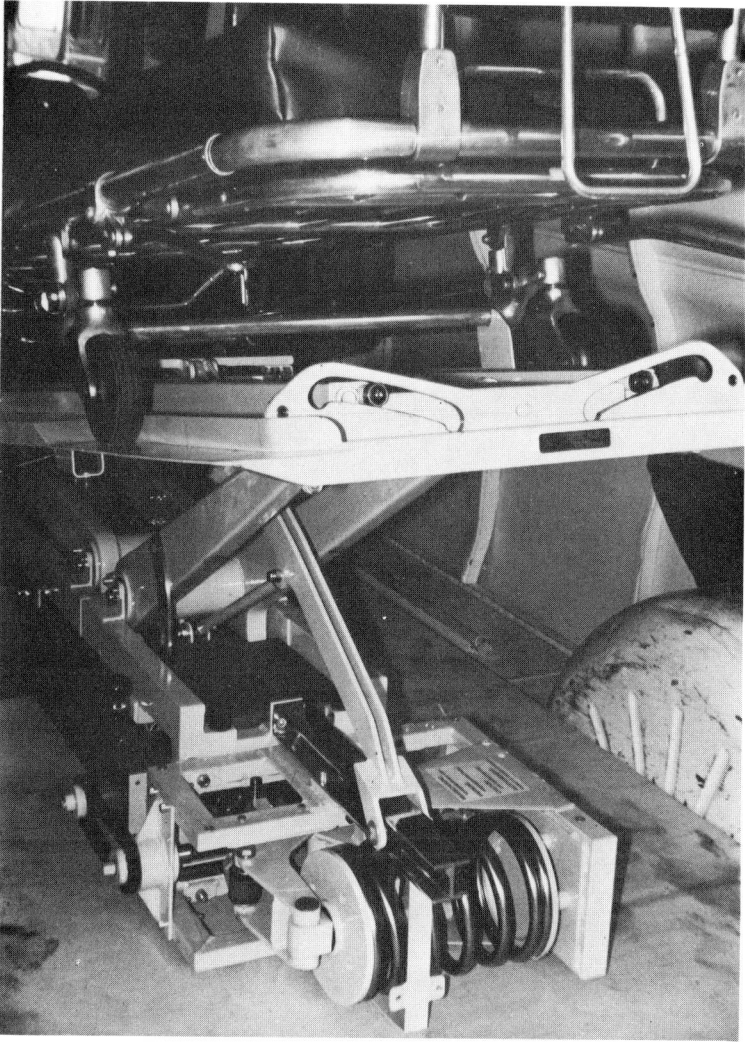

Fig. 20.7. A close up of the Laura Vico Vleugelbrancard (Floating Stretcher) showing the platform, lever system, electric motor, chain drive and spring unit exposed to view. (By courtesy of F W Equipment Ltd.)

ACKNOWLEDGEMENTS

I would like to acknowledge the assistance of the following in the preparation of this chapter: the British Red Cross Society and Mrs J Fawcett, Staff Officer National Headquarters; the Chief Ambulance Officer of the City of Bath Ambulance Service, Mr R A Fysh; the Chief Ambulance Officer of London Ambulance Service, Mr W E Cooke, OBE; the Chief Officer of the County Borough of Brighton Ambulance Service, Mr E R Kimber; Dennis Motors Ltd, of Guildford, Surrey; FW Equipment Ltd, of Bradford.

REFERENCES

Cullen (1967), Mortality of the Ambulance Ride, *Brit. med. J.*, **3**, 438.

Ministry of Health Working Party on Ambulance Training and Equipment (1967), Parts 1 and 2. London: HMSO.

National Research Development Corporation (1969), *Ogle Report on Emergency Ambulances.* NRDC.

Pichard (1970), The Effects of Acceleration and Vibration on Sick Persons During Transport, *Revue des Corps de Santé*, **11**, 611.

Snook (1972a), Automatic Traffic Light Control, *'Fire' Journal of the British Fire Services*, **65**, 3.

Snook (1972b), Medical Aspects of Ambulance Design, *Brit. med. J.*, **3**, 574.

Snook (1972c), The Use of Flashing Beacons, *Fire Protection Review*, **5**, 214.

Snook (1974), *Medical Aid at Accidents.* London: Update Publications.

Snook (1976), Ambulance ride: fixed or floating stretcher, *Brit. med. J.*, **2**, 405.

Stoors (1970), Transport of Sick New Born Babies, *Brit. med. J.*, **3**, 328.

21

The Coroner

PETER HATCH

This chapter deals with legal enquiries into sudden deaths but only in broad outline since these investigations are conducted differently in different parts of the world, sometimes by lawyers, sometimes by medical graduates (from GPs to forensic pathologists) and sometimes by both. In England a death by accident must be the subject of a public inquest, usually with a jury, and there is no provision for written evidence, whether by sworn affidavit or signed statement, as a substitute for personal attendance of witnesses. Other countries adopt a less formal procedure and it may be helpful to give some reference to the English system (which goes back to 1177 AD) as many others are derived from it.

WHEN THE FIGHT IS LOST

Inevitably in emergency care some casualties succumb to the accident before help arrives or die despite all that is done. Those involved will be extremely lucky as well as skilful if they can work in this field very long before they make the acquaintance of the coroner, or his equivalent elsewhere. The very nature of the work dealt with in this book, by its call on modern techniques, and in particular, mobility of equipment, can cause an apparent conflict to arise between the medical practitioner and the coroner unless something is understood about the latter's viewpoint. Even some doctors who deal often with the coroner never get out of their initial view that he is officious, obstructive, critical and best avoided. If one has to deal with the coroner, however, it would seem best to try to understand his approach to his necessary function, to meet the difficulties which this may place in one's way and even to turn them to advantage.

Emergencies do not arise in neat textbook fashion, except perhaps on these pages where the relevant factors are selected for purpose of example. In attending the scene of an incident the first and paramount aim is the saving of life, but it cannot be the only aim, as certain other obligations must not be overlooked. Taking an extreme example, if four occupants of a car which is in risk of bursting into flames appear to be dead, obviously the team will remove them rapidly if at all possible, in the hope that some or all can be revived. If they cannot, the coroner will be involved. He will certainly want to know who was taken from the driver's position. If no one can tell him he will be critical. This is because it is his duty to ascertain such facts—for the very good reason that the dependants of the three others may be able to claim compensation from an insurance company if they can prove the driver was in fact driving within the terms of his policy. Even the question whether a particular person had been using a safety belt before being removed from the vehicle by rescuers is now of interest to insurers and may in the near future be a factor influencing the payment or the scale of damages.

Insurance claims that become claims for damages in the courts are of little help or use to those concerned with emergency services who may quite understandably say they are not going to let considerations of these matters affect their conduct when dealing with accidents. It would not be right, however, to adopt the same attitude to the coroner. He can actually help. Whenever there is a fatality then an inquest will be held as soon as possible, in public, and will probably be reported in the press. This can provide permanent, official, and reasonably efficient publicity for the emergency service. If facilities are short then the best man to convince of this fact is the coroner. One remark from him, or one rider from a coroner's jury is worth twenty letters to the treasurer of a local authority. Do not expect the coroner to be recruited to your cause or to become a campaigner, at least in his public utterances, since he is a law officer and must remain as free of bias towards good causes as towards private interests.

No coroner will ask that you hesitate in your emergency work or refrain from doing something you consider necessary because of what he might say. Be satisfied of your own competence before undertaking this work and then do what you believe to be necessary. Time and again the seemingly hopeless case who looks certain to be a candidate for the coroner has somehow survived with emergency care. Sometimes the doctor's professional knowledge tells him there is no hope. This must not be allowed to influence the situation, with the doctor saying to himself, 'This man is going to die in any case; if he dies after I perform surgery the coroner may blame me'. Coroners are not as unknowledgeable as is generally supposed. For example a man with a displaced fracture of the femur is trapped in a vehicle. If he is left long without reduction of the fracture he may die from fat embolism two or three days later. If he has other injuries and has lost blood he is not a promising subject for amputation of a foot or arm which may be holding him in the vehicle. He may die from a cause immediately connected with the surgery. No doctor should be hesitant of his own position in attempting the surgery. The decision is his to make and if made on a professional basis then it is merely a matter of letting the record show this. Some would ask, 'Why put it on the record at all? Why does not the coroner just say death was due to the injuries and leave the doctor out of it?' If you are ever in this position your viewpoint is a subjective one and therefore unreliable. If in the example given the pathologist found that loss of blood during the amputation was the final cause of death then he would have to say so to the coroner. This may underline the fact, for example, that plasma ought to be more readily available to meet such cases. The doctor's proper course, in the unlikely event that he feels he needs self protection in such a case is to see that the pathologist has a written report containing the reason for the urgency of the surgery; this he will readily understand and in turn will make clear in his report.

If one appreciates that the coroner's function is merely to record the facts, and that to investigate a doctor's actions is not the same as to criticise them, then the coroner will not loom so large as a person to resent.

RULES AND REGULATIONS

Whatever the emergency there are some routines which the trained operator will follow because he knows they make sense, such as the doctor excluding air from a syringe before an injection, or a fireman confining a fire before trying to remove a victim. The coroner too has his basic rules which must not be broken, and he regards these as merely common sense.

The first rule worthy of mention is that dead bodies must not be moved around the country. This is because the law puts a duty on the coroner for the area where the death occurred to undertake the enquiries as to its cause. Coroners are surprisingly busy people. It may take three minutes for a death to occur and ten hours (or two hundred times as long) to investigate that death. To ensure that every death which requires it is investigated there is one coroner for each district, and the death must be reported to him and to him alone. Some highly populated districts may have a coroner for twenty square miles; elsewhere a coroner's district may cover a thousand square miles, but in each area there is no doubt which coroner is responsible.

If bodies, i.e. persons **known** to be dead, are moved from one coroner's district to another then the system breaks down and coroners complain. There are no objections to moribund patients being moved to a hospital where if emergency measures are successful they may continue to receive intensive care, but if all help fails in the ambulance, on the way to a hospital which is outside the district where the injuries were received, then the correct thing to do is certify DOA which, it should be pointed out, means 'dead on arrival' and not 'dead on admission'.

When there are several deaths from one incident, some at the scene and others DOA, or after arrival at hospital, then there is a procedure for the two coroners to decide between them which is to hold the inquest on the several deaths. It is unlikely that either of them will appreciate their decision being anticipated, and usually the first death in time is taken as the deciding factor.

The coroner is involved once a death has occurred. All deaths which are not from natural causes (so therefore all road fatalities) must be reported to the coroner who must hold an inquest in the case of road, rail and air deaths. It is for the coroner to decide not only whether there is to be a post mortem examination (almost invariable with accident victims) but also who is to do this. The coroner cannot pay a fee to doctors for services rendered before the case becomes a coroner's case, or even for a written report unless he has asked for it (usually through the coroner's officer). Some coroners take the view that it is improper for them to discuss a case with a person who may be, or will be, a witness at an inquest, and require all messages and queries to be relayed through the coroner's officer. The correct way to find out a post mortem result is to ask the pathologist if he has, or can get, the coroner's authority to disclose it. A doctor cannot issue a death certificate in a coroner's case unless, being satisfied as to the cause of death, he initials the certificate on the back to say he has reported the death to the coroner.

It may be useful to add a word about your position as a participant at an emergency. If the incident becomes the subject of an inquest then although attending the scene for one particular purpose you may find yourself in a different capacity, as a witness giving evidence at the inquest. Don't shirk this duty, for instance by telling the police you did not notice something they are investigating. A full enquiry can lead to measures being taken which improve road safety. If there have been many victims and much confusion at the scene, try to make notes afterwards of things you did or saw which others are unlikely to have seen. Obviously if these things appear to you to be important you will pass them on to an investigating officer before you leave the scene. Small, apparently unimportant things can sometimes later assume more significance. The making of your own notes also helps you to be critical and to ask yourself next time, given the same set of circumstances if you would do things in the same order. Particularly do inquests bring out the fact that if a routine is the more rigorously adhered to the more urgent the emergency, it achieves better results than to abandon routine and have to say afterwards that things were so urgent there wasn't time for it. Over all lies your duty as a citizen to give evidence of things you know, and the trained operative with a privileged right to attend emergencies has an even greater duty to assist a proper investigation. If inquests have to be attended, explain well in advance to the coroner's officer the nature of your commitments as coroners prefer to work as part (albeit the head!) of a team working together to the same end.

THE CORONER'S OFFICER

Whenever you have dealings with the coroner it will usually be through the coroner's officer. If you have some idea of his job, he will at least spring fewer surprises and cause you less inconvenience.

The sort of fatalities with which we are concerned will all be inquest cases, on the following general routine:

Certifying death

This involves a doctor on the scene or at a reception hospital.

Identification

This includes viewing of the body by the coroner. This may require time for the identifying witnesses to travel and involve evidence from those earliest on the scene, if mutilation has occurred, or of effects found with the body, e.g. door keys, etc.

Opening of inquest

Usually this begins with medical evidence of the cause of death in order that the body can be disposed of by burial or cremation, after the coroner has issued the disposal document.

Preparation of evidence

This includes taking of statements at the scene, or later if fuller statements are needed; taking photographs at the scene; and making expert examinations by vehicle examiners, forensic officers, and others. If witnesses are injured and still in hospital this can hold up the inquest.

Calling of inquest

The witnesses whose statements have been seen by the coroner, and whom he requires, are warned to attend, and a jury summoned.

Holding of inquest

Evidence is given in full before the jury, and solicitors or sometimes barristers attend for interested parties to take notes and cross examine.

The verdict

In addition to the medical cause of death this gives the means of death. It should be noted that a coroner's jury, unless making a finding of murder or other criminal charge, are not allowed to attribute blame in an accident. This last point is the most misunderstood of all and causes people to leave an inquest thinking it a waste of time. They should perhaps stop and consider what really has been achieved:

the facts have been established and the jury have made all the conclusions which, in fairness to all concerned, can be made without holding a trial. In other words, the coroner is concerned with facts. If the facts speak for themselves then conclusions are superfluous; if not then it is dangerous to draw conclusions from them.

GENERAL OBSERVATIONS

The preceding pages are addressed to the qualified doctor who is part of a team and may seem to suggest that the role of other team members is less important. This is only because the object of the operation is to get medical help to the victim. The passer-by who holds a light or who stops traffic is just as much a participant. Some general views on teamwork from a coroner who has seen the emergency service working in his area for ten years may be of interest.

At its best the emergency service is one of the finest contributions that those taking part can make to their community. It is concerned with human beings who are utterly dependent on the goodwill, knowledge and technique of their fellow men. It is likely to remain for this reason either unpaid or underpaid since the satisfaction of a job well done is reduced to a mundane level when it comes to claiming 'turning-out fees' or mileage allowances; and most of those involved would sooner see money spent on more equipment than on pay. One of the most expensive aspects of equipment is the communications system which in the ideal situation is on standby 365 days a year. At this point even the disabled with no special skills can be drawn into the organisation in manning a listening post or doing the paper work. Don't think that the scheme can be run without paper work. Consider the situation of a hospital Secretary who is asked to authorise the emergency service to draw anything a doctor requests from his stores. He cannot agree. But if he knows the emergency service has a voluntary secretary who will fill in and send him an incident report stating what equipment or supplies were used, where they were obtained, and by whom they were taken then he has something to go on. If this is backed up with a card index system indicating the contribution in vehicles, manpower or equipment provided by different sources then it may be easier to obtain official funds from those sources when they can see the importance of their contributions.

Voluntary contributions of this kind may seem a little removed from the urgent on-the-spot help that is at the centre but in those inquests where the service has been involved it becomes clear to the observer that it is teamwork which gets results and creates efficiency. If you go to an incident and only contribute a pair of hands to lift a vehicle off a patient you have made a vital contribution. If your special skills are called on then you have contributed to the team which saves lives, and you can feel privileged to be a member of it.

As the material things in life increase, and public and personal standards of responsibility decline, you may expect there will be more work for you to do. If you are there to do it you will not merely ease the work of the coroner but make a substantial contribution to the welfare of your community.

22

Evaluation as a Function of Organisation—Projection of a Model Emergency Service

ALFRED DOOLEY

PREAMBLE

The evaluation of emergency care has for many years been a matter of concern to workers in this field, to the Medical Commission on Accident Prevention (MCAP) and to Government departments. The subject was brought to the forefront following Government rejection of a recommendation in 1974 of the House of Commons Employment and Social Services Sub-Committee of the Expenditure Committee on Accident and Emergency Services that Government finance should be made available to GP schemes for the purchase of equipment and radiotelephones and for insurance of doctors attending accidents (Recommendation 11, Fourth Report, 1974, HMSO, London). In 'Observations on the Fourth Report' (Cmnd 5886, 1975, HMSO, London) it was stated: '. . . the Departments do not feel able to allocate from the limited funds available to its resources to an area where the benefit is not as yet proven. Nevertheless the DHSS have suggested that the MCAP should undertake a survey of GP emergency schemes and has offered to contribute to the cost of research.' In a further DHSS statement (Health Trends, May 1975) the enquiry was broadened to include ambulance training: 'The Department has asked the MCAP to evaluate the efficacy of various GP schemes for coping with road accidents and of the training given to ambulance men in handling victims of road accidents'.

In May 1975 the author was brought in by MCAP to conduct

a Pilot Study on as broad a basis as was possible within the limited funds available from purely MCAP sources. These funds were exhausted by June 1976, since when the work has continued on a voluntary basis, support for an extended study having been refused by DHSS.

The insistence on proof of benefit from developments in emergency work presented a considerable problem. Documentation was found in general to be uneven and fragmented, and data recovery and processing methods sometimes archaic. **By necessity and taking into account the urgent need for results, use was made of the best information available in the search for quantifiable criteria which could lead to definitive conclusions.** The study is in process of being completed prior to publication elsewhere. Meantime what is attempted in this chapter is to provide a picture in breadth and perspective of what has emerged and what, in the author's view, may be projected for the future. The extent to which benefit may be capable of 'proof' will ultimately depend on monitoring facilities built into the Service and on the underlying logic on which statistical inferences are drawn. Nevertheless a tentative assessment of the effect of activities studied and of the scope for general improvement in emergency care is made in discussion at the end of this chapter.

THE BROAD VIEW

As this volume amply demonstrates, organised human activity depends increasingly on information. The nature of the activity and the way it is organised determine the scope and purpose of the required information and provide incentive and justification for the effort of providing it. They will also define limits within which information will be cost-effective.

In order usefully to discuss the recording, storage, processing and recovery of information in the field of rescue and emergency care it is therefore necessary to consider at some length the nature and organisation of this activity. In so doing it would not be appropriate in this short review to attempt to survey the present "state of the art" in its many manifestations—this is done in specific areas in other chapters. Nor would it be proper to draw comparisons between or express judgements on particular schemes.

The author's brief but far ranging incursion into this field during the year 1975/76 served not only for detailed study of specific activities but also, and perhaps more importantly, for obtaining a bird's eye view of this field of work. A strong impression has emerged that improvement in emergency care will (and has in some areas) come from taking a broad and comprehensive view in which different approaches are seen as complementary rather than alternative and rescue and emergency care is regarded as a combined operation. In fact the time seems ripe for developing rescue/emergency care as an integrated service within which progress is made on a broad front, through effective coordination and monitoring of existing operations and the constant appraisal and introduction of methods of improvement.

Such development will depend for its initiation on little more than an acceptance by Government Departments of the premise that rescue/emergency care is a combined operation: the problem of 'evaluation' of specific activities which has bedevilled the subject over a number of years will be resolved in the normal course of events as effective information systems are built into the coordinating machinery. **Evaluation will become routine monitoring rather than research.**

The first step is seen as the initiation of **Area Emergency Service Coordinating Committees** by means of a joint circular from the Department of Health and Social Security and the Home Office. Without in any way insisting on ideal solutions this circular includes a hypothetical model or projection to provide a scenario for such committees. The elements of such a model are suggested in what follows: most of the items are to be found either singly or severally in schemes already operating. Generally there is lacking in practice today the cementing effect of adequate coordination and documentation as well as the concept of advance on a broad front.

The **Model Emergency Service** is postulated as a combined operation of police, fire service, ambulance, general practitioners and hospitals managed by representative Area Emergency Service Coordinating Committees with recognition and support from Area Health Authorities in the form of clerical and data processing facilities (under the umbrella of Community Health). There is also representation from trades unions and other organisations who have a contribution to make in preparing the way for advances in training, re-grading and remuneration.

Terms of reference of these Committees are framed around the **overall objective: to raise the standard of the Service by all practicable means.** These will vary according to Area conditions and facilities. A considerable fund of experience in many aspects of the work is now available through bodies such as the Medical Commission on Accident Prevention and is put at the disposal of Area Committees.

For the purpose of presentation and discussion the functions of the Committees may be separated into

Coordinating
Deploying
Monitoring
Training

although in practice these interrelate and overlap.

Coordination rests initially on agreement on aims and methods ensured by broad representation on the Committees. Day to day coordination requires frequent review of performance by a small executive committee. This depends on feed back from the monitoring system dealt with later: this system provides information on the work load and how it is dealt with in such a form that rational decisions may be taken.

Coordination has a more specific and more immediate meaning in regard to mobilising the service following a 999 or other emergency call. An agreed callout procedure is essential, chosen on the basis of best available communications facilities in relation to need. In the projected Model the **callout function is the responsibility of police control.** This is mainly because of their capacity using computer-backed communications equipment to direct police mobiles to the sites of emergencies and thereby obtain rapid assessment of required aid on which correct deployment of support depends. This in no way delays despatch of the emergency ambulance, 999 calls being simultaneous to police and ambulance control. Following assessment of need by police at the scene, if necessary, procedure is put in motion to mobilise the doctor covering the zone. Subsequently the doctor maintains liaison with ambulance control by radiotelephone.

Police control is linked by direct line to the Accident and Emergency Departments of hospitals serving the Area. This makes it possible to warn these departments of impending arrival of casualties when severe or moderate injuries are reported. This procedure, established as routine, also ensures that when major accidents or 'disasters' occur, resulting in many casualties, hospitals are alerted at the earliest moment in the normal course of events and medical aid is mobilised as required.

Police training is extended to cover assessment of aid required following rapid inspection of accident conditions and injury. The procedure is preferred to that based on assessment by ambulance control because this has then to be based on lay information given by the 999 caller to control. Delayed assessment until the ambulance arrives at the scene will be acceptable only when victims are trapped but in such cases this will probably have been mentioned in the 999 call and action already taken.

Other aspects of the coordinating function stem from the concept of emergency work as one service as compared with a stepwise process involving independent rather than interdependent bodies. This concept is apparent when in special circumstances the police escort ambulances, doctors travel with patients and ambulance personnel stay on in A & E Departments with their patients. **The keynote of the Model Service is expressed in continuity of care and responsibility with a common interest in providing the highest possible level of care throughout.**

A particular area taken care of in the Model is the Ambulance Service—A & E Department relationship. Close cooperation is essential in the patients' interest, the ideal being the acceptance by the A & E personnel of emergency ambulance work as a field extension of A & E work. Progress in this direction is accelerated by joint training schemes, by location of emergency ambulances with their advanced trained crews at hospitals and by the installation of adequate on-going information systems.

Deployment. In discharging their many responsibilities as the arm of the civil authority the **police** have a continuously deployed mobile force controlled (and therefore located and directed) using up-to-date communications techniques. Road accidents involving personal injury are one of these responsibilities. Police participation in the Emergency Service is therefore logical and essential. It involves no changes in deployment but brings into full use an existing facility.

On the other hand the **emergency ambulance function** in the projected Model Service is provided by first-tier advanced trained personnel manning specially equipped ambulances normally located at hospitals (See Chapter 1). This arrangement represents a composite solution to a number of problems. First, it resolves the organisational difficulty of giving advanced training in a service in which emergency calls may be only 5 to 10 per cent of the work load, the main bulk of the work being transportation of out-patients and admissions. In a normal single tier system full value is not obtained from advanced training because personnel so trained take their turn in the transportation rota. On the other hand the alternative 2-tier system in which advanced trained crews are deployed solely on emergency calls can, if these crews operate from ambulance stations as is normal, result in subjecting these men to almost perpetual standby and very little action. Emergency calls of all types (accident and medical) serviced by typical ambulance stations away from city-scale conurbations appear to average between 15 and 25 per month per station. It would hardly be realistic to have highly trained crews standing by in ambulance stations to meet this level of call-frequency and with no alternative occupation.

Deploying emergency ambulances and crews in such a way that most of them are seconded to hospitals overcomes this difficulty as well as having other advantages. Crews are of course fully operational under the direction of ambulance control by radio and bleep system. Waiting time is usefully occupied by on-going advanced training in hospital departments under the direction of consultants in A & E and anaesthetics departments. At a certain level of training the crews represent valuable additional manpower for such tasks as taking bloods and keeping records. Above all, mutual confidence and understanding are established between A & E Department personnel and ambulance crews. Full information on the condition and previous treatment of patients is transmitted both verbally and on record sheets filled in by ambulance crews for each patient (see later under monitoring). Co-ordination of the functions of the emergency ambulance service and A & E Departments is thus substantially advanced.

This arrangement is of course effective only to the extent that suitable hospitals are available in relation to distances and road networks. In many cases ambulance stations are already located in the same towns as suitable hospitals. Where this is not the case surveys are initiated by the Emergency Coordinating Committee to ascertain the limits of practicability of this approach using frequency/time to scene distributions as a basis for decisions. Without drawing hard and fast boundaries or sacrificing flexibility, zones will be found, probably on the periphery of each Committee area, which will be regarded as outside the normal range of hospital-based ambulances and served by outlying ambulance stations which cope with both emergency and transportation work. **In these zones arrangements are made to call out General Practitioners to provide emergency medical care at the scene when need arises.** The callout procedure is such that this need is assessed and the doctor deployed sufficiently quickly to enable him to attend the scene without delaying ambulance operation, it being laid down that only in very exceptional circumstances will the ambulance wait for the doctor.

Emphasis is put on assessment of need to prevent recurrent waste of doctors' time through being called out to treat minor injuries. However, equal importance is attached to speed of assessment since mobilisation has to be achieved in time to allow the doctor to reach the scene before the ambulance has departed with the patient—if anything a more frustrating result than unnecessary callout. For reasons discussed earlier, assessment of need and subsequent callout are carried out by police as an extension to their normal functions in relation to accidents and emergencies.

Operational performance as monitored by the information service is kept under constant review by the Coordinating Committees. Such factors as availability of doctors in relation to the incidence of emergencies in particular zones are closely watched and necessary adjustments made. Disposition of doctors in relation to ambulance station location is also kept under review: for example it may not be sensible to have doctors setting off from the same place as ambulances when the latter will normally have some minutes start while assessment is made. However in this situation the radiotelephone link between doctor, ambulance control and ambulance provides coordination and enables a rendezvous to be arranged if desirable.

Monitoring requires the installation of an information recovery system with four main functions:

First, to monitor service activities in logistical terms; for example deployment of forces in relation to incidence of calls and effectiveness of callout procedures and communications.

Second, to provide information on each patient in a form such that continuity is secured in recording injury, condition and treatment from the scene to hospital discharge. The self-evident objective here is primarily to provide accident surgeons with information on the patient to save time, avoid confusion and assist diagnosis.

Third, to enable various aspects of the Service such as communications, resuscitation and other procedures and training to be separately audited.

Fourth, to provide a means for monitoring the overall long-run outcome of the Service in terms of saving life and suffering. This function would previously have been called 'evaluation' but since the Emergency

Coordinating Committees are committed to a continuous process of development in which progress is regularly assessed as a matter of routine, the term 'monitor' is preferred.

The first three of these four objectives are achieved through a single data recording and recovery process initiated in the ambulance phase, developed in successive hospital departments and processed by the Committee secretariats. It is probable that coordination and deployment of the Emergency Service along lines generally similar to those postulated above are necessary prerequisites to setting up such a process. **Until these apply it may be unrealistic to expect any one of the services concerned to take the responsibility for recording and providing the required information.** Indeed, in a fragmented service it has been observed that such information may be disregarded even when made available: for example ambulance reports may be consigned to A & E Department waste-paper baskets.

Given acceptance of the need, practicability and value of information recovery, decisions are required on variables to be recorded and in what form, bearing in mind the objectives. A clear distinction is made between information required for organisational purposes, i.e. essential details of call with type of emergency, times of call and of deployment of services, location, C V of patient and so on, and that required to give A & E Departments the best chance to treat the patient, such as condition of patient as found, during first aid and in transit, and that required for on-going treatment and possible later audit.

Difficulties in keeping and using records stem primarily from deficiencies in organisation. Not even the best designed forms will be completed unless there is conviction that the information is required, will be used and, by rapid feedback, be seen to be used. To emphasise the point again, it could therefore be futile to call for data recovery systems in advance of positive action to provide an integrated service.

In the Model Service the form used is on size A 4 (295 × 210 mm) write-through material to give four copies. The upper half is completed by ambulance crews. It includes first, organisational information about the callout and the patient, second, principal features of injury to and condition of the patient and third, a record of resuscitation and first aid procedures carried out.

The lower half is completed in hospital A & E and other departments. It provides a record of condition of patient and medical aid given from entry to hospital to discharge or transfer.

This form is designed on the 'box' principle so that the majority of the information is recorded using ticks in 'boxes' covering appropriate ranges of predetermined variables. Such forms have been in use in certain advanced ambulance schemes for some years and experience is available on design and use. A similar format applied to hospital A & E departments represents a major change from almost completely open manuscript-type sheets to multiple question/answer type forms. Specified rather than random information is recorded and handwriting no longer gives trouble.

Processing is facilitated by precoding recorded variables, code numbers being printed alongside boxes on the forms. Subsequent transfer to punch cards, disc or tape, or otherwise depending on storage and processing facilities, therefore involves minimal labour. In this connection it is envisaged that a mini or micro computer will be available in each Committee office to allow close control over programming and rapid feedback of results. This prospect is offered by the current rapid development in computer technology through which the availability of office-scale equipment will rise, and the cost will fall dramatically. By this means computer processing will be brought closer to the source of information and will be achieved by people on the spot rather than by specialists at a distance.

Disposal of copies of the record form is: one copy to each of ambulance control, hospital A & E department, hospital medical records office and Emergency Committee office. In case of transfer to another hospital a photocopy is sent with the patient.

This information system with other aspects of the emergency service is under continuous review and development by Emergency Coordinating Committees. The application of modern information recovery methods to hospital accident and emergency work is only now beginning as experimental schemes are being introduced by pioneers such as Rutherford and Maynard in Belfast. For reasons already discussed their broader application depends on unification of the service rather than on development of techniques.

The fourth function of the information system is to monitor the overall outcome of the service in terms of saving life and reducing suffering. This is a rationalisation of the evaluation theme which has run through consideration of emergency work for many years and has resulted in delayed decisions. Specifically, evaluation of general practitioner schemes was required before a decision on Government recognition and support could be made, this leading to the author's Pilot Study. With hindsight and a knowledge of the level of documentation available and of the range of clinical variables, one could perhaps subscribe to the view of physicists and philosophers that 'you must not ask questions if you know it is impossible to find the answer!'

The evaluation of benefit to patients from particular activities on the basis of ambulance and hospital records faces two main difficulties. First, the paucity and lack of continuity of records: this will be corrected as integration of the service is achieved along lines suggested above. But the second difficulty is deep and fundamental: it is that of quantitatively assessing clinical benefit to individual patients. **Classifications of injury and degree of injury do not lend themselves to quantification.** Assessments therefore inevitably have a large subjective element and conclusions are not definitive. In addition there is difficulty in finding suitable 'control' series for comparison, necessary since evaluation implies assessment relative to a datum or to an alternative system.

To by-pass these difficulties inherent in studies based on morbidity, a method has been developed in the Medical Commission Pilot Study which transfers the focus of attention and study from ambulance and hospital records to police and coroners' records. This is made possible by limiting information used to the fatal end of the injury distribution pattern and using this to indicate the shape of this pattern and the level of emergency care.

The reasoning underlying this method is in process of publication elsewhere. Suffice it to say here that it depends on the premise that for statistical purposes, saving of life is **the** crucial index of the effectiveness of rescue and emergency care: and that saving of life means keeping alive a maximum possible number of severely injured victims who have survived the impact of the accident (or other emergency) up to the time that trained help arrives as provided by the Emergency Service. Certainly a proportion of these victims will have injuries such that survival will be highly improbable. But there will also be a marginal number whose survival will be dependent on the effectiveness of the Service at each stage of the rescue and care process.

The long-run frequency of survival/non-survival will be reflected in fatality statistics in the number of patients who die later, i.e. subsequent to arrival of aid, at the scene, en route to hospital or in hospital. Obviously the number dying instantly (who were dead when aid arrived) could not be affected by the level of care but this number relative to those dying later is used to locate the latter within the injury distribution pattern.

Care indices based on this approach must of course be related to accident conditions. These vary widely and it might be thought that clinical variables have merely been exchanged for accident variables. In practice classification of accident conditions has to cope with a smaller number of better defined variables than are accident injuries. For the purpose of ensuring 'like with like' comparisons it is necessary only to define a limited number of characteristic groups of accidents such as pedestrian–vehicle, single vehicle, 2-vehicle and so on, with subdivision for type, speed and other factors. Limitation to fatalities also greatly reduces the volume of information required as well as eliminating difficulties of classification of injury: **death is definitive.**

Problems associated with recording and recovering the required information are greatly reduced by the fact that the authority taking responsibility for this function, for reasons legal and unconnected with emergency care, are the police. Police work is based on information: everything is recorded as a matter of routine and in accessible form. In the case of accidents resulting in death with which this method is concerned the police have a particular function in assembling definitive information for coroners' inquests. This will include details required for the emergency care index which are principally time of death in relation to time of accident and the conditions under which the accident occurred. **All the information required for monitoring emergency care according to this method will therefore, subject to police cooperation, be available from a single source.**

At the time of writing this method is in process of development under the aegis of the Medical Commission on Accident Prevention. Nevertheless in the Model as here projected care indices so obtained are computed at annual intervals for use of the Area Emergency Coordinating Committees and for inclusion as an addendum to deaths from accidents in OPCS Monitor (Office of Populations, Censuses and Surveys–Government Statistical Service). A yardstick is thus made available for the comparative monitoring of emergency services on a national scale.

Training. A programme of training for all participating services in their particular functions within the Emergency Service is continuously under review by the Coordinating Committees. In all cases this has to be a combination of background knowledge and either transmitted or actual practical experience.

The substantial numbers of **police** deployed in a given area and whose function in emergency care is the assessment of need, attend regular lecture/demonstrations by doctors and ambulance instructors experienced in emergency work, on accident injury and certain types of medical emergency. Special emphasis is put on factors found to be important for prognosis. The proceedings are kept informal with ample provision for questions and discussion.

Development of the **Emergency Ambulance Service** previously described involves advanced theoretical and practical training of selected ambulance personnel within departments of hospitals to which the ambulance units are seconded. Curricula are drawn up with suitable tests and examinations leading to award of a certificate of qualification. Training is at a level such that the techniques of endotracheal intubation, intravenous infusion and defibrillation may be added to the normal range of resuscitation and first aid procedures. There already exists a substantial fund of experience of such training in the United Kingdom of which the Medical Commission has knowledge (See Chapter 1). Location of emergency ambulances and their crews at hospitals greatly facilitates the training process both organisationally and financially since crews remain operational during training. The latter could in fact be said to be continuous under these conditions so that the need for refresher courses is diminished.

Courses in emergency procedures, diagnosis and treatment are arranged for general practitioners and hospital medical and surgical staff involved in the work of the Service. The programme includes regular seminars for discussion of information on cases treated fed back from the record system.

DISCUSSION

The Model Emergency Service projected here as a view of the shape of things to come represents in summary form the outcome of the author's Pilot Study in this field during 1975/76. It is a synthesis of a number of pioneer schemes and practices which have been demonstrated to be practicable in their particular environment and to have withstood the test of time.

The MCAP was at pains to set up this study as independent,

impartial and all-embracing. In the selection of an investigator previous experience in this field was a disqualification: a new look was required and this, it is hoped, has been achieved. In particular it is thought that the implications of certain activities in relation to the whole have been realised to an extent perhaps not fully appreciated by specialists working within their own environmental constraints. An example of this is the way in which advanced ambulance training is organised and the resulting service deployed at Frenchay, Bristol (see Chapter 1): these methods seem suitable for general application and have been incorporated into the Model Service.

The efficacy of GP schemes and their role in the emergency field were, as indicated by Parliamentary and Government reactions referred to at the outset to this chapter, the questions which triggered off this study. It was natural that in pursuing this aspect of the subject a detailed investigation was made of the pioneer scheme of this type, the North Yorkshire Road Accident After Care Scheme (RAAC) initiated in 1967 by Dr K C Easton (Chapter 6). Its structure, methods and records were studied in depth covering a period of $3\frac{1}{2}$ years to mid-1975. Police, ambulance, hospital and GP records were examined and at the completion of the study an assessment of overall benefit was made using the method described above under Monitoring. At that stage comparison data were limited and application was made to DHSS for financial support to extend the investigation on a national scale. This having now been rejected, further limited work is being done in selected areas on a voluntary basis with a view to obtaining more definitive comparison data.

Pending the completion of this work and in view of the impending publication of the present volume it would appear reasonable to give some indication of the inferences tentatively drawn from data already available using the method based on mortality data. **According to this criterion the level of emergency care in the RAAC Scheme area was significantly higher than that in an adjoining rural area, and than that obtaining nationally in rural areas.** In extrapolating from this conclusion special attention should be paid to the relatively highly integrated structure and methods of this scheme as representing a combined operation of all services.

The further development of such a scheme towards a full Area Emergency Service as envisaged in the hypothetical Model would be expected to reinforce and extend the overall effectiveness and benefit of the operation. What would be the likely extent of the benefit were such a service to be available nationally?—this is the 64 000 dollar question the author is repeatedly pressed to answer. In attempting an answer great care has to be taken in defining a datum or base line for comparison, it being clear that schemes and activities of all kinds, whether improvement in normal practice such as basic ambulance training and improvement of hospital facilities, or in special scheme activities such as GP and hospital based schemes and advanced ambulance training, have probably raised the overall level year by year. The level at any given time will however vary area by area according to the set-up existing in each area.

Against this background and on the basis of data available to date, and taking reduction of mortality as an index of improvement, **there would appear to be scope for preventing something of the order of 20% of total RTA deaths through the introduction of Area Emergency Services as projected in the Model.** This figure could be higher or lower in particular areas according to the prevailing level of emergency care.

This perspective immediately raises questions of ways and means through which an objective of this magnitude may be attained. In the field of emergency care, at any rate in the UK, the initiative has been left to individuals, with Government departments remaining largely aloof. This is in sharp contrast with road accident prevention, in which the Department of the Environment (DOE) and the Home Office with collaboration of the Association of Chief Police Officers, play an active part, as exemplified by the collection of elaborate statistics on road accidents resulting in injury (in the Stats 19 form) by the police for subsequent processing by DOE. These statistics are almost entirely concerned with how and why the accident happened. The outcome so far as the victim is concerned has little notice: severity of injury is recorded as 'killed', 'seriously injured' or 'slightly injured'. There is in fact nothing recorded on which to monitor rescue and emergency care, comparable with the extensive data recorded on the circumstances of the accident. Arrangements are currently in hand by DOE to revise Stats 19 and to link police and hospital accident records. This development could present an opportunity for DHSS to take a positive attitude in the emergency field by ensuring that 'time to die' and other data from police and hospital records are made available in a form suitable for monitoring emergency service activities.

Above all, some initiative must surely be forthcoming from DHSS along lines postulated earlier in this chapter to encourage a collective approach to emergency work and to provide back-up facilities for Area organisation. This should link up logically with planning arrangements for coping with major accidents and disasters, where differences in scale should not fundamentally alter organisation and method. Experience in a number of existing schemes in dealing with actual major accidents resulting in large numbers of casualties strongly supports the view that such schemes form a foundation on which to build plans for mobilising the services required to cope with the range of foreseeable incidents.

APPENDIX A

Products and Suppliers

Product	Supplier
Althesin	Glaxo Laboratories Ltd, Greenford Road, Greenford, Middlesex UB6 OHE
Ambu	Ambu International Ltd, 10 Station Road West, Canterbury, Kent CT2 8AN
Aramine	Merk Sharp and Dohme Ltd, Hertford Road, Hoddesdon, Hertfordshire EN11 9BU
Brook Airway	BOC Medishield Ltd, Elizabeth Way, Harlow, Essex
Camp Collar	S H Camp and Co Ltd, East Portway, Andover, Hampshire SP10 3NL
Cardiff Inhaler	BOC Medishield Ltd, Elizabeth Way, Harlow, Essex
Dextran 40, 70, 110, 150 also: Dextraven 110, 150 Lomodex 40, 70	Fison's Ltd, Pharmaceutical Division, 12 Derby Road, Loughborough, Leicestershire LE11 OBB

Product	Supplier
Dextraven 110, 150	Fison's Ltd, Pharmaceutical Division, 12 Derby Road, Loughborough, Leicestershire LE11 0BB
Dopram	Robins A H Co Ltd, Red Kiln Way, Horsham, Sussex
Entonox	BOC Medishield Ltd, Elizabeth Way, Harlow, Essex
Fortral	Winthrop Laboratories, Sterling Winthrop House, Surbiton, Surrey KT6 4PH
Haemaccel	Hoechst Pharmaceuticals, Hoechst House, Salisbury Road, Hounslow, Middlesex TW4 6JH
Humotet	Wellcome Medical Division, the Wellcome Foundation Ltd, Ravens Lane, Hertfordshire HP4 2DY
Kelocyanor	Rona Laboratories Limited, Cadwell Lane, Hitchin, Hertfordshire SG4 0SF
Ketalar	Parke, Davis and Company, Usk Road, Pontypool, Gwent NP4 8YH
Kleenex	Kimberly-Clark Ltd, Larkfield, Maidstone, Kent
Laerdal	Laerdal Products, Stavanger, Norway. Marketed in the UK by Vickers Ltd, Medical Engineering, Priestley Road, Basingstoke, Hampshire RG24 9NP

Product	Supplier
Lomodex 40, 70	Fison's Ltd, Pharmaceutical Division, 12 Derby Road, Loughborough, Leicestershire LE11 OBB
Macrodex	Pharmacia (Gt Brt) Ltd, Paramount House, 75 Uxbridge Road, London W5 5SS
Micropore	3M (UK) Ltd, 3M House, Wigmore Street, London W1A 1ET
Min-E-Pac	BOC Medishield Ltd, Elizabeth Way, Harlow, Essex
Narcan	Winthrop Laboratories, Sterling Winthrop House, Surbiton, Surrey KT6 4PH
Penlon	Longworth Scientific Instrument Co Ltd, Abingdon, Berkshire
Penthrane	Abbott Laboratories Ltd, Queenborough, Kent ME11 5EL
Space Blanket	F W Equipment Co Ltd, Whitehall Props, Town Lane, Wyke, Bradford, Yorkshire
Stockinette for Collars	Seton Products Ltd, Tubiton House, Medlock Street, Oldham, Lancashire
Uvistat	WB Pharmaceuticals Ltd, PO Box 23, Bracknell, Berkshire RG12 4YS
Valium	Roche Products Ltd, PO Box 2LE, 15 Manchester Square, London W1A 2LE

Product	*Supplier*
Venflon cannula	Smith and Nephew Ltd, Bessemer Road, Welwyn Garden City, Hertfordshire

APPENDIX B

Rank Identification in the Emergency Services

Principal ranks and markings in the emergency services.

AMBULANCE

METROPOLITAN
OR AREA
AMBULANCE
OFFICER

ASSISTANT
METROPOLITAN
OR AREA
AMBULANCE
OFFICER

DIVISIONAL
AMBULANCE
OFFICER

ASSISTANT
DIVISIONAL
AMBULANCE
OFFICER

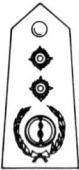 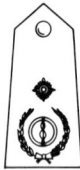 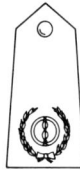 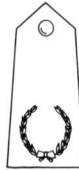

SUPERINTENDENT   STATION OFFICER   SUB-OFFICER

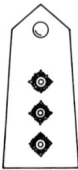 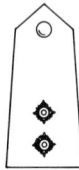 

478

FIRE SERVICE

CHIEF OFFICER

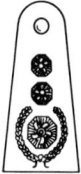

ASSISTANT
CHIEF OFFICER

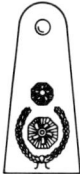

SENIOR
DIVISIONAL
OFFICER

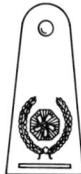

DIVISIONAL
OFFICER

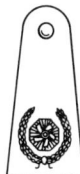

ASSISTANT
DIVISIONAL
OFFICER

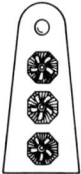

STATION OFFICER

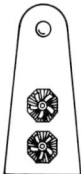

SUB-OFFICER

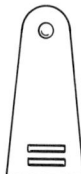

LEADING FIREMAN

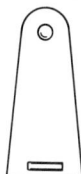

POLICE

CHIEF
CONSTABLE

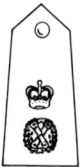

ASSISTANT CHIEF
CONSTABLE

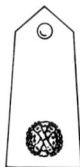

CHIEF
SUPERINTENDENT

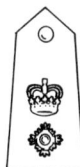

SUPERINTENDENT

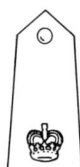

CHIEF
INSPECTOR

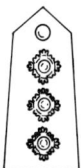

INSPECTOR

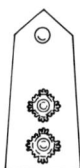

SERGEANT

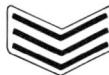

CONSTABLE

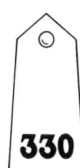

Index

481